Practical Paediatric Nutrition

INSTITUT
15, COTSWOLD ROAD
SUTTON
SURREY, SM2 5NG

Institute of Cancer Research Library

Practical Paediatric Nutrition

E. M. E. Poskitt MA, MB, BChir, FRCP
Senior Lecturer in Child Health, University of Liverpool,
Honorary Consultant Paediatrician, Royal Liverpool Children's Hospitals

Butterworths
London Boston Singapore Sydney Toronto Wellington

All rights reserved. No part of this publication may be reproduced or transmitted in any form or by any means, including photocopying and recording, without the written permission of the copyright holder, application for which should be addressed to the Publishers. Such written permission must also be obtained before any part of this publication is stored in a retrieval system of any nature.

This book is sold subject to the Standard Conditions of Sale of Net Books and may not be re-sold in the UK below the net price given by the Publishers in their current price list.

First published 1988

© Butterworth & Co. (Publishers) Ltd., 1988

British Library Cataloguing in Publication Data

Poskitt, E. M. E. (Elizabeth M. E.)
  Practical paediatric nutrition.
  1. Children. Nutrition. Health aspects
  I. Title
  613.2′088054

ISBN 0-407-00408-4

Library of Congress Cataloging in Publication Data

Poskitt, E. M. E. (Elizabeth M. E.)
    Practical paediatric nutrition / by E.M.E. Poskitt.
      p. cm.
    Includes bibliographies and index.
    ISBN 0-407-00408-4 :
    1. Nutrition disorders in children. 2. Children–Nutrition.
  I. Title.
    [DNLM: 1. Child Nutrition. 2. Infant Nutrition. 3. Nutrition Disorders–in infancy & childhood.   WS 115 P855p]
  RJ399.N8P67   1988
  618.92′39–dc19
  DNLM/DLC
  for Library of Congress   87-36844
                                                             CIP

Photoset by Butterworths Litho Preparation Department
Printed and bound in Great Britain by
Anchor Brendon Ltd., Tiptree, Essex

Preface

It is my aim, in writing this book, to present a unified view of paediatric nutrition which will be of practical use to those working with children, particularly those dealing with clinical problems in hospitals and in the community. The book is not intended to be a manual of practical procedures. Neither is it a book of diets nor a manual of nutritional biochemistry. Excellent books cover these fields, and I hope I have given them due credit in the references.

Whether or not the book achieves its aim of being practical will be a reflection of the author's conceit and the reader's judgement. Suffice it to say that it was my intention to avoid discussion of basic nutritional science except where it linked directly with clinical problems.

It may be asked why, in a book entitled *Practical Paediatric Nutrition*, basic growth charts and comprehensive tables of recommended dietary allowances are not included. The limitations of these sorts of reference data and their national variations are discussed in the text. Growth charts recognized locally are usually available to those working in paediatrics or in nutrition. Recommended dietary allowances are quoted in the book, but they, too, vary from country to country. All inclusive reference data tend to produce highly detailed tables and graphs which have little practical value when compressed on to the pages of a book this size.

I have also deliberately avoided great detail in the practical nutritional management of some of the chronic, less common, children's conditions. In much of Britain, conditions such as inborn errors of metabolism are managed in regional paediatric centres as well as district general hospitals. Those who lack the back-up services or who are themselves inexperienced in managing these conditions would be wise to seek help and advice from their regional centre rather than to seek the answer from a book. But I hope this book will provide a guide to basic management as support for others' experienced advice. The expertise developed in regional centres is enormous and we should not be clinically too proud to ask for help – it is the children who will suffer.

The main point of a preface must be to express thanks to those who otherwise go uncredited. I am deeply grateful for the ideas and stimulation often provided unknowingly by the colleagues with whom I am in day-to-day contact. Special thanks must go to those who have been kind enough to read and/or advise on parts of this book: Campbell Davidson, David Heaf, Tom McKendrick, Tony Nunn, Colin Smith and Christine Clothier and the Dietetic Department at the Royal Liverpool Children's Hospitals (Alder Hey). Nevertheless, I must take full responsibility for any inaccuracies in the text and for the views expressed.

My greatest thanks remain for those stalwarts who have put up with the typing and processing of endless scruffy annotated redrafts with cheerfulness, remarkable speed and incredible skill in deciphering minute pencilled hieroglyphics: Jenny Leonard and, above all, Joan Gleave.

E. M. E. Poskitt

Contents

1 Clinical nutritional assessment 1
2 Nutrition in pregnancy and its effects on the fetus 15
3 Breast feeding 24
4 Formula feeding 41
5 Low-birthweight infants 51
6 Weaning 73
7 Failure to thrive 80
8 Protein-energy malnutrition 96
9 Mineral deficiencies 114
10 Vitamin deficiencies 130
11 Problems of vegetarian and unusual diets 153
12 Nutrition and the teeth 161
13 Inborn errors of metabolism 167
14 Intolerant reactions to food 185
15 Gastrointestinal disorders 191
16 Parenteral nutrition – intravenous feeding (IVF) 218
17 Renal problems 230
18 Diabetes 239
19 Obesity and anorexia nervosa 254
20 Adolescence 275
21 Children's nutrition and later health 282
  Appendix 289
  Index 291

Chapter 1
Clinical nutritional assessment

We all need food. Some need more than others. The nutrient requirements of individuals are affected by age, sex, size, rate of growth, activity, the environment and individual differences as yet unexplained. On average, males have higher energy requirements than females of the same weight and age. Small bodies – owing to larger surface area – have higher energy requirements per unit weight than large bodies. The temperature of the environment influences the need to use energy to keep warm or to sweat and thus affects needs. Yet in childhood, the main variations in nutrient requirements relate to changing size and rates of growth.

The extent to which individuals are adequately supplied with food is represented by their nutritional status. Because of high nutrient requirements per unit weight and dependence on adults for the provision of food, children are more likely to suffer inadequate nutrition than adults. Energy deficiency is readily apparent in slow weight gain or weight loss, wasting, poor linear growth and diminished activity. Deficiency of other nutrients may be much more difficult to detect.

Assessing nutritional status: What does the diet tell us?

It might be thought that the adequacy of an individual's nutrition could be judged from dietary intake. However, adequate dietary records are difficult to achieve, and individual needs are so variable that it is difficult to know how to interpret even reasonably reliable records (Marr, 1971). The recommended daily amounts (RDA) of most nutrients are the amounts judged sufficient for the nutritional needs of the *majority* of the population but with built-in safety margins (10–15% or more of estimated requirements) added. Defined thus, RDA will be greatly in excess of the minimal dietary needs of most individuals and the majority of individuals probably eat less than the RDA for many nutrients and yet remain totally normally nourished. By contrast, the RDA for energy is the 50th centile of expected requirements for the population, but even so the RDA for energy currently recommended by the World Health Organization (WHO) and many governments may be above present-day average needs. Several studies have shown that the majority of children in Britain have intakes of energy below the RDA and yet thrive (Durnin *et al.*, 1974; Whitehead, Paul and Cole, 1982). Moreover, there is great inter-individual variation in normal nutrient needs, especially for energy. In any group of children or adults, those in the group with the lowest energy intakes have only about half the daily intake of those eating most and yet they are well and

Table 1.1 Recommended daily amounts of food energy and some nutrients for UK children (DHSS, 1979)

Age group	Boys Energy (MJ (kcal))	Protein (g)	Calcium (mmol (mg))	Iron (µmol (mg))	Girls Energy (MJ (kcal))	Protein (g)	Calcium (mmol (mg))	Iron (µmol (mg))
Months:*								
0–3	2.2 (530)	13	15 (600)	107 (6)	2.1 (500)	12.5	15 (600)	107 (6)
3–6	3.0 (720)	18	15 (600)	107 (6)	2.8 (670)	17	15 (600)	107 (6)
6–9	3.7 (880)	22	15 (600)	107 (6)	3.4 (810)	20	15 (600)	107 (6)
9–12	4.1 (980)	24.5	15 (600)	107 (6)	3.8 (910)	23	15 (600)	107 (6)
Years:								
1	5.0 (1200)	30	15 (600)	125 (7)	4.5 (1100)	27	15 (600)	125 (7)
2	5.75 (1400)	35	15 (600)	125 (7)	5.5 (1300)	32	15 (600)	125 (7)
3–4	6.5 (1560)	39	15 (600)	143 (8)	6.25 (1500)	37	15 (600)	143 (8)
5–6	7.25 (1740)	43	15 (600)	179 (10)	7.0 (1680)	42	15 (600)	179 (10)
7–8	8.25 (1980)	49	15 (600)	179 (10)	8.0 (1900)	47	15 (600)	179 (10)
9–11	9.5 (2280)	57	17.5 (700)	214 (12)	8.5 (2050)	51	17.5 (700)	214 (12)
12–14	11.0 (2640)	66	17.5 (700)	214 (12)	9.0 (2150)	53	17.5 (700)	214 (12)
15–17	12.0 (2880)	72	15 (600)	214 (12)	9.0 (2150)	53	15 (600)	214 (12)

* For details of nutrient requirements in infancy *see* chapters on infant feeding.

thrive (Widdowson, 1947). Thus RDAs cannot be used satisfactorily to assess the adequacy of nutrition in individuals. Their main purpose is for planning diets, particularly for populations where food loss in processing means that overestimating is almost essential.

Table 1.1 presents British RDA for some nutrients in relation to the ages of children. Requirements for vitamins and minerals are itemized in Chapters 9 and 10. Varying size of children at different ages should be considered, and *Table 1.2* presents estimated *minimum* requirements for health and normal growth related to units of body weight. Values for 'minimum' requirements are mostly theoretical but probably exaggerate rather than underestimate minimum requirements in most cases. The variations between RDA of different national governments highlight the difficulties posed when trying to use these recommendations (*Table 1.3*).

Table 1.2 Estimated minimum dietary needs/kg/day of infants and children according to age*

Age	Infant (weeks from conception)		Child				Adolescent 15 Years	
			Months		Years		Male	Female
	28†	40	5	12	5	10		
Energy:								
kJ	630	530	357	420	340	260	252	231
kcal	150	126	85	100	80	62	60	55
Protein (g)‡	3.0	1.5	1.4	1.2	1.0	0.8	0.7	0.6
Water (ml)	200	150	120	100	80	50	30	30
Sodium (mmol)	3–4	2.5	1.0	1.0	0.5	0.5	0.5	0.5

* Fomon, 1974; Widdowson, 1981a; Whitehead, Paul and Cole, 1982.
† Requirements very uncertain and depend on clinical state (*see* Chapter 5).
‡ Assuming protein of high dietary value.

Table 1.3 Examples of range of RDA in 7–9-year-old girls published by different national bodies

	DHSS*	FNB†	FAO/WHO‡
Energy:			
MJ	8.0	10.1	9.2
kcal	1900	2400	2190
Protein (g)	47	34	25
Calcium:			
mmol	15	20	10–12.5
mg	600	800	400–500
Iron:			
μmol	179	179	90–179
mg	10	10	5–10

* Department of Health and Social Security, 1979.
† Food and Nutrition Board, 1980.
‡ Joint FAO/WHO ad hoc Expert Committee, 1973.

4   Clinical nutritional assessment

Apart from actual nutrient needs changing with age, the diets of children vary since children's dependence and ability to cope with food varies according to their age and their neurological and physical development. *Table 1.4* outlines developmental changes relevant to children's ability to cope with their food. Neonates have no teeth, no chewing skills, and are unable to put food to their mouths, but they do have well-developed sucking and swallowing reflexes. Their high total body water and poor renal concentrating capacity demand high fluid intakes. Thus milk, with its varied nutrient content, is a very appropriate food. When fluid requirements per unit body weight are less, fluid diets become too voluminous and low in nutrient density to be satisfactory: hence the need to wean.

Table 1.4 Developmental 'milestones' important in nutrition

Age	Achievement
Fetus:	
14 weeks	Swallowing movements
17–20 weeks	Beginning of rooting/sucking movements
28–29 weeks	Sucking reflex
34–35 weeks	Co-ordination of swallowing and sucking
Infant and child:	
12 weeks	Swallows rather than protrudes food placed on anterior tongue
20 weeks	Drinks from held cup with biting movements
28 weeks	Feeds self biscuit, rusk, etc.; beginning to make chewing movements; teeth may begin to erupt
7 months	Shuts mouth and shakes head to refuse food
9 months	Finger feeds readily
10 months	Drinks from cup but throws away
12 months	Grabs at spoon, unable to get food to mouth
15 months	Can supinate and control spoon, replaces cups
18 months	Dawdles and plays with food

Nutritional assessment

Normal body composition

Table 1.5 indicates the changes in body composition that occur with age in childhood. Changes in nutrient requirements per unit weight in childhood both depend on, and influence, these changes. Newborn infants have high total body water, with increased extracellular water compared with older children. Body fat increases rapidly in the first months of life to reach very high levels at 4–6 months, and then gradually falls during the next few years. Growth of both lean and fat tissue is rapid at birth but falls dramatically in the first year, especially in the first 6 months, remains at fairly steady levels in early childhood and then accelerates briefly for girls at puberty and over a more prolonged period for boys at puberty (*Figure 1.1*).

Nutritional state can be assessed clinically, anthropometrically and biochemically. These methods are complementary rather than alternative. Some nutritional problems have specific clinical features, others are more readily diagnosed biochemically. Some, such as energy deficiency, may be most apparent from anthropometric changes.

Table 1.5 Age-related changes in body composition*

Age:	Fetus weeks			Infant months		Child years		Adult
	26	33	40	4	12	5	10	
				Whole body				
Water (%)	86	80	72	60	59	60	60	60
Fat (%)	1	6	14	26	24	18	17	12 (men) 25 (women)
				Fat-free mass				
Water (%)	87	85	84	82	78	74	72	72
Protein (%)	10	12	14	15	19	20	20	21

* Fomon, 1974; Widdowson, 1981b; Lentner, 1981.

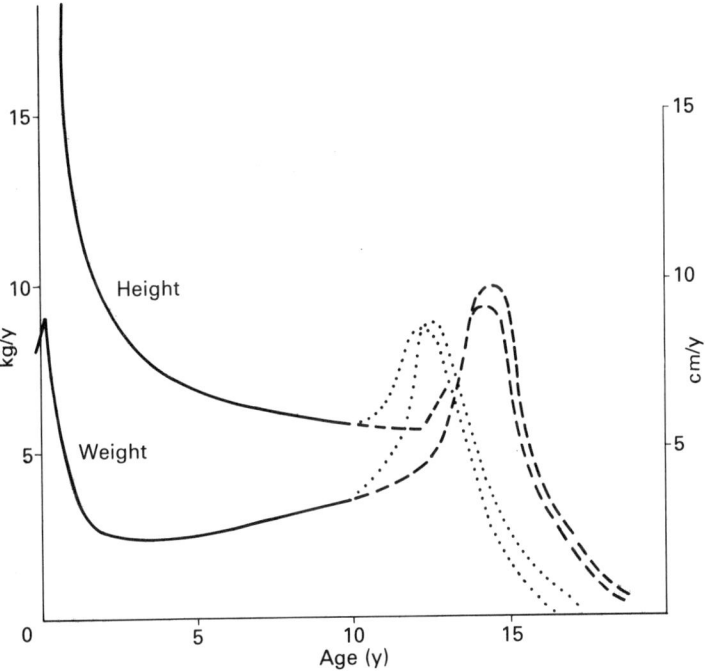

Figure 1.1 50th centile height and weight velocity (repeated whole-year increments) for boys and girls (Tanner and Whitehouse, 1966). ———, boys and girls (much the same in prepubertal age group); . . ., height and weight, girls; – – –, height and weight, boys.

Clinical nutritional assessment

The clinical features of nutritional deficiency are legion. *Tables 1.6* and *1.7* outline the main clinical points to be noted in the assessment of nutritional status. Some clinical signs are non-specific, for example wasting. Others, such as the signs of rickets or the presence of Bitot's spots in vitamin A deficiency, are much more

Table 1.6 Clinical assessment of nutritional states – integument and epithelia

Skin:	Colour: anaemia, bruising, petechiae, pigmentation Texture: dry, scaly, ulcerated, hyperkeratotic Dehydration with loss of skin turgor; oedema Xanthelasmata
Nails:	Lines of growth arrest Koilonychia
Hair:	Thickness; curliness; colour; pluckability
Eyes:	Xerosis conjunctivae; Bitot's spots Xerophthalmia Cataracts: visual acuity Arcus senilis. Kayser–Fleischer ring
Mouth:	Angular stomatitis; bleeding, swollen gums Glossitis; colour of tongue; loss of papillae
Teeth:	Stage of eruption, presence of caries Discoloration

Table 1.7 Clinical assessment of nutritional status – other physical signs

Musculo-skeletal system:	Posture. Hypotonia: distended abdomen; delayed walking. Wasting: loss of gluteal and axillary muscle and fat. Bony deformity, rickety rosary, craniotabes, bowing of legs, swollen metaphyses
Abdomen:	Hepatomegaly. Splenomegaly. Ascites
Cardiovascular system:	Bounding pulse; cardiac size; oedema. Blood pressure
Central nervous system:	Affect: apathy; depression; confusion; psychosis. Peripheral neuritis. Evidence of subacute combined degeneration of cord

specific. History and clinical examination are essential for assessment of nutritional state in individuals, but the detailed history and examination necessary are rarely feasible when the nutritional problems of populations are being assessed. Anthropometric methods are more practical for nutritional assessment of large populations, but should be combined with clinical and biochemical assessment if they are to be diagnostically accurate.

Anthropometric assessment

A number of anthropometric procedures used to assess nutritional status, and comments on the difficulties or inaccuracies of each procedure, are outlined below. Sophisticated instruments are available for measuring weight, length and fatness, but simple equipment can be constructed and used accurately, provided effort is expended in standardizing methods.

Table 1.8 Commonly used anthropometric techniques

Measurement	Equipment	Method
Weight	Platform scales Beam balance Spring balance Electronic balance	Minimal clothing. Repeat measurements in same clothing, same time of day. Good equipment should give results: ±5 g for infants ±50 g for older children
Length/height	Measuring table 0–2 years Stadiometer over 2 years Flat board, two measurers, foot board and rigid, accurate tape	Lie child flat or stand straight against wall. Hold head so canthi of eyes and upper margin external auditory meatus in same horizontal/vertical plane. Gently stretch. Feet at right angles to foot board or ground
Skull circumference	Rigid plasticized or metal tape	Measure around greatest circumference (excluding ears!)
Mid upper arm circumference	Rigid plasticized or metal tape	Circumference of arm in horizontal plane half-way between tip of acromion and olecranon with arm (left) hanging by side
Skinfolds	Skinfold calipers	See Chapter 19. Raise skinfold between index finger and thumb. Apply calipers to base of fold. Reading made when needle stationary. Usually mean of several (3) measurements.

Table 1.9 Anthropometric techniques: application

Measure	Accuracy	Usefulness
Weight	Can be very accurate but depends on equipment used (electronic or beam balances preferable)	Basic measurement of nutritional assessment. Non-specific indicator of health and nutrition. Trends over time more useful than single measure. Should be related to height and age
Length/height	Can be very accurate. Not easy to get accurate measurements in infants or in young standing children because of natural lordotic posture	Indication of long-term health and nutrition. Does not decrease and thus cannot reflect short-term problems. Serial measurements more useful than single measurements. Influenced by genetic and hormonal factors as well as nutrition
Skull circumference	Fairly accurate	Most useful in early infancy when rate of change rapid. Probably only influenced by severe malnutrition, thus disproportion between normal skull circumference and low body weight may indicate poor nutrition rather than other growth restriction
Mid upper arm circumference	Simple. Fairly accurate	Indicates lean and fat tissue of upper arm. Fair indicator of overall nutrition. Useful 1–5 years when age not accurately known since more or less constant measurement over that age period. Affected by oedema. Most useful combined with skinfolds
Skinfolds	Difficult to obtain consistent results, especially between observers	Only clinically practical direct assessment of fatness (see Chapter 19)

8 Clinical nutritional assessment

Interpretation of anthropometry
Interpretation of anthropometric results can be difficult and is often a source of great controversy between nutrition workers. Weight, height and skull circumference can be related to national or international growth standards. Most national and international growth standards describe cross-sectional studies of growth of populations. Longitudinal growth studies show much sharper changes in growth rate both in early infancy and at puberty (*Figure 1.2*). Serial anthropometry is more valuable than a single set of measurements since rates of growth are better indicators of nutritional adequacy (given the limitations of the growth standards) than growth achieved so far. This is particularly true for height, since children do not shrink and nutritional deficiency of recent onset may encompass stature within the normal range despite currently deficient growth velocity.

   Waterlow and Rutishauser (1974) used relative stature as an indicator of the duration of malnutrition and define various patterns of poor nutrition depending on the relation of weight and height to normal values (*Figure 1.3*). Indices derived from anthropometric parameters can be used for comparison of groups of varying age. They are particularly useful if developed as percentage expected value for age (*Table 1.10*). Results should always be interpreted carefully. For example, many weight for height indices are biased towards diagnosing tall for age children as overweight and short for age, but not wasted, children as underweight (Cole, 1979). This relative heaviness or lightness may be a reflection of the normal patterns of growth of tall and short children, rather than an indication of underlying nutritional excess or deficiency (*see* Chapters 8 and 19).

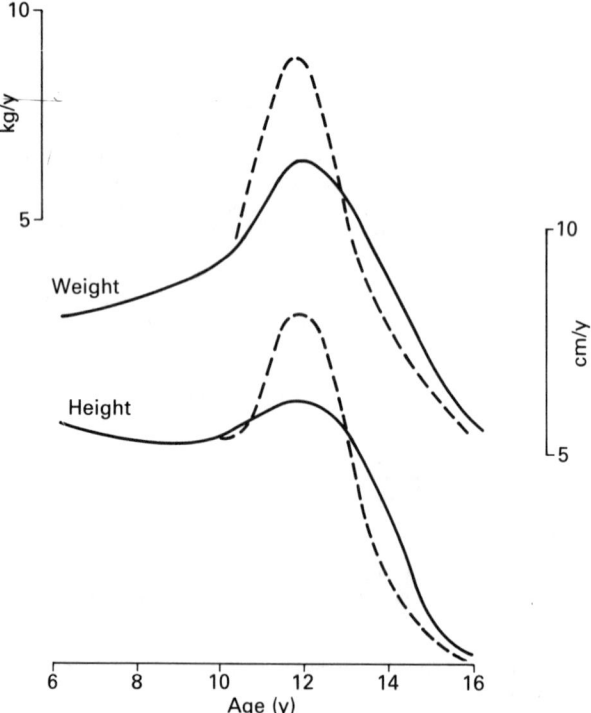

Figure 1.2 Contrast in 50th centile single whole year increments in growth (——, cross-sectional) and repeated whole-year increments (- - - -, longitudinal) for pubertal growth spurt in girls.

	Weight >80% expected	Weight <80% expected
Height >90% expected	NORMAL	WASTED
Height <90% expected	SHORT	STUNTED

Figure 1.3 Interpretation of weight and height for age

Table 1.10 Interpretation of anthropometric measurements (*see also* Chapters 8 and 19)

Weight	Centile for age[1]	Plot on standard weight for age centile charts[2] or tables[3]
	SD score	Difference of actual weight from mean for age ÷ standard deviation (SD) for weight for age[3]: positive or negative value according to whether weight for age above or below mean
	Centile weight for height	Compare with charts of expected weight for height[3,4]
Height	Centile for age	As with weight centile for age
	SD score	As for weight SD score[2–4]
Skull circumference	Centile for age	Compare with standard centiles[5,6]
Mid upper arm circumference (MUAC)	Centile for age, relatively age independent	Compare with centile tables[7] See Chapter 8. Normal values more or less constant, 1–5 years
Skinfold thickness	Centile for age: triceps and subscapular	Plot against centiles[7–9]: interpretation difficult since 'normal' range not defined. Values >75th centile may be abnormal at some ages.
	Estimation % body fat	Use nomograms or derived formulae (*see* Chapter 19). *Not* precise
MUAC and triceps skinfold	Mid upper arm muscle circumference (MAMC)	$MAMC = MUAC - (triceps\ skinfold \cdot \pi)$ or $= MUAC - \left[\left(\dfrac{triceps}{2} + \dfrac{biceps}{2}\right) \cdot \pi\right]$

1. Gestational age must be taken into account with premature infants.
2. Tanner, Whitehouse and Takaishi (1966).
3. Vaughan (1979).
4. WHO (1983).
5. Smith (1977).
6. Gairdner and Pearson (1971).
7. Frisancho (1974, 1981).
8. Tanner and Whitehouse (1962).
9. Tanner and Whitehouse (1975).

Anthropometric indices can be used to estimate body composition from derived formulae developed in experimental studies (*see* Chapter 19). These estimates are not precise. They are not interchangeable and the results of studies where groups have been assessed nutritionally by one method cannot be compared directly with those from studies of groups assessed by different methods or against different standards.

Biochemical assessment

Table 1.11 lists haematological and biochemical indices of nutritional status. Specialized biochemical studies of vitamin and mineral status are included in later

Table 1.11 Laboratory assessment of nutritional status

Haematology:	* Haemoglobin
	* Blood film appearances
	Mean corpuscular volume
	Mean corpuscular haemoglobin concentration
	White cell count and differential: lobulation of neutrophil nuclei
	Reticulocyte count
	Platelet count
	Bleeding and clotting time
	Partial thromboplastin time
	Prothrombin time
Biochemistry:	
Blood	* Glucose, urea, sodium, potassium, chloride
	* Total protein and albumin
	Vitamin A and retinol binding protein (RBP)
	Folic acid
	Vitamin B_{12}
	Total ascorbic acid and white or red blood cell ascorbic acid levels
	25-OH-vitamin D
	Vitamin E levels
	Serum iron, transferrin, total iron binding capacity, ferritin
	Zinc, copper, magnesium
	Calcium, phosphate, alkaline phosphatase
	Cholesterol: high and low density lipoprotein cholesterol
	Fasting triglycerides
	Amino acids
Urine	Amino acid profile
	* Protein
	Creatinine
	Ascorbic acid; thiamine

* First-line tests.

chapters. There is, sadly, no simple biochemical investigation for overall assessment of the nutritional status of individuals. Even for individual nutrients, blood levels often give little indication of nutrient distribution in the body. Total body analysis might indicate body composition and the size of nutrient stores, but this procedure has been used rarely (Widdowson and Spray, 1951) and is obviously not possible for living subjects! Biochemical assessment of nutrition thus depends on the distribution, in health and disease, of the nutrients being studied and the amount by which their distribution is affected by other metabolic changes. For example, estimation of serum calcium gives little information on the calcium content of bone or the adequacy of calcium nutrition since calcium stores are large and serum calcium levels are influenced by gastrointestinal and renal function and by hormones such as vitamin D and parathormone, as well as by actual calcium intake.

Does nutrition matter?

Good nutrition is necessary for optimal growth in childhood. Yet large size is admirable, but not essential to survival. It may even be a disadvantage if food is short, since a large body, on average, requires more food than a small one. Apart from growth, however, specific nutritional deficiencies affect all aspects of body function.

What is implied by 'good nutrition'? Adequacy of diet but not overindulgence is part of good nutrition. Diet can rarely be separated from other advantageous or disadvantageous environmental factors. Thus good nutrition should be defined in terms of the individual and for that individual's needs. For populations dietary adequacy or inadequacy should be assessed against whether the population is from a 'Westernized' country with low levels of activity and little infection, or a developing country with (for example) high energy needs for fetching water, tilling ground, herding cattle (all activities in which quite small children may partake) and with a heavy load of infection. In addition dietary adequacy should be considered against the long-term effects. Will the diet, although leading to optimal childhood growth and health, contribute to the diet-related diseases of adult life?

The importance of nutrition in childhood can be interpreted indirectly from morbidity and mortality statistics. Death and illness from infection are particularly common at ages when malnutrition is most prevalent (Puffer and Serano, 1973). Undernourished children are particularly at risk of death or complications from measles and diarrhoea even in developed, relatively affluent, countries. Undoubtedly the contributions of infection and environmental deprivation (*see* Chapter 8) to the *development* of malnutrition as well as the *consequences* of malnutrition, confuse the association. Nevertheless, there is a direct effect of malnutrition on many immunological mechanisms which lowers the ability of these children to combat a wide variety of infections (Chandra, 1983). Thus nutrition is critical in the survival and health of young children particularly those in otherwise disadvantaged environments.

Overnutrition also contributes to morbidity and mortality but here the connection is even less direct than for undernutrition since the increased morbidity and mortality is largely seen in middle life even though overnutrition may have begun in childhood. The 'diseases of Western civilization' such as atherosclerosis, some cancers and obesity are widely regarded as consequences of diets of affluence. However, the presumed effects of such diets are chronic and cumulative and date back perhaps over decades. The evidence for the dietary link is almost entirely developed from retrospective studies, although a few useful prospective studies have taken place or are doing so (*see* Chapter 21).

For both the immediate effects of undernutrition and the long-term effects of overnutrition, dietary intake is only one factor influencing health. An unhygienic background leads to greater likelihood of infection amongst small children, undernourished or otherwise. Death from infection amongst children who fail to thrive in Britain is not as inevitable as it seems amongst children in developing countries, probably in part due to the availability of clean water, a lower prevalence of parasitic infestations and less bacterial contamination of foods. The risks of overnutrition to adult longevity are probably less amongst those who do not smoke and who partake in moderate activity and consume diets higher in fibre and polyunsaturated fatty acids than is customary in 'Western' diets (*see* Chapter 21). Dietary 'balance' or the distribution of nutrients within the total intake is as important as the overall quantity of the diet.

The importance of other factors in influencing the impact of diet is shown by the demonstration that mean dietary intakes by British children (and others in developed countries) are less than they were 20–40 years ago and yet children in this country are, on average, taller, fatter and less likely to die of infection than ever before (Whitehead, Paul and Cole, 1982). Better environmental hygiene, warmer homes and reduced activity must all contribute to this.

12 Clinical nutritional assessment

We have discussed the dietary influences on physical growth and physical health. Does nutrition also have a part to play in the development of optimal brain growth and mental and intellectual health and achievement? Once again it is difficult to separate the effects of inadequate nutrition from the effects of poor nurture and inadequate stimulation. When undernutrition occurs independent of other disadvantages it is usually only for short periods, and it seems likely that its effects will be proportionately less.

It used to be thought that tissues grew by periods of cell multiplication and then cell growth. The overlap between the two periods was slight, and catch-up growth could occur only by cell growth and not by cell multiplication if the early period of cell multiplication had passed (Winick and Noble, 1966). This theory has been gradually eroded by demonstrations that the period of cell multiplication overlaps extensively with cell growth in most tissues and may even continue beyond the period of increase in cell size. The concept of 'critical periods' for growth now recognizes that tissues have much greater flexibility for timing catch-up growth than was previously thought. In the brain, Dobbing (1981) has demonstrated that increase in brain cell number continues well into the second year of life, although the period for very rapid brain cell multiplication takes place early in intrauterine life (20 weeks' gestation) before 'intrauterine malnutrition' is likely. Opportunity for catch-up brain cell multiplication is thus possible in young children provided that the malnourishing period is relatively short lived. Nevertheless, prolonged malnutrition is associated with reduced skull size implying reduced brain growth. Computed tomography in 1–4 year-old children with severe protein-energy malnutrition showed that severe malnutrition is accompanied by some cerebral atrophy (Househam and de Villiers, 1987). All the children described were severely malnourished and, although this is not stated, had probably had prolonged malnutrition. Interestingly, in these children the cerebellum did not show the same

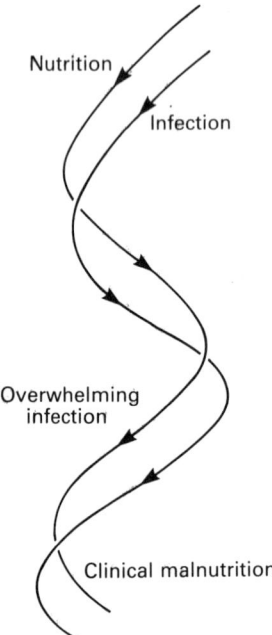

Figure 1.4 Downward progression of interaction of poor nutrition and infection.

atrophy as other areas of the brain. Cerebellar growth takes place over a relatively short period around birth and cerebellar cell multiplication may have been more or less complete before malnutrition developed in these children.

Does reduced cerebral growth mean reduced intellect? Here again improved understanding of the determinants of intellectual achievement has altered views on the likely effects of malnutrition on cerebral function. It is now widely recognized that environmental and emotional deprivation may have profound effects in inhibiting the development of normal cerebral function. Dobbing (1981) stated that, 'the importance of nutrition in the whole ecology of underprivilege may be no greater than that of any other of its myriad components'. Given appropriate stimulus and love, children with fewer brain cells may achieve more than those with normal brain cell number but less effective nurture. Nevertheless, prolonged malnutrition can influence intellectual function (Stoch and Smythe, 1967) often in relatively subtle ways.

Nutrition matters for health, both physical and mental, of children. But nutrition is only part of the nurture, that is the whole act of rearing, of children. There is a vicious declining spiral of disadvantage involving infection, nutrition and other aspects of nurture which entwines too many of the world's children (*Figure 1.4*). It is amongst these children, weakened by malnutrition and made unwell by infection, that, even if brain growth were unaffected by malnutrition, the exploring and learning experiences of childhood would be deficient. And if the weakness and apathy of these children is compounded by lack of interest or stimulus from malnourished, ill and infected parents, the children's disadvantages will only increase. Hence the need to ensure good nutrition for all.

References

CHANDRA, R. K. (1983) Nutrition, immunity and infection: Present knowledge and future directions. *Lancet*, **i**, 688–691

COLE, T. J. (1979) A method of assessing age and standardised weight for height in children seen cross sectionally. *Annals of Human Biology*, **6**, 249–268

DEPARTMENT OF HEALTH AND SOCIAL SECURITY (1979) Recommended daily amounts of food energy and nutrients for groups of people in the United Kingdom. *Reports on Health and Social Subjects,* No. 15. London: Her Majesty's Stationery Office

DOBBING, J. (1981) The later development of the brain and its vulnerability. In *Scientific Foundations of Paediatrics*, edited by J. A. Davis and J. Dobbing, pp. 744–758. London: William Heinemann

DURNIN, J. G. V. A., LONERGAN, M. E., GOOD, J. and EWAN, A. (1974) A cross-sectional nutritional and anthropometric study, with an interval of 7 years on 611 young adolescent school children. *British Journal of Nutrition*, **32**, 169–179

FOMON, S. J. (1974) *Infant Nutrition*, 2nd edn. Philadelphia: W. B. Saunders

FOOD AND NUTRITION BOARD (1980) *Recommended Dietary Allowances*, 9th edn. Washington, DC: Washington National Academy of Sciences

FRISANCHO, A. R. (1974) Triceps skinfold and upper arm muscle size norms for assessment of nutritional status. *American Journal of Clinical Nutrition*, **27**, 1052–1058

FRISANCHO, A. R. (1981) New norms of upper limb fat and muscle areas for assessment of nutritional status. *American Journal of Clinical Nutrition*, **34**, 2540–2545

GAIRDNER, D. and PEARSON, J. (1971) A growth chart for premature and other infants. *Archives of Disease in Childhood*, **46**, 783–787

HOUSEHAM, K. C. and DE VILLIERS, J. F. K. (1987) Computed tomography in severe protein energy malnutrition. *Archives of Disease in Childhood*, **62**, 589–592

JOINT FAO/WHO AD HOC EXPERT COMMITTEE ON ENERGY AND PROTEIN REQUIREMENTS (1973) *World Health Organization Technical Reports,* Series No. 522

LENTNER, C. (ed.) (1981) Geigy Scientific Tables, 8th edn. Vol. I: *Units of Measurement, Body Fluids, Composition of the Body, Nutrition.* Basel: Ciba-Geigy

MARR, J. W. (1971) Individual dietary surveys: purposes and methods. *World Review of Nutrition and Dietetics,* **13,** 105–164

PUFFER, R. R. and SERANO, C. V. (1973) *Patterns of Mortality in Childhood.* Scientific Publications No. 262. Pan American Health Organisation. Washington: World Health Organisation

SMITH, D. W. (1977) *Growth and its Disorders.* Philadelphia: W. B. Saunders

STOCH, M. B. and SMYTHE, P. M. (1976) 15 year developmental study on effects of severe undernutrition during infancy on subsequent physical growth and intellectual functioning. *Archives of Disease in Childhood,* **51,** 327–336

TANNER, J. M. and WHITEHOUSE, R. H. (1962) Standards for subcutaneous fat in British children. Percentiles for thickness of skinfold over triceps and below scapula. *British Medical Journal,* **i,** 446–450

TANNER, J. M. and WHITEHOUSE, R. H. (1975) Revised standards for triceps and subscapular skinfolds for British children. *Archives of Disease in Childhood,* **50,** 142–145

TANNER, J. M., WHITEHOUSE, R. H. and TAKAISHI, M. (1966) Standards from birth to maturity for height, weight, height velocity and weight velocity for British children in 1965. *Archives of Disease in Childhood,* **41,** 454–471

VAUGHAN, V. C. (1979) Growth and development. In *Nelson Textbook of Pediatrics,* 11th edn., edited by V. C. Vaughan, R. J. McKay and R. E. Behrman, pp. 10–46. Philadelphia: W. B. Saunders

WATERLOW, J. C. and RUTISHAUSER, I. H. E. (1974) Malnutrition in man. In *Early Malnutrition and Mental Devleopment,* edited by J. Cravioto, L. Hambraeus and B. Vahlquist, pp. 13–26. Stockholm: Almquist and Wiksell

WHITEHEAD, R. G., PAUL, A. A. and COLE, T. J. (1982) Trends in food energy intakes throughout childhood from one to 18 years. *Human Nutrition: Applied Nutrition,* **36,** 57–62

WIDDOWSON, E. M. (1947) A study of individual children's diets. *MRC Special Reports Series No. 257.* London: Her Majesty's Stationery Office

WIDDOWSON, E. M. (1981a) Nutrition. In *Scientific Foundations of Paediatrics,* 2nd edn., edited by J. Davis and J. Dobbing, pp. 41–53. London: William Heinemann Medical Books

WIDDOWSON, E. M. (1981b) Changes in body proportions and composition during growth. In *Scientific Foundations of Paediatrics,* 2nd edn., edited by J. Davis and J. Dobbing, pp. 330–342. London: William Heinemann Medical Books

WIDDOWSON, E. M. and SPRAY, C. M. (1951) Chemical development *in utero. Archives of Disease in Childhood,* **26,** 205–241

WINICK, M. and NOBLE, A. (1966) Cellular response in rats during malnutrition at various ages. *Journal of Nutrition,* **89,** 300–306

WORLD HEALTH ORGANISATION (1983) *Measuring Change in Nutritional Status.* Geneva: World Health Organisation

Chapter 2
Nutrition in pregnancy and its effects on the fetus

The extent to which maternal nutritional problems affect the health and growth of the fetus is controversial. Low birth weight, prematurity and high perinatal mortality rates are common in countries where poor maternal nutrition is also common. Yet poor maternal nutrition is rarely an isolated problem. Poorly nourished mothers usually live in societies where women perform most of the agricultural work – even late in pregnancy – and have burdensome domestic rituals such as fetching water from sources many miles from their homes. Infectious diseases are prevalent and may affect fetal growth and pregnancy outcome. Antenatal care may be non-existent.

Even in developed societies the majority of women who are poorly nourished come from disadvantaged homes and often avoid antenatal care and continue to smoke and consume alcohol in pregnancy. Their infants are at risk of growth problems for many reasons. The areas of ignorance and confusion that exist about the effect of maternal nutrition on the fetus are consequently understandable.

There are, however, some conditions where maternal inadequacy or excess of particular nutrients does have a definite relationship to problems in the fetus and newborn infant. Vitamin and mineral deficiencies are particularly likely to be reflected in fetal deficiency states (*Table 2.1*). Circulating levels of many nutrients, including vitamins and minerals, change in pregnancy. Alterations in levels usually reflect changes in binding to proteins, or in mobilization and storage, rather than deficiency states. For example, levels of water-soluble vitamins are generally lower in the blood of pregnant women compared with non-pregnant women. These lower levels are only rarely associated with clinical abnormality in mother or fetus (Metcoff, 1985). Where maternal deficiency does exist, problems in the infants will be exacerbated by breast feeding since deficiencies acquired *in utero* remain uncorrected by postnatal nutrition.

Vitamin deficiencies

Thiamine deficiency

Where mothers are thiamine (vitamin B_1) deficient, infants are born thiamine deficient also. If they are fed thiamine-deficient maternal milk they are likely to develop infantile beri beri presenting as cardiac failure or sudden infant death at a few months of age (*see* Chapter 10).

Table 2.1 Maternal nutritional deficiency or excess known to affect the fetus

Nutritional problem	Effect on fetus or neonate
Vitamin deficiencies:	
B_1	Infantile beri-beri
B_6	Convulsions
B_{12}	Megaloblastic anaemia
Folate	Increased abruptio placentae, prematurity, fetal abnormality
D	Hypocalcaemic convulsions, neonatal rickets, poor tooth enamel
Mineral deficiencies:	
Iodine	Deafness, mental retardation, spastic cerebral palsy; hypothyroid goitre and cretinism
Zinc	Low birth weight
Excessive intakes:	
Alcohol	Fetal alcohol syndrome
Vitamin A	Fetal abnormality
Vitamin B_6	Pyridoxine withdrawal convulsions
Abnormal nutrient metabolism:	
Hyperglycaemia – diabetes	Large immature infants, neonatal hypoglycaemia, increased fetal wastage
Hyperphenylalaninaemia (PKU)	Microcephaly, cerebral palsy, congenital heart disease
Low zinc absorption (acrodermatitis enteropathica)	Intrauterine growth retardation, fetal abnormality

Vitamin D deficiency

Infants born to mothers with osteomalacia may present clinically as neonatal rickets with low birth weight, craniotabes, bony deformity, respiratory distress due to softness of the ribs and often convulsions secondary to hypocalcaemia. Defects in dental enamel may become apparent later (Cockburn et al., 1980). Maternal milk will also be low in vitamin D.

Vitamin B_{12}

Vitamin B_{12} is not well mobilized from maternal tissues during pregnancy. Thus the fetus is dependent on maternal diet for B_{12}. Deficiency of vitamin B_{12} is only likely to be a problem amongst strict vegans (see Chapter 11) and women with pernicious anaemia or malabsorption syndromes. Fetal deficiency may not be apparent initially but unless the deficiency is corrected postnatally, anaemia and, more dangerously, sub-acute combined degeneration of the cord will develop in the next 12–18 months.

Folic acid

Serum folate levels fall in pregnancy but this probably reflects true diminution in folate stores since folate-responsive megaloblastic anaemia is common in pregnancy. Folate deficiency is exacerbated by the demands of fetal growth on maternal reserves in multiple pregnancies, the readiness with which folic acid deficiency develops under stress, drugs, alcoholism, and malabsorption.

The effects of maternal folate deficiency on the fetus are not fully understood. Several conditions giving rise to maternal folate deficiency (anti-convulsant treatment; alcoholism) are associated with poor fetal growth and congenital abnormality. Yet fetal alcohol syndrome and fetal anticonvulsant syndrome show no association with folate levels in the mother. Folate supplementation has been associated with decreased prevalence of ante-partum haemorrhage; abruptio placentae; stillbirth; premature delivery; and poor fetal growth amongst women in poor urban environments. Folate supplementation may even be the relevant nutrient in the prevention of spina bifida and anencephaly (Laurence et al., 1981) by pre- and post-conception vitamin supplementation (see below). Yet the relatively higher fetal than maternal blood levels offer some protection to the fetus in maternal folate deficiency since maternal megaloblastic anaemia is not inevitably accompanied by fetal folate deficiency.

It is advisable to give folate supplements to those mothers in whom there is a predisposition to deficiency: those with haemolytic anaemia, those taking anticonvulsants, those addicted to alcohol, and those carrying multiple pregnancies.

Mineral deficiencies

As with vitamins, plasma levels of minerals change during pregnancy and it is difficult to judge when true deficiency is present (Metcoff, 1985). Recommendations for trace element requirements during pregnancy are largely speculation.

Iodine

Maternal iodine deficiency has been recognized for a long time as affecting the fetus, although until recently it was thought that iodine deficiency only affected the fetus through fetal hypothyroidism and cretinism secondary to the thyroid deficiency. There are two populations of abnormal children (endemic cretins) born to iodine-deficient mothers. Some children have a bloated appearance with dry skin and coarse features and are thyroid deficient, short and mentally retarded (myxoedematous cretins). Others are deaf, mentally retarded and with spastic cerebral palsy (neurological cretins) but euthyroid. In early fetal life iodine appears important for normal cerebral development and particularly for normal development of the inner ear and the eighth nerve. Deficiency results in neurological cretinism. In later fetal life the main need for iodine is to maintain normal thyroid development and thyroid hormone synthesis. Without adequate thyroid hormone, brain development and growth of fetus and infant are affected and myxoedematous cretinism results. Intramuscular iodized oil 4 ml to mothers prior to conception is effective in preventing endemic cretinism (Pharoah, Buttfield and Hetzel, 1971).

Zinc

Zinc deficiency in the mother is associated with poor fetal outcome. Stillbirth, abortion, low birth weight and increased prevalence of congenital abnormality have been suggested as consequences of maternal zinc deficiency although the natural fall in the circulating zinc level in pregnancy may confuse normal low plasma zinc levels with deficiency. Meadows *et al.* (1981) have demonstrated low levels of muscle and leucocyte zinc in mothers delivering small-for-dates infants. Supplementation of women with definite problems in zinc balance – such as acrodermatitis enteropathica (*see* Chapters 9 and 15) – with zinc sulphate greatly reduces the prevalence of pregnancy complications and fetal abnormality.

Less clear-cut relationships between maternal and fetal nutrition

Energy

It has been estimated that pregnancy demands an increased daily energy intake approximating to 840 kJ (200 kcal) averaged throughout pregnancy. In early pregnancy the increased needs are for increase in size of the reproductive organs, increased blood volume and fat deposition. In late pregnancy the increased energy is required for rapid fetal growth and increased resting metabolic rate (Forsum, Sadurkis and Wager, 1985). Fat deposited in early pregnancy may be mobilized to meet fetal needs. However, most studies of the intakes of pregnant women suggest that the women do *not* necessarily increase their energy intakes. Early pregnancy particularly may be associated with increased efficiency of energy utilization and, in many parts of the world, late pregnancy may be marked by reduced energy expenditure in activity (Whitehead, Lawrence and Prentice, 1986).

Energy-restricted intakes for obese pregnant women are undesirable as, particularly in late pregnancy, fetal growth may be restricted. Weight reduction of obese women should be encouraged before or after pregnancy (and lactation).

The effect of maternal energy and/or protein deficiency on growth and development of the fetus are the focus of considerable debate. This is perhaps because it is difficult to separate poor maternal nutrition from other adverse socio-economic factors that affect fetal growth. One study where maternal malnutrition was a relatively isolated adverse factor was in the now classical study of the effects of poor nutrition on fetal growth during the Dutch Famine Winter of 1944–45 (Smith, 1947). Previously well-nourished pregnant women were subjected to quite severe famine in parts of Holland in late 1944 and early 1945. The famine was followed by plenty as relief was sent into the famine areas very rapidly in May 1945.

Weights of infants born to mothers pregnant during the famine showed that infants born to mothers in the last trimester of pregnancy at the height of the famine had an average of 9% reduction in birth weight. Length and skull circumference were also reduced but less dramatically. However, there was great variation in response of mothers to the famine so that the lowered birth weight was only apparent as a population mean. Some mothers actually lost weight during pregnancy yet produced infants weighing 3.5 kg or over (above average normal birth weight).

A more severe famine in Leningrad in 1942 resulted in a reduction in mean birth weight of over 500 g (Antonov, 1947). Yet even this weight reduction is small compared with the 50% weight reduction occasionally seen in otherwise apparently well newborn infants and vaguely attributed to 'malnutrition'.

Thus maternal food intake, of which energy is probably the critical factor, can influence fetal weight at term. However, maternal needs are dependent not only on the basic requirements of mothers and of their fetuses, but also on energy output in activity. Where women are labouring in fields until delivery higher energy intakes are needed in pregnancy than for women who can rest frequently, travel by car and undertake no heavy work during late pregnancy. Major economic and sociological changes are required in many countries before women will be able to achieve energy balance in late pregnancy. Yet action to reduce the work of women in late pregnancy may be a much more effective way of improving fetal growth than by energy supplementation of mothers at risk of producing small babies.

Energy supplementation of women in poorly nourished populations has a modest effect on fetal weight if supplementation is directed at women at risk of producing underweight infants (Viegas et al., 1982a). Supplementing whole populations with energy supplements has little noticeable effect since the women at greatest risk form only a small proportion of the total number (Viegas et al., 1982b). Even with selected supplementation, the mean improvement in birth weights of infants born to supplemented mothers is only 100–300 g greater than the mean weight of infants born to matched unsupplemented mothers. This difference is not dissimilar from the difference of 200–500 g weight reduction in mean fetal weight of malnourished populations compared with well-nourished populations. Food supplements may also have a significant effect on birth weight of infants born to women who smoke in affluent countries where clinical malnutrition is not common (Metcoff et al., 1985).

Protein

It is important that any food supplements for pregnant women lead to an overall balanced diet. Rush, Stein and Susser (1980) found increased length of gestation and reduced proportion of low birth weight infants with balanced protein-energy supplements given to a poor black urban population of pregnant women. High protein supplements led to an excess of very early premature births and significant growth retardation before 37 weeks' gestation. The explanation for these effects of high protein supplements is not clear but high-protein, low-energy intakes have been associated with severe birth weight depression elsewhere (Grieve et al., 1979).

Vitamins

Although the numbers were too small to reach significance, data from the Dutch Famine studies suggested that poor maternal nutrition in early pregnancy was associated with increased central nervous system abnormalities. In a large study, Smithells, Sheppard and Schorah (1976) assessed levels of various vitamins in women in early pregnancy and found an association between neural tube defects in the fetus and below average levels of serum folate, red cell folate, white blood cell vitamin C and riboflavin in the first trimester. Further work has shown that pre-conceptual and pregnancy supplementation with multivitamin preparations for women with a family history of neural tube defects reduces the incidence of neural tube defects in the offspring when compared with similar women not receiving supplementary vitamins (Smithells, 1982). Since the original studies used a multivitamin preparation, it is not yet clear which, or whether, one particular vitamin is the preventive agent. Studies are in progress.

The protective effect of vitamin supplementation against central nervous system abnormalities is unusual in that there is no evidence that women giving birth to infants with neural tube defects are *deficient* by recognized standards, in particular vitamins. Thus they must accrue some benefit from intakes of vitamins above normal requirements. It is not known whether these women or their fetuses have unusual metabolic requirements needing increased levels of vitamins or co-enzymes, or whether the presence of increased vitamin levels can counteract other abnormal metabolism, or even whether safe levels of vitamins in pregnancy are underestimated. Some of the carefully controlled studies now being conducted will probably elucidate these matters further. *Table 2.2* indicates groups of women for whom dietary supplementation in pregnancy may be advisable.

Table 2.2 Possible indications for dietary supplementation in pregnancy

Supplement	Groups that might benefit
Energy (with or without protein)	Recognized 'at risk' groups with evidence of undernutrition
Vitamins:	
Combined supplement	History, or family history, of infants with neural tube defects. Those known to be at risk of vitamin deficiency; malabsorption states
A	Where xerophthalmia prevalent
B_1	Where beri-beri prevalent
B_{12}	Pernicious anaemia, Crohn's disease, strict vegans
D	Women from Indian Subcontinent, Muslim Middle East and Horn of Africa resident in Northern Europe
Folic acid	Multiple pregnancies, poor social circumstances, high prematurity rates
Minerals:	
Iron	Where there is evidence of maternal iron deficiency
Zinc	Acrodermatitis enteropathica
Iodine	Areas of endemic goitre and endemic cretinism
Selenium	Areas of prevalent Keshan disease

Fetal malnutrition: 'Placental insufficiency'

Infants small for gestational age are often described as showing fetal 'malnutrition'. These infants are low weight for gestational age and are sometimes divided into two categories: the 'disproportionate' infants with relative sparing of brain growth, skull circumference and length, and the 'proportionate' group where skull circumference, length and weight are all equally retarded. The former group are considered the result of malnutrition in late pregnancy. The latter group indicate prolonged intrauterine growth retardation for a variety of reasons (*Table 2.3*).

In practice infants are not easily segregated into the two groups described. We find that most small-for-dates infants amongst the deprived urban population fall into a more or less proportionately growth-retarded group. A large proportion of weight in the newborn comes from the weight of the head. Thus it may be more appropriate to seek evidence of truly disproportionate growth amongst infants within the normal range of birth weight since, if the head is normal size, the total weight, despite a small body, may be within the normal range.

Malnutrition in the mother, particularly in late pregnancy, can affect fetal growth sufficiently to make the infant 'small for dates'. However, as discussed, the degree of weight reduction is on average small and only occurs with severe maternal food restriction. Yet in all countries some 'malnourished' infants are born to mothers

Table 2.3 Causes of intra-uterine growth retardation ('small for dates' infants)*

Maternal causes:	
Domicile at high altitude	Low socio-economic status
Severe malnutrition	Smoking
Chronic illness, especially:	Drugs: anticonvulsants, alcohol
Essential hypertension	Mother at extremes of child-bearing age
Chronic renal disease	Excessive physical exercise
Abnormal uterus	
Hyperpyrexia	
'Pre-eclamptic toxaemia'	
Placental causes:	
Abnormal cord insertion	Placental malaria
Low lying placenta	Placental infarction
Partial placental abruption	
Fetal causes:	
Multiple births	Chromosomal abnormality
Intrauterine infection	Other severe congenital abnormality
Genetic small size	

* There is considerable overlap in the classification of causes.

who appear to have eaten adequately in pregnancy. The infants are underweight, short – although usually less restricted in length than weight – and thin. They are prone to hypothermia and hypoglycaemia. Typically brain growth is relatively less severely affected than other aspects of growth, and skull circumference is more appropriate for gestational age than weight or length. Bone deposition is affected and the skull bones are soft and malleable and the fontanelle large. Postnatally these infants show good appetites and accelerated weight gain and growth so that catch-up to the normal growth centiles is usual.

The smaller for gestational age the infant, the more likely it is that pathological rather than nutritional factors have restricted growth, particularly if ultrasound studies suggest that the fetus has been growing poorly since early pregnancy. However, for those with last-trimester growth retardation and no recognized pathological cause a diagnosis of placental insufficiency is often made. These infants usually have small placentae which are often gritty and infarcted.

A diagnosis of 'placental insufficiency' tells us little of the true aetiology of the poor fetal growth and may only serve to disguise our ignorance of placental function and the factors controlling fetal growth. A large proportion of placental tissue is derived from fetal tissue. Thus it is not surprising that a small, poorly grown fetus has a small poorly grown placenta. Is fetal growth restricting placental growth or placental size restricting fetal growth?

The placenta grows proportionately more rapidly than the fetus in the second trimester and reaches maximum weight at about 33 weeks' gestation. Placental villous surface area and vascularity probably continue to increase until late gestation (Gluckman and Liggins, 1984). In pre-eclamptic toxaemia infarction of the placenta may greatly reduce its functional area.

Placental size influences fetal growth by a variety of means. The fetus is dependent on placental function for nutrition and oxygenation and ultimately survival. A small fetus with a small placenta has little chance for the excessive nutrient intake needed for catch-up growth. Reduced placental function for gestational age will restrict fetal growth even further. This is a concept of critical importance when considering the practicalities of the safest time to deliver growth-retarded fetuses. The fetus whose growth is restricted by 'placental insufficiency' is particularly at risk during labour when placental delivery of oxygen to the fetus is compromised by uterine contractions. Yet the fetus is small and at risk of the complications of low birth weight if delivered. Sometimes, it is argued, these infants should be allowed to grow a little more *in utero* before expediting delivery. This can be a mistake. If placental function is restricting growth it will continue to do so, and the fetus will only become relatively more growth retarded with time. Size and nutrient demands may outstrip placental function and sudden intrauterine death or death during parturition is not uncommon. The fetus with growth restriction due to failing placental function has more hope of survival *ex utero* than *in utero*.

It should not be forgotten that the placenta itself has nutritional demands. In sheep the utero-placental tissue consumes about 50% of the oxygen and 66% of the glucose supplied by the maternal circulation to the uterus. The proportions in the pregnant woman may be similar. Yet the uteroplacental tissue seems to use little of the amino acid supply to the uterine circulation. This may perhaps explain why linear growth is less affected than fat deposition in the fetus affected by 'placental insufficiency' and certainly explains why these fetuses are usually polycythaemic since the low oxygen tension of intrauterine life is even lower when supply is limited and uteroplacental needs have to be met (Battaglia and Hay, 1984).

The fetus is protected from non-nutritional environmental hazards more than it will be after birth. Even so other factors influence growth besides the placenta's ability to deliver oxygen and nutrients. Genetic and hormonal factors are important, although growth hormone and thyroid hormone have little effect at this stage in life whereas insulin is an important growth promoting hormone. And mother's socio-economic environment will be reflected in both the delivery of drugs, alcohol and nicotine to the placenta and in changes in uterine blood flow with changes in posture, hormonal milieu and, perhaps, emotion. As at every stage in life, nutrition cannot be totally separated from other aspects of nurture. This may be advantageous to the fetus by protecting against disaster resulting from a single adverse environmental factor. It is, however, very disadvantageous to those studying fetal nutrition or trying to make definitive statements about the influence of maternal nutrition on the fetus!

References

ANTONOV, A. M. (1947) Children born during the siege of Leningrad in 1942. *Journal of Pediatrics*, **30**, 250–259

BATTAGLIA, F. C. and HAY, W. W. (1984) Substrate requirements for fetal and placental growth and metabolism. In *Fetal Physiology and Medicine*, 2nd edn., edited by R. W. Beard and P. W. Nathanielsz, pp. 601–628. London: Butterworths

COCKBURN, F. *et al.* (1980) Maternal vitamin D intake and mineral metabolism in mothers and their newborn infants. *British Medical Journal*, **281**, 11–14

FORSUM, E., SADURKIS, A. and WAGER, J. (1985) Energy maintenance costs during pregnancy in healthy Swedish women. *Lancet*, **i**, 107–108

GLUCKMAN, P. D. and LIGGINS, G. C. (1984) Regulation of fetal growth. In *Fetal Physiology and Medicine*, 2nd edn., edited by R. W. Beard and P. W. Nathanielsz, pp. 511–557. London: Butterworths

GRIEVE, J. F. K., CAMPBELL-BROWN, M. and JOHNSTONE, F. D. (1979) Dieting in pregnancy: a study of the effect of a high protein low carbohydrate diet on birthweight in an obstetric population. In *Carbohydrate Metabolism in Pregnancy and the Newborn,* edited by M. W. Sutherland and J. W. Stowers, pp. 518–533. Berlin: Springer-Verlag

LAURENCE, K. M., JAMES, M., MILLER, M. H., TENNANT, G. B. and CAMPBELL, H. (1981) Double blind randomised controlled trial of folate treatment before conception to prevent recurrence of neural tube defects. *British Medical Journal,* **282,** 1509–1511

MEADOWS, M. J. et al. (1981) Zinc and small babies. *Lancet,* **ii,** 1135–1137

METCOFF, J. (1985) Maternal–fetal nutritional relationships. In *Pediatric Nutrition,* edited by G. C. Arneil and J. Metcoff, pp. 56–108. London: Butterworths

METCOFF, J. et al. (1985) Effect of food supplementation (WIC) during pregnancy on birth weight. *American Journal of Clinical Nutrition,* **41,** 933–947

PHAROAH, P. O. D., BUTTFIELD, I. H. and HETZEL, B. S. (1971) Neurological damage to the fetus resulting from severe iodine deficiency during pregnancy. *Lancet,* **i,** 308–310

RUSH, D., STEIN, Z. and SUSSER, M. (1980) A randomized controlled trial of prenatal nutritional supplementation in New York City. *Pediatrics,* **65,** 683–697

SMITH, C. A. (1947) Effects of maternal undernutrition upon the newborn infant in Holland 1944–45. *Journal of Pediatrics,* **30,** 229–243

SMITHELLS, R. W. (1982) Diet and congenital malformations. In *Nutrition in Pregnancy* edited by D. M. Campbell and M. D. G. Gillmer, pp. 155–165. London: Royal College of Obstetricians and Gynaecologists

SMITHELLS, R. W., SHEPPARD, S. and SCHORAH, C. J. (1976) Vitamin deficiencies and neural tube defects. *Archives of Disease in Childhood,* **51,** 944–950

VIEGAS, O. A. L., SCOTT, P. H., COLE, T. J., EATON, P., NEEDHAM, P. G. and WHARTON, B. A. (1982a) Dietary protein energy supplementation of pregnant Asian mothers at Sorrento, Birmingham. II: Selective during third trimester only. *British Medical Journal,* **285,** 592–595

VIEGAS, O. A. L., SCOTT, P. H., COLE, T. J., MANSFIELD, H. M., WHARTON, P. and WHARTON, B. A. (1982b) Dietary protein energy supplementation of pregnant Asian mothers at Sorrento, Birmingham. I: Unselective during second and third trimesters. *British Medical Journal,* **285,** 589–592

WHITEHEAD, R. G., LAWRENCE, M. and PRENTICE, A. M. (1986) Incremental dietary needs to support pregnancy. In *Proceedings of the XIII International Congress of Nutrition,* edited by T. G. Taylor and M. K. Jenkins, pp. 599–603. London: John Libbey

Chapter 3
Breast feeding

Breast feeding has had varied popularity over the centuries. Much of the historical literature on infant feeding recommended that infants were not fed colostrum, were given foods other than breast milk, or were not suckled until days – or even weeks – postpartum (Wickes, 1953; Fildes, 1986). Happily for most infants, these views went largely unnoticed by mothers until this century, since the majority of women had little access to books and could not read. Following the Second World War, however, there was a dramatic decline in the prevalence of breast feeding in Britain such that, by the 1960s, only a small minority of infants were breast fed for any length of time (Neligan, 1978). Since the mid-1970s a resurgence of breast feeding has meant that in some parts of Britain over 75% of infants leave maternity hospitals wholly breast fed. Many continue to be breast fed for 4 months or more (Martin and Monk, 1982). Recent data shows that the upsurge in the prevalence of breast feeding in the 1970s has not continued. The prevalence of breast feeding in 1985 in Britain was almost the same as in 1980 (DHSS, 1988).

There are strong social-class influences on feeding practices in Britain. Breast feeding is most prevalent amongst the educated and professional middle classes. Formula feeding remains the predominant feeding method amongst lower social class women in deprived urban areas and, perhaps surprisingly, amongst many immigrant groups (Evans *et al.*, 1976).

Physiology of breast feeding
Prolactin
The main hormone concerned with preparing the breast for milk production and then secretion of milk after delivery is prolactin. Prolactin levels rise in late pregnancy and usually peak around the time of delivery. Placental oestrogen and progesterone inhibit milk secretion during pregnancy but the fall in these hormones with delivery allows prolactin to exert a milk-secreting effect (Howie, 1985). This is enhanced by the neuro-endocrine pathway whereby suckling stimulates further prolactin secretion. Stimulation of the areolar area by suckling sends nerve impulses to the mother's brain and ultimately to the hypothalamic area where stimulation of prolactin secretion via the anterior pituitary is induced. After each episode of suckling, prolactin levels rise, reaching a peak 30–45 minutes after initiation of the feed. Values then fall gradually over the next few hours. Frequent suckling maintains high levels of prolactin whereas infrequent suckling produces wide swings in circulating levels. Prolactin responses to night-time suckling tend to be higher than those due to daytime suckling. Night feeding is thus important for maximal breast-milk production (Glasier, McNeilly and Howie, 1984).

The neuro-endocrine pathway for prolactin secretion is affected by drugs and also, to some extent, by emotion. Pain, anxiety and insecurity all contribute to less effective prolactin secretion (Jelliffe and Jelliffe, 1978).

In well-nourished mothers, breast-milk output can be maintained at adequate levels for several months, *once established,* despite relatively low prolactin levels. Mothers who wish to breast feed for prolonged periods (6 months or more) and poorly nourished mothers, must keep up high-frequency suckling and high prolactin levels in order to maintain adequate milk output.

Oxytocin

The other hormonal mechanism governing breast feeding is oxytocin release which stimulates the 'let-down' reflex. Contraction of myoepithelial cells causes ejection of milk from the breast tissue alveoli into the terminal ducts which the infant then drains by sucking. Again, stimulation of the oxytocin reflex occurs by stimulation of the areolar area at suckling. Nerve impulses to the posterior central nucleus of the hypothalamus induce oxytocin release from the posterior pituitary. Sensory contact with the infant through sight or sound can also stimulate this reflex. Production of oxytocin is readily stimulated or inhibited by emotional responses. Lack of confidence, fear for the baby, pain and discomfort can all lead to poor oxytocin response and consequent inability of the infant to obtain milk from the breast (Jelliffe and Jelliffe, 1978).

Practical problems with breast feeding

It is not always recognized that the mechanics of sucking and obtaining milk from the breast are different from those of sucking from the bottle. Unfortunately, many mothers are more familiar with the sight of infants bottle feeding than breast feeding. In traditional societies, experienced women often give specific help and support to postpartum women in order both to allow mothers to rest following birth of the baby and to help and advise mothers with breast feeding and caring for their infants. In Britain and other developed countries it is becoming more common to have selected women – midwives or lay volunteers – attached to maternity units to help and advise mothers on the techniques of breast feeding. Their services can be invaluable (Gunther, 1973; Jones and West, 1985).

Sucking from a bottle is achieved by alternate compression and release of the narrow section of the teat against the roof of the mouth. In breast feeding infants must get their jaws around the areola as by compressing this, milk is ejected from the terminal lacteals under the areola into the nipple and thus into the mouth. Sucking on the nipple will be totally ineffective. This 'latching on' to the aerola may be a problem for some infants (Fisher, 1981). Mothers with large, well-developed breasts must pay particular attention to keeping their infant's nostrils clear of breast tissue, otherwise the infants cannot breathe and suck, so they breathe by opening their mouths and sucking ceases. Pushing an infant's cheeks back towards the breast may only stimulate the rooting reflex (whereby the newborn infant turns to light touch around the mouth), so the infant turns towards the pushing hand.

Sore nipples are common early in lactation. If possible, lactation should continue despite this problem since it is often a transient stage and may be related to infants sucking vigorously but obtaining little milk. Reducing stimulation to the breast by decreasing the frequency of suckling is likely to lead to reduced breast-milk production. Where cracked nipples are due to thrush infection, both mothers' nipples and infants' mouths require treatment since mothers and infants may be reinfecting one another.

Many infants seem very hungry at 6–7 days of age and again at 4–6 weeks of age (Wickes, 1952). They appear unsatisfied by breast feeding. This cycle of increasing appetite leading to increased frequency of feeding and thus greater stimulation of milk production provides its own resolution, and mothers must be encouraged to suckle infants frequently if the infants appear hungry and dissatisfied.

Establishing breast feeding

Table 3.1 lists the main antecedents of successful breast feeding. Early frequent suckling is vitally important (de Chateau and Winberg, 1978; Salariya, Easton and Cater, 1978). Where the clinical state permits, mothers should suckle their infants immediately after delivery. Oxytocin secretion will encourage contraction of the

Table 3.1 Antecedents of successful breast feeding

Mother:	Healthy, well nourished, eating and drinking adequately, breast fed previous infants successfully, observed infants being breast fed, was breast fed herself, confident in her ability to breast feed
Infant:	Healthy, mature, hungry and vigorous sucker
Circumstantial:	Early onset of suckling, frequent suckling early in puerperium, suckling frequently at night

uterus in the third stage of labour. The process of suckling will also promote hormonal stimulation of breast-milk production. Infants should then be suckled many times both during the day and night in the first few days of their lives, although the duration of suckling need only be short. Healthy infants may take 90% of the feed volume in the first 4 minutes' sucking at each breast (Lucas, Lucas and Baum, 1979). Once breast feeding is established, well-nourished women can usually maintain good milk output feeding their infants only five or six times daily. Poorly nourished women may need to suckle much more frequently in order to maintain adequate milk production.

Why breast feed?

Table 3.2 lists the advantages of breast feeding. The main advantage must be the protection breast feeding provides against infection. Women in all countries should be encouraged to breast feed since this protection is advantageous to infants even in

Table 3.2 Advantages of breast feeding

Composition of milk:
  Appropriate for infants' needs.
  Better absorption of fats, minerals and vitamins than formula milks.
  Contains enzymes, hormones, prostaglandins which may be important for growth and development especially of gastrointestinal tract

Protection against infection:
  Clean food source.
  Anti-infective properties: cellular, humoral (*see Table 3.3*)

Cheap

Convenient (when mother and baby together)

Infant regulates supply of food by demand

Successful breast feeding indicates effective mother–infant bonding

---

relatively hygienic Western societies. In developing countries, it is immoral to encourage mothers to feed their newborn infants by methods other than breast feeding.

Protection against infection

Where it is relatively easy to obtain clean water and where there is proper sterilizing equipment, it is less important that breast feeding provides a relatively clean source of food for young infants. In much of the world it is impossible to sterilize feeding utensils adequately and to store milk under cool conditions. Thus many artificial milk sources are inevitably contaminated and present an unacceptable risk of infection to young infants. Breast feeding is the only 'safe' method of infant feeding in such circumstances. Yet breast milk is not sterile. It may contain several thousand organisms per ml, but it also contains protective factors which make it unlikely that infants will acquire symptomatic infection from the bacteria in their mothers' milk (Goldman *et al.*, 1982). These protective factors are of major importance to infants in disadvantaged environments but also exert significant effects on infants from more satisfactory home environments (Jelliffe and Jelliffe, 1978; Yoshioka, Ideki and Fujiia, 1983; Duffy *et al.*, 1986).

Table 3.3 lists the main anti-infective factors in human milk.

Cellular factors

The cell count of human milk is approximately 4×10^9 cells/l in milk early in lactation (Rolles and Cussens, 1980). The cells are macrophages, lymphocytes and neutrophils. The role of the cells in milk is closely linked with that of immunoglobulin A (IgA), mainly present in the secretory form. Rapid transfer of lymphocytes from Peyer's patches in the maternal gut or from the respiratory tract to the breasts facilitates transfer of protection against maternal gut and respiratory pathogens to infants. The macrophages in milk act as scavengers in infants' gastrointestinal tracts, phagocytosing bacteria already damaged by other factors in the milk. Immunoglobulin A contained within them is released during phagocytosis.

Table 3.3 Anti-infective properties of human milk

Cellular:
  Macrophages
  Lymphocytes
  Neutrophils
Humoral:
  Secretory immunoglobulin A
  Lactoferrin
  Other nutrient binding proteins
  High polyunsaturated fatty acid content
  Low buffering capacity
  Lysozymes
  Interferon
  Complement factors
  Lipases

Humoral factors

Secretory IgA forms about 50% of the high protein content of colostrum (the secretion produced by the breast in the first days postpartum) and continues to be present in smaller quantities in milk (around 10% total protein) even when lactation continues into the second half of the first year of life. Secretory IgA is resistant to digestion in the gastrointestinal tract and can be detected in the stools of breast-fed babies. It probably acts by adhering to the gastrointestinal mucosa and thus prevents adhesion of pathogenic organisms, many of which adhere to mucosa in order to exert their pathogenic effect. It functions as an 'antiseptic intestinal paint'. Human milk usually contains specific factors active against other organisms infants are likely to encounter, especially respiratory syncytial virus and rotavirus. Even if these factors do not totally protect against infection, the course of infection with organisms such as rotavirus is likely to be modified (Duffy *et al.*, 1986). Breast feeding is thus protective against organisms that commonly affect infants in relatively affluent environments as well as disadvantaged environments.

Lactoferrin in milk binds iron closely and thus both facilitates iron absorption and prevents gut organisms utilizing intestinal iron for their own multiplication. Vitamin and mineral binding proteins also facilitate absorption and prevent vitamins and trace elements being available for bacterial multiplication. Lysozyme has a non-specific effect against bacteria and interferon a non-specific effect against viruses. The acid pH and low buffering capacity of human milk, together with specific oligosaccharides which associate with casein (bifidus factor), encourage the growth of *Lactobacillus bifidus* and discourage colonization of the infant gut by Gram-negative bacilli and other organisms (Yoshioka, Ideki and Fujiia, 1983; Duffy *et al.*, 1986).

Composition

The first 'milk' produced by the breast is colostrum. This is secreted in small quantities in late pregnancy and then in larger quantities in the first days postpartum. Volumes remain small – perhaps 120 ml per day.

The composition of colostrum differs from that of mature milk since it is much richer in proteins, especially immunoglobulins and lactoferrin, trace elements and vitamin A. *Table 3.4* outlines some of the constituents of colostrum. It is not possible to be specific about composition since, as milk secretion begins after delivery, the composition of colostrum is altered by dilution with real milk. The high concentrations of immunoglobulin and lactoferrin in colostrum are probably significant in protection of the neonate from pathogenic organisms. Specific roles for the other nutrients present in high quantities in colostrum are less obvious.

Table 3.4 Composition (units/l) of colostrum compared with mature human milk (DHSS, 1977)

	Colostrum	Mature human milk
Energy:		
kJ	Very variable	2940
kcal		700
Total protein (g)	100	11
Secretory IgA (g)	54	1.5
Lactoferrin (g)	14	1.5
Casein:whey ratio	16:84	40:60
Fat (g)	29	42
Saturated:polyunsaturated	41:59	50:50
Lactose (g)	53	70
Vitamin:		
A (µg)	1260	600
D (µg)	18	6
Sodium (mmol)	21	6.5
Chloride (mmol)	17	12
Calcium (mmol)	8	9
Phosphate (mmol)	5	5
Iron (µmol)	28	14

The composition of mature human milk is much more appropriate for the nutrition of human infants than that of unmodified cows' milk (*see Table 4.1*). When standard infant formulas consisted of relatively unmodified cows' milk, many infants suffered, and some died, from the complications of formula, rather than breast, feeding. Modern highly modified formulas are much safer and there is little evidence that the composition of human milk is *quantitatively* more appropriate for infants than standard formulas based on cows' milk. *Qualitatively*, however, this is not the case. There are still important compositional differences between human and formula milks which are advantageous for breast-fed infants. Not the least of these are the anti-infective properties already described. Other factors specific to breast milk also facilitate absorption of some nutrients.

Fat
The fat content of human milk varies with maternal nutritional status, the time of day, the stage of a feed and the duration of lactation. Fat levels are highest in well-nourished women after the main meal of the day, towards the end of a feed and in the first months of lactation (Jelliffe and Jelliffe, 1978; Harzer *et al.*, 1983).

Normal term infants absorb about 95% of breast-milk fat but only about 85% of fat from unmodified cows' milk. Absorption of fat from modern formulas is better than that from unmodified cows' milk, but less good than that in breast milk. Pancreatic lipase is low in newborn infants and fat absorption is more dependent on lingual lipase secreted at suckling than at other ages (Fink, Hamosh and Hamosh, 1984). Breast milk contains a bile salt stimulated lipase which facilitates fat digestion.

The small size of the fat globules in breast milk also speeds digestion through presenting a large surface area to volume ratio for enzymatic action. The high unsaturated fatty acid composition of human milk fat also encourages absorption. Where saturated fatty acids are present in human milk triglycerides, they occupy the middle binding position in the glycerol molecule so that lipolysis of peripheral fatty acids allows the saturated fatty acids to be absorbed as 2-monoglycerides – a form in which their absorption is more efficient than as non-esterified fatty acids (Fomon, 1974).

Protein
Human milk protein is predominantly lactalbumin with a relatively low proportion of casein. The low casein content of human milk gives it a rather transparent appearance when compared with cows' milk. Mothers should not be allowed to think (as they sometimes do) that the thin appearance of their milk makes it inadequate for nutrition of their infants. Human milk contains amino acids in roughly the proportion they are required for synthesis of human protein except that there are higher levels of taurine, cysteine and tryptophan than would seem necessary. Cysteine is an essential amino acid for young infants since absent cystathionease and a relative deficiency of cystathione synthetase prevent synthesis of cysteine from the methionine. The high levels of taurine are less easy to explain, although young infants conjugate bile acids with taurine. In the absence of taurine, glycine conjugation occurs instead. Taurine is necessary for retinal development in kittens but it is not known whether it is important for human retinal development. Why tryptophan levels are high in human milk is not known.

Lactose
The only carbohydrate present in mammalian milks is lactose. Lactose does not occur in other naturally occurring plant or animal tissues. It may be argued that the presence of lactose in milk is due to its high solubility as a sugar. It provides a source of energy, yet conserves water. Calcium absorption may be facilitated by lactose since calcium lactate is a relatively soluble form of calcium. Galactose derived from lactose is utilized in the synthesis of brain lipids, but sufficient galactose can be synthesized in the body for normal brain development even if infants are fed lactose-free milks. Thus there are no totally satisfactory explanations for the uniqueness of lactose in milk.

In neonates, lactose is incompletely absorbed and bacterial digestion leads to acid stools and sometimes the presence of reducing substances in the stool. The neonatal capacity to absorb lactose improves over the first week, but infants fed human milk continue to have rather acid stools owing to the low buffering capacity of the milk. The growth of lactobacilli in the large bowel is facilitated by the acid environment, whereas the growth of potentially pathogenic Gram-negative organisms is inhibited.

Minerals and vitamins
The iron content of breast milk is low, but iron absorption is facilitated by the presence of lactoferrin. Similar patterns of absorption apply to a number of other

nutrients. Folic acid and vitamin B_{12} have specific binding proteins which aid their absorption. Proteins which bind zinc and other minerals act similarly (Sandström, Cederblad and Lönnerdal, 1983).

Human milk appears particularly low in vitamin D. Rickets is not common in breast-fed infants in the first months of life unless their mothers are also deficient in vitamin D. Excellent calcium absorption facilitated by the high lactose content of human milk may reduce the vitamin D requirement of young infants.

Bonding

One advantage often claimed for breast feeding is that it promotes mother–infant 'bonding'. This aspect may have become exaggerated in the excitement over the rediscovery of bonding 10–15 years ago. Budin (1907) in Paris at the beginning of this century pointed out that the care of sick malnourished infants who required bottle feeding and mother–child separation sometimes resulted in physically healthy infants rejected by their mothers who had not been involved in their care. Clearly breast feeding and mother–child separation are incompatible. Differences can be shown between the way breast-feeding and bottle-feeding mothers handle their infants a few days after birth, but it is doubtful if these differences have long-term significance. The attitude of a mother who chooses to breast feed may, by selection, be different from that of a mother who chooses to formula feed. Thus it may not be breast feeding *per se* that causes the differences in mother–child interaction. Successful breast feeding probably does reinforce the mother–child bond where perhaps this is initially tenuous. Moreover, successful breast feeding is 'an outward and visible sign' of effective mother–child interaction. Breast feeding will fail without stimulation of neuro-endocrine responses by maternal emotional responses to sight and suckling of the infant.

It is important to keep the relation of bonding and breast feeding in proportion. Mothers may, for reasons beyond their control, fail to feed their infants successfully at the breast. They may suffer considerable guilt and feelings of failure. If these are heightened by suggestions that, because they cannot breast feed, they will fail to bond successfully with their infants they may become so stressed that they no longer enjoy caring for their infants. It is clearly unrealistic to suggest that the mother–child relationship of bottle-fed infants is inadequate. The grief of women who fail to breast feed successfully must be acknowledged so that appropriate support and counselling can be given when necessary.

Disadvantages of breast feeding

The main medical disadvantage of breast feeding is the difficulty in ascertaining the volumes of milk that infants are ingesting. This is of little importance if infants are well and thriving, but becomes fundamental to making a diagnosis with infants who fail to thrive. Infants who fail to thrive primarily due to inadequate breast-milk intake and those who have little appetite and failure to thrive for other reasons may be difficult to distinguish. If it is important to know how much an infant is receiving from the breast, test weighing can be performed, but this is not a particularly accurate procedure (Whitfield, Kay and Stephens, 1981; Stothers, 1982). Infants are weighed in clean nappies, fed to satisfaction at the breast and then weighed again with the same nappies (*Figure 3.1*). Milk ingested should be indicated by the

32 Breast feeding

(a) Infant weighed accurately in clean nappy

(b) Infant fed to satisfaction

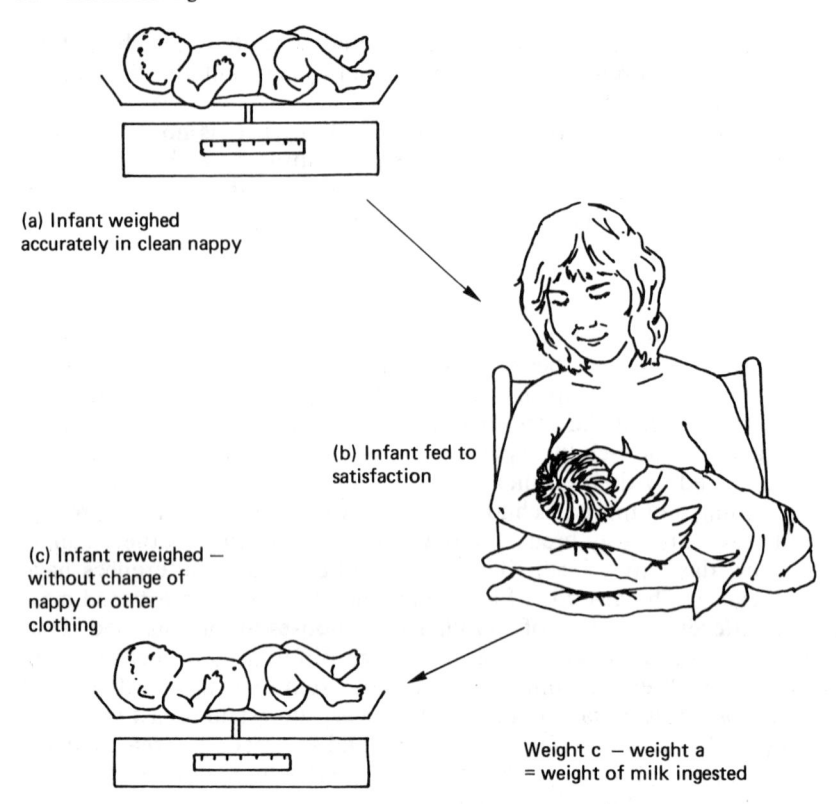

(c) Infant reweighed — without change of nappy or other clothing

Weight c − weight a = weight of milk ingested

Figure 3.1 Test weighing feeds to estimate breast-milk output.

difference between the two weights. Test weighing must be continued over 24 hours of breast feeding since infants often take a lot from the breast early in the day and then may take relatively little milk until evening. Other methods of estimating breast milk output are suitable for research purposes, but not practical for most clinical settings (Coward *et al.*, 1979).

Failure to thrive at the breast

Some infants present with severe failure to thrive secondary to inadequate breast-milk production. Often these babies are quiet and lethargic rather than fretful and obviously hungry. Those who express their hunger by crying may be offered water if they have only recently been suckled. Many of their mothers are well-educated women who know that breast feeding is best for their infants and that obesity is not good and who are therefore reluctant to accept that their thin, quiet, well-behaved infants are not getting sufficient milk (Evans and Davies, 1977). The infants appear satisfied, perhaps because other aspects of nurture are so caring and adequate that they compensate for the lack of food. Some are too poorly nourished to have energy for crying.

Recognition of the desperate plight of these infants may only come when their mothers visit relatives or baby clinics. The infants are wasted and under weight for age. They are constipated, passing small, greenish, dry stools secondary to their gross underfeeding. Occasionally they may be described as having green diarrhoea. This 'diarrhoea' describes small quantities of green liquid consisting of bile and mucus passed in starvation – 'starvation stools'. The infants may suck vigorously at the breast, but test weighing demonstrates ingestion of totally inadequate volumes of milk.

It is not usually possible to resurrect adequate breast-milk secretion for these infants to thrive on breast feeding alone. If the infant is aged 10 weeks or more, early introduction of solids and continuation of breast feeding may accelerate growth. With younger infants, complementary formula feeding will be necessary. Complete change to full volume formula feeding is the more satisfactory solution for the infant since with supplementary feeds, infants are liable to receive only token additions to their inadequate breast-milk intake. As the mothers introduce formula milk, the stimulus to breast milk production from their infants' hunger declines further.

It is often difficult to explain to mothers of infants failing to thrive at the breast that their milk output is insufficient. A tactful approach is needed. It may be helpful to reassure mothers that the main advantages of breast feeding come in the first days or weeks of life hence failure at a later stage is less depriving or disadvantageous for infants. They may insist on continuing breast feeding but must give full complements as well. Suckling infants after, or in between, *adequate* formula feeds is very acceptable since it may provide some nutrition and protection for the infant if mother is still producing milk. It usually provides a lot of satisfaction both to mothers and to infants. The resolution of feeding problems in infancy usually evolves more from mothers' attitudes and beliefs than from rigid instructions from doctors.

Do breast-fed infants need water?
Often infants with failure to thrive at the breast are being given significant amounts of water by bottle as well as suckling at the breast. The practice of feeding water to young infants seems to have developed in the late 1960s when it was recognized that dehydration and starvation exacerbated neonatal jaundice and when hypernatraemia was common due to feeding unmodified cows' milk formula. This practice has persisted, and breast-fed infants are liable to be offered water in the middle of the night or in between '3–4 hourly' feeds in maternity hospitals. Mothers continue offering water at home.

There seems to be no indication for giving normal breast-fed infants water. In early lactation, infants should be allowed to suckle for a few minutes if restless since this stimulates greater milk production. Breast feeding should not follow the clock but infants' demands, except that infants sleeping more than 4 hours during the day in early lactation should be woken and suckled to stimulate breast-milk production. In later lactation, if infants seem hungry (or thirsty) they should be put to the breast since without suckling according to need, supply will never equate with demand. Breast-fed infants in Southern Israel in the summer showed no evidence of dehydration despite absence of water supplements. Thus water supplements to normal healthy breast-fed infants in Northern Europe seem likewise unnecessary (Goldberg and Adams, 1983).

Neonates receiving phototherapy for hyperbilirubinaemia have increased water loss both through the exposed skin and into the gastrointestinal tract due to the effects of bilirubin breakdown products in the gut. Such infants should be given 10–20% extra fluid as milk or water *whilst receiving phototherapy*.

Breast-milk jaundice

This is a common problem which causes no difficulty in itself but which generates a lot of concern amongst medical personnel since jaundice due to other causes in young infants may indicate serious underlying disease. Breast-milk jaundice is consequently often over-investigated in order to exclude other possibilities. The maternal worry thus engendered may inhibit satisfactory lactation or persuade mothers that their breastmilk is not good enough for their infants and encourage them to change to formula feeding.

Breast-milk jaundice presents as an unconjugated hyperbilirubinaemia usually at its peak in the second week of life. It rarely reaches dangerous levels since the peak bilirubin is about 250 μmol/l and generally settles to around 200 μmol/l or less by the end of the second week. The hyperbilirubinaemia may be secondary to rapid absorption of long-chain fatty acids in the milk and a high breast milk lipase content. Fatty acid absorption is rapid, and this inhibits bilirubin uptake by the liver, causing an unconjugated hyperbilirubinaemia (Odell, 1981). A more recent suggestion is that high glucuronidase activity in some breast milks breaks down conjugated bilirubin secreted into the gut via the bile duct leading to increased reabsorption of unconjugated bilirubin. The effect of this is to present the immature liver with a much greater load of bilirubin for conjugation. Hyperbilirubinaemia results (Gourley and Arend, 1986).

Infants with breast-milk jaundice are usually gaining weight rapidly and thriving despite their hyperbilirubinaemia. Thriving provides an important clinical difference from the other causes of late hyperbilirubinaemia (infection, hypothyroidism, neonatal hepatitis syndrome) where infants fail to thrive and feed poorly.

Vitamin K deficiency

Infants are born with low vitamin K levels. Formula milks are now supplemented with vitamin K and levels rise quite rapidly in bottle-fed infants. In breast-fed infants vitamin K levels remain low and there is considerable risk of haemorrhagic disease of the newborn with bruising and/or bleeding from gastrointestinal tract or umbilical stump, usually in the first week of life. Factors II, VII, IX and X are deficient. Prothrombin time and activated partial thromboplastin time will be prolonged.

All infants, irrespective of how they are expected to be fed, should be given 1 mg natural vitamin K analogues (e.g. Konakion; Roche) by mouth or intramusculary immediately after birth. Occasionally infants – usually breast fed – present with haemorrhagic disease of the newborn after the first week of life despite therapeutic vitamin K at birth (Shearer, *et al.*, 1982). Any infant presenting with easy bruising or bleeding in early life should be given a second dose of vitamin K if there is no other obvious explanation for the bleeding tendency (Verity, Carswell and Scott, 1983).

Drugs in breast milk

Many drugs are transmitted to the infant in breast milk. The amounts ingested by infants are usually low since the concentrations of most drugs in milk are equivalent to plasma levels. Some drugs are actively secreted into milk and are contraindicated during lactation or, when treatment of the mother is essential, lactation is contraindicated (Committee on Drugs, 1983).

The breast-fed infants of mothers who are receiving drugs not thought to be transmitted in significant amounts should be observed for possible side effects. Occasionally idiosyncratic and allergic responses occur to drugs which are only present in the milk in minute quantities. The types of drugs to be used cautiously or not at all are listed below:

1. Drugs to be avoided in lactation or which contraindicate breast feeding:
   (a) Because of undesirable effects at any dosage: cytotoxic drugs, folate antagonists, immunosuppressive agents, radioactive drugs and treatments.
   (b) Because of relatively high levels in milk and undesirable effects: lithium, tetracycline, benzodiazepines, isoniazid, gold, rifampicin, indomethacin, ethambutol, chloramphenicol, nalidixic acid, cimetidine, non-warfarin anticoagulants.
   (c) Because of previous hypersensititivity reaction by infant – e.g. penicillin, aspirin.
   (d) Because of inhibitory effect on lactation: bromocriptine, contraceptive agents, chlorthiazides.
2. Drugs to be prescribed only when infant can be observed for possible unwanted effects: anticonvulsants, alcohol, laxatives, opiates, sympathomimetics.
3. Drugs to be avoided in certain circumstances:
   (a) Sulphonamides in hyperbilirubinaemia because of displacement of bilirubin from albumin binding sites.
   (b) Drugs that can precipitate haemolysis if infant has glucose-6-phosphate dehydrogenase deficiency.
   (c) Aspartame (commercial sweetener) with phenylketonuric infants.

Infections transmitted in breast milk

Breast milk is not sterile, but the risks to infants from bacteria in their own mother's milk are few since the milk almost certainly carries secretory IgA protective against these bacteria. Viruses in milk are more likely to cause infection. This is particularly likely if the milk is fed as banked, but not pasteurized, milk to infants other than the mother's own. Cytomegalovirus infection may be acquired from milk where mothers have either primary infection, or reactivation of infection, during lactation (Dworsky et al., 1983). In the latter case it is likely that the mothers' own infants were infected transplacentally and have either acquired cytomegalovirus infection already or acquired resistance to it before birth. Maternally acquired immunoglobulin G may provide protection for the infant when there is maternal reactivation.

Hepatitis B virus can also be acquired through breast milk, particularly if the mother's blood shows H Be Ag. However, the greatest risk to these infants is from ingestion of maternal blood at delivery. Infants of such mothers should be given hepatitis B immunoglobulin immediately at delivery followed by a full course of active hepatitis B immunization soon after this. Maternal hepatitis B carriage is *not* a contraindication to breast feeding. Formula-fed infants of hepatitis B carrying mothers are also likely to acquire the infection at, or shortly after, birth from close contact with their mothers.

Infants born to mothers infected with HIV may have acquired the infection transplacentally. If not, they may become infected by viral transmission in milk. Until there is some chance of successful immunization or treatment for AIDS it would seem that HIV-positive women in developed Westernized countries should be advised to formula feed their infants (DHSS, 1988). HIV is common in some areas of the developing world, most notably East and Central Africa. The relative risk of mother–child transmission in breast-fed and non-breast-fed infants in these countries and the chances of HIV-infected children developing acquired immune deficiency syndrome (AIDS) are not known. Risks for morbidity and mortality from artificial feeding may be greater for these infants than the risks of acquiring HIV infection, so breast feeding should probably continue. This is an area of great ignorance at the present time.

Breast-milk banking

The advantages of breast milk, particularly for sick infants and relatively large low birthweight infants, are such that there is a need to provide milk for infants who have to stay in hospitals without their mothers or who require tube feeding because of immaturity or sickness. Breast-milk banks have been established in association with many special care nurseries and neonatal surgical units. Mothers who have infants in these units, or who have more milk than their own infants require, express milk either manually or by breast pump and then deliver it to the bank. Milk that drips from the contralateral breast during feeding can also be collected. Some mothers produce 50–100 ml of 'drip' milk daily, but the quality of drip milk is less satisfactory than that of milk produced by manual or pump expression. 'Drip' milk should not be fed without some 'fortification'.

Mothers who produce milk for these banks provide a tremendous service. There are, however, problems associated with storing the milk in ways that make it not only safe but also immunologically and nutritionally useful to infants (DHSS, 1981).

Breast milk obtained under hygienic conditions can be stored at 4°C for 24 hours with safety. Most units culture this raw milk before it is fed to infants. Milk containing more than 10^5 organisms/ml is discarded or processed. Raw milk stored at 4°C loses most of its constituent cells since these adhere to containers and do not tolerate storage well. Milk stored in polypropylene containers shows a significant decrease in lysozyme and lactoferrin content after 24 hours. That stored in polyethylene containers loses much of its specific secretory IgA antibodies to *E. coli* somatic antigen. The rate at which lipase activity declines is not clear. Some fat is lost through adherence to containers, particularly if the milk is then fed by slow nasogastric or orogastric drip.

Breast milk can also be pasteurized and stored for some weeks. A rapid rise in temperature to 62.5°C and then holding this temperature for 30 minutes reduces the bacterial colony count of milk to nil in over 95% of samples. Milk pasteurized in this way is stored deep frozen until needed. All cells and much of the lipase, lactoferrin and secretory IgA activity are probably lost. Lysozyme seems fairly well preserved but pasteurization seriously impairs the overall antibacterial effects of human milk. Antiviral factors may be more resistant.

Where milk is 'raw' and remains unused after 24 hours, it can be deep frozen. If frozen rapidly in small volumes immediately after expression nutrient quality is preserved quite well for at least a week (Reynolds *et al.*, 1982).

Carriers of hepatitis viruses, cytomegalovirus or HIV should not be used as milk donors. Preferably no milk should be pooled. If milk is pooled, fewer than ten donations should be used in one pool. Recent concern over AIDS has led to government recommendations that *no* unpasteurized milk should be banked.

Banked human milk may be low in some nutrients, notably energy. This is particularly so for drip breast milk. Banked human milk may be fortified to meet the needs of infants. Before starting such a complicated procedure, it is wise to ensure that at least some of the benefits of human milk (anti-infective properties, facilitated nutrient absorption) are preseved in the banking and fortifying process, otherwise the effort of supplementing the milk is not worth while. Supplements of medium-chain triglycerides, phosphate and partially skimmed human milk can be added to increase energy, phosphate, protein and mineral intake.

Growth of breast-fed infants

There have been innumerable studies trying to assess the relative growth of breast- and formula-fed infants. Every possible result seems to have been obtained. Some studies suggest that formula-fed infants grow best, some that breast-fed infants grow best and some show no difference. Many factors other than the type of milk used determine the growth of infants. However, many breast-fed infants undoubtedly grow exceedingly well and growth can be just as rapid as that of the most rapidly growing formula-fed infants.

Recent studies from Cambridge and the Gambia have shown that initial growth of both breast- and formula-fed infants is more rapid than previously represented by growth centiles. This had been recognized 30 years previously (Wickes, 1952). Growth tends to slow in the third and fourth months of life as a natural process and not due to inadequacy of the milk diet (Whitehead, Paul and Cole, 1981; Whitehead and Paul, 1981; Butte *et al.*, 1984). Energy requirements/kg body weight/day are particularly low between 4 and 6 months. The volumes of milk mothers who have not weaned their infants produce at 4–6 months lactation support satisfactory growth levels, although the volumes appear inadequate using previous interpretations of infants' energy requirements and growth rates.

The addition of non-milk foods to the diet of breast-fed infants is likely to reduce the vigour of infants' suckling and decrease the stimulus to milk secretion. Breast-milk output declines rapidly when most women in developed countries introduce weaning foods since they usually decrease the frequency of suckling as they introduce weaning diet. In more traditional societies, women who continue to breast feed during weaning may still suckle their infants frequently. Breast milk output may remain around 500–600 ml in the second half of the first year.

Prolonged breast feeding

Practical advice to breast-feeding mothers suggests that infants should be introduced to solids from 3 months at the earliest, but by 6 months at the latest (DHSS, 1988). Some totally breast-fed infants continue to grow exceedingly well in the second 6 months of life when breast milk alone is usually insufficient (Ahn and MacLean, 1980). The mothers of infants who are successfully totally breast fed after the age of 6 months are generally women who have shown particular dedication to breast feeding and who have practised and maintained high-frequency suckling and thus continue to stimulate secretion of large volumes of milk in the second 6 months of life (Florack *et al.*, 1984). The infants have received no food nor fluid other than breast milk. Although it has been stated that women produce a maximum of 800 ml of milk per day, many mothers can produce much more milk than this under appropriate circumstances. One mother feeding triplets has been recorded as secreting more than 3 litres of milk per day (Saint, Maggiore and Hartmann, 1986). *Table 3.5* outlines the factors contributing to successful prolonged lactation.

Table 3.5 Factors contributing to successful prolonged lactation

Well-nourished mother eating well
Hungry vigorous infant
High-frequency suckling maintained through first 6 months of infant's life
Night-time feeding continued
No supplementary milk, water or diet given
Mother non-smoker
Mother not taking hormonal contraceptives

The mothers we have just described who feed their infants on breast milk alone successfully after 6 months are fairly exceptional. Energy deficiency in the second 6 months of life due to inadequate milk intake from the breast and delayed weaning is one of the more important causes of poor growth in infancy. The relatively low levels of iron, vitamins and trace elements in breast milk may fail to meet requirements for totally breast-fed infants after 6 months of age. Thus infants who are breast fed for prolonged periods are likely to fail to thrive and to develop iron-deficiency anaemia and vitamin D deficiency (unless adequately exposed to summer sunlight). Trace element deficiencies are also likely, although these may be difficult to demonstrate.

Despite the inadequacy of breast milk alone to meet requirements of the majority of infants after 6 months of age, breast feeding and weaning foods should be fed together for as long as practical. This is particularly important for infants of mothers in traditional disadvantaged societies where weaning foods are likely to be low in protein. The 500–600 ml/day of breast milk usually secreted by these mothers at this stage in lactation can make a significant contribution to infants' protein needs. Energy requirements at the age of a year are met by about 1500 ml of milk, but protein requirements can be satisfied by approximately 1 litre of milk (if milk were still the only food consumed).

Improving breast-feeding 'statistics'

It has been commented that in 1970 supplying formula milk for the infants in Chile who were not breast fed required the equivalent of the annual milk production of 32 000 Chilean cows. It was estimated that 78 600, out of a potential 93 200, tons of breast milk were 'unrealized' owing to formula feeding (Berg, 1973). These statistics can be repeated the world over. Apart from being economically wasteful, this prevalence of formula feeding has disastrous effects on the health of infants in developing countries.

The dangers of infection to formula-fed infants and the expense of formula feeding are less significant in Britain but the arguments still apply. All those concerned for the health of children should do everything in their power to encourage breast feeding of young infants (DHSS, 1988). The advertisement of formula milks, even if not banned as in some countries, should be discouraged. Commercial publicity given to new mothers needs to be scrutinized carefully and critically. Education of the general public is necessary to encourage breast feeding as the natural and expected way for young infants to be fed (Richards, 1982). Facilities for mothers to breast feed in public places must be increased and it must become generally more acceptable for women to use their breasts for their biological purpose. Breast feeding is too often regarded as 'not quite decent', something that takes place behind closed doors. This must change.

References

AHN, C. H. and MacLEAN, W. C. (1980) Growth of the exclusively breast fed infant. *American Journal of Clinical Nutrition*, **33**, 182–192

BERG, A. (1973) *The Nutrition Factor*, p. 90. Washington: The Brookings Institution

BUDIN, P. (1907) *The Nursling*. London: Caxton Printing Company

BUTTE, N. F., GARZA, C., O'BRIAN SMITH, E. and NICHOLS, B. L. (1984) Human milk intake and growth in exclusively breast fed infants. *Journal of Pediatrics*, **104**, 187–195

COMMITTEE ON DRUGS (1983) The transfer of drugs and other chemicals into human breast milk. *Pediatrics*, **72**, 375–383

COWARD, W. A., WHITEHEAD, R. G., SAWYER, M. B., PRENTICE, A. M. and EVANS, J. (1979) New method for measuring milk intakes in breast fed babies. *Lancet*, **ii**, 13–15

DE CHATEAU, P. and WINBURG, J. (1978) Immediate postpartum suckling contact and duration of breast feeding. *Journal of Maternal and Child Health*, **3**, 392–395

DEPARTMENT OF HEALTH AND SOCIAL SECURITY (1977) *The Composition of Mature Human Milk*. Reports on Health and Social Subjects, No. 12. London: Her Majesty's Stationery Office

DEPARTMENT OF HEALTH AND SOCIAL SECURITY (1988) *Present Day Practice in Infant Feeding: Third Report*. Report on Health and Social Subjects, No. 32. London: Her Majesty's Stationery Office

DEPARTMENT OF HEALTH AND SOCIAL SECURITY (1981) *The Collection and Storage of Human Milk*. Report on Health and Social Subjects, No. 22. London: Her Majesty's Stationery Office

DUFFY, L. C., RIEPENHOFF-TALTY, M., BYERS, T. E., LA SCOLEA, L. J., ZIELEZNY, M. A., DRYJA, D. M. and OGRA, P. L. (1986) Modulation of rotavirus enteritis during breast feeding. *American Journal of Diseases of Children*, **140**, 1164–1168

DWORSKY, M., YOW, M., STAGNO, S., PASS, R. F. and ALFORD, C. (1983) Cytomegalovirus infection of breast milk and transmission in infancy. *Pediatrics*, **72**, 295–299

EVANS, N., WALPOLE, I. R., QURESHI, M. V., MEMON, M. H. and EVERLEY-JONES, H. W. (1976) Lack of breast feeding and early weaning in infants of Asian immigrants to Wolverhampton. *Archives of Disease in Childhood*, **51**, 608–612

EVANS, T. J. and DAVIES, D. P. (1977) Failure to thrive at the breast: an old problem revisited. *Archives of Disease in Childhood*, **52**, 974–975

FILDES, V. A. (1986) *Breasts, Bottles and Babies*, p. 403. Edinburgh: Edinburgh University Press

FINK, C. S., HAMOSH, P. and HAMOSH, M. (1984) Fat digestion in the stomach: stability of lingual lipase in the gastric environment. *Pediatric Research*, **18**, 248–254

FISHER, C. (1981) Breast feeding: a midwife's view. *Journal of Maternal and Child Health*, **6**, 52–57

FLORACK, B., OBERMANN-DE BOER, G., KAMPEN-DONKER, M., VAN WINGEN, J. and KROMHOUT, D. (1984) Breast feeding, bottle feeding and related factors. *Acta Paediatrica Scandinavica*, **73**, 789–795

FOMON, S. J. (1974) *Infant Nutrition*. Philadelphia: W. B. Saunders

GLASIER, A. S., McNEILLY, A. S. and HOWIE, P. W. (1984) The prolactin response to suckling. *Clinical Endocrinology*, **21**, 109–116

GOLDBERG, N. M. and ADAMS, E. (1983) Supplementary water for breast fed babies in a hot and dry climate – not really a necessity. *Archives of Disease in Childhood*, **58**, 73–74

GOLDMAN, A. S., GARZA, C., NICHOLS, B. L. and GOLDBLUM, R. M. (1982) Immunological factors in human milk during the first year of lactation. *Journal of Pediatrics,* **100,** 563–567

GOURLEY, G. R. and AREND, R. A. (1986) β-glucuronidase and hyperbilirubinaemia in breast fed and formula fed babies. *Lancet,* **i,** 644–646

GUNTHER, M. (1973) *Infant Feeding.* Harmondsworth: Penguin Books

HARZER, G., HAUG, M., DIETERICH, I. and GENTNER, P. R. (1983) Changing patterns of human milk lipids in the course of lactation and during the day. *American Journal of Clinical Nutrition,* **37,** 612–621

HOWIE, P. W. (1985) Breast feeding – a new understanding. *Midwives Chronicle and Nursing Notes,* **99,** 184–192

JELLIFFE, D. B. and JELLIFFE, E. F. P. (1978) *Human Milk in the Modern World.* Oxford: Oxford University Press

JONES, D. A. and WEST, R. R. (1985) Lactation nurse increases duration of breast feeding. *Archives of Disease in Childhood,* **60,** 722–774

LUCAS, A., LUCAS, P. J. and BAUM, J. D. (1979) Pattern of milk flow in breast fed infants. *Lancet,* **i,** 1139–1141

MARTIN, J. and MONK, J. (1982) *Infant Feeding 1980.* London: Office of Population Censuses and Surveys

NELIGAN, G. (1978) Breast feeding: reversing the decline. *Journal of Maternal and Child Health,* **3,** 23–28

ODELL, G. B. (1981) *Neonatal Hyperbilirubinaemia,* p. 67. New York: Grune and Stratton

REYNOLDS, G. J., MEADE, H. J., BROWN, B. J., FITZGERALD, J. S., ISHERWOOD, D. M. and LEWIS-JONES, D. I. (1982) Simplified banking of human milk. *British Medical Journal,* **284,** 560

RICHARDS, M. P. M. (1982) Breast feeding and the mother–infant relationship. *Acta Paediatrica Scandinavica* (Suppl.), **299,** 33–37

ROLLES, C. J. and CUSSENS, L. (1980) Cells in human milk. *Archives of Disease in Childhood,* **55,** 969–972

SAINT, L., MAGGIORE, P. and HARTMANN, P. E. (1986) Yield and nutrient content of milk in eight women breast feeding twins and one woman breast feeding triplets. *British Journal of Nutrition,* **56,** 49–58

SALARIYA, E. M., EASTON, P. M. and CATER, J. I. (1978) Duration of breast feeding after early initiation and frequent feeding. *Lancet,* **ii,** 1141–1143

SANDSTRÖM, B., CEDERBLAD, A. and LÖNNERDAHL, B. (1983) Zinc absorption from human milk, cow's milk and infant formula. *American Journal of Disease in Childhood,* **137,** 726–729

SHEARER, M. J., BARKHAN, P., RAKIN, S. and STIMMLER, L. (1982) Plasma vitamin K_1 in mothers and their newborn babies. *Lancet,* **ii,** 460–463

STOTHERS, J. K. (1982) Accuracy of routine clinical test weighing. *Archives of Disease in Childhood,* **57,** 810

VERITY, C. M., CARSWELL, F. and SCOTT, G. L. (1983) Vitamin K deficiency causing infantile intracranial haemorrhage after the neonatal period. *Lancet,* **i,** 1439

WHITEHEAD, R. G. and PAUL, A. A. (1981) Infant growth and human milk requirements. *Lancet,* **ii,** 161–163

WHITEHEAD, R. G., PAUL, A. A. and COLE, T. J. (1981) A critical analysis of measured food energy intakes during infancy and early childhood in comparison with current international recommendations. *Journal of Human Nutrition,* **35,** 339–348

WHITFIELD, M. F., KAY, R. and STEPHENS, S. (1981) Validity of routine clinical test weighing as a measure of the intake of breast fed infants. *Archives of Disease in Childhood,* **56,** 919–921

WICKES, I. G. (1952) Rate of gain and satiety in early infancy. *Archives of Disease in Childhood,* **27,** 449–456

WICKES, I. G. (1953) A history of infant feeding. *Archives of Disease in Childhood,* **28,** 151–158, 232–240, 332–340, 416–422, 495–502

YOSHIOKA, H., IDEKI, K. and FUJIIYA, M. (1983) Development and differences in intestinal flora in the neonatal period in breast fed and bottle fed infants. *Pediatrics,* **72,** 317–320

Chapter 4
Formula feeding

Infants who are not breast fed require infant formula. In the recent past, infant formulas were basically cows' milk reconstituted by adding water and sugar to dilute the high electrolyte and protein content of cows' milk when compared with human milk, whilst maintaining adequate energy density. These unmodified cows' milk formulas caused many problems (*see below*). Modern formulas, which have only been in widespread use in Britain since 1975, are more appropriate in quantitative composition than unmodified cows' milk based formulas (DHSS, 1980a) but are still very different in quality from breast milk (*Table 4.1*). Formulas lack the anti-infective properties of human milk and facilitated absorption of fat, minerals and vitamins. They also lack the enzymes, hormones and prostaglandins present in human milk.

Table 4.1 Composition (units/l) of human milk, cows' milk based and soya protein based formulas and cows' milk*

	Human milk*	Standard infant formulas†	Soya formulas†	Cows' milk
Energy:				
kJ	2940	2720–2940	2800–2850	2800
kcal	700	650–700	670–680	670
Protein (g)	11	15–19	18–22	35
casein:whey	40:60	82:18–32:68	–	82:18
Fat (g)	42	24–38	36–38	36
Saturated:unsaturated	50:50	40:60–63:37	ND	63:37
Carbohydrate (g)	70	69–86	67–68	49
Sodium (mmol)	6.5	6.5–13.5	8–13	23
Chloride (mmol)	12	11–16	10–11	28
Calcium (mmol)	8.8	9–18	14–16	30
Phosphate (mmol)	5	10–18	9–14	32
Iron (µmol)	13.5	116–125	116–125	9
Vitamin A (µg)	600	610–1000	≈850	400
Vitamin C (mg)	38	55–69	≈68	15
Vitamin D (µg)	6	10–11	≈12	0.2

* Fomon, 1974; DHSS, 1977; Lucas, 1986.
† Manufacturer's literature to provide range of values encompassed by standard formulas.
ND, no data.

Modern, modified, cows' milk formulas

Table 4.2 outlines the qualitative composition of the main milks used in Britain. Manufacturers modify their products fairly frequently, and if there is concern about the effects or lack of a nutrient in a child it is important to check current constituents of formula milks with the manufacturers.

Table 4.2 Qualitative composition of standard infant formulas used in Britain

Formula	Manufacturer	Protein source	Fat source	Carbohydrate source
1 Highly modified formulas (whey>casein; UFA>SFA)				
Premium	Cow & Gate	C, W	M, V	L
SMA Gold Cap	Wyeth	C, W	B, V	L
Osterfeed	Boots/Farley	C, W	M, V	L
2 Highly modified protein but intermediate fat (whey>casein; SFA>UFA)				
Aptamil	Milupa	C, W	M, V	L
3 Predominantly cows' milk protein (casein>whey; UFA>SFA)				
SMA White Cap	Wyeth	C	B, V	L
Ostermilk Complete	Boots/Farley	C	M, V	L, MD
Ostermilk Two	Boots/Farley	C	M, V	L, MD
Babymilk Plus	Cow & Gate	C	M, V	L
4 Predominantly cows' milk protein and saturated fat (casein>whey; SFA>UFA)				
Milumil	Milupa	C	M, V	L, MD, A

A = amylose
B = beef fat
C = cows'-milk protein
L = lactose
M = milk fat
MD = maltodextrins
SFA = saturated fatty acids
UFA = mono- and poly-unsaturated fatty acids
V = vegetable oils
W = demineralized whey

All modern cows' milk based formulas for sale in Britain as feeds for normal, healthy, full-term infants are greatly modified with reduced protein and electrolytes and added vitamins and iron compared with cows' milk (DHSS, 1988). The most highly modified formulas are those where the proportion of curd and whey protein has been 'humanized' (i.e. made comparable in quantity of nutrients to breast milk) and in which the fats are predominantly mono- or poly-unsaturated fatty acids similar in pattern to those of full-term human milk, but of vegetable origin. These are probably the most appropriate milks for very young infants, although there is nothing about their formula that makes them in any way unsuitable for older infants. It is perfectly reasonable for mothers to keep their infants on these highly modified formulas until they change to 'doorstep' milk at 1 year.

The less modified milks are those where the protein composition is basically that of cows' milk with high curd to whey ratio and/or the fat is predominantly saturated fatty acid. There is no reason to change infants to these less highly modified formula feeds, although many mothers and health visitors appear to feel that these milks are more satisfying to older infants. If digestion and absorption of fat and protein were less efficient, the infants' gastrointestinal tracts might empty less readily thus increasing the duration of satiety after a meal. There is no substantial evidence that this is so. 'Satisfaction' following feeding probably reflects mothers' or attendants' views on feeding more than it represents actual differences in satiety felt by the infants.

Modern cows' milk based formulas represent considerable developments in understanding of infant nutrition arising from recognition of the problems of cows' milk feeding. They are far from the 'Full Cream National Dried' formulas widely sold 20 years ago. Protein content is greatly reduced but, where casein predominates, the different amino acid composition necessitates slightly higher protein in the cows' milk based formulas than in human milk in order to meet requirements for cysteine. More recently, some manufacturers have added taurine to these milks since this is another amino acid present in high concentration in human milk (Rassin, Sturman and Gaull, 1978). The importance of the high taurine levels in human milk is not understood. Work in animals suggests that taurine may be important in brain and retinal development. Taurine-containing bile salts may emulsify fats more effectively than glycine-containing bile salts. It is unlikely that adding taurine to formulas to make composition similar to human milk is harmful, and it may be beneficial.

The fat of cows' milk is predominantly saturated fatty acids. Polyunsaturated fatty acids are better absorbed than the saturated fats of butter. This has led manufacturers to alter the fat composition of cows' milk based formulas to 'humanize' them. Vegetable fats high in polyunsaturated fatty acids are added after removal of butter fat. Quantitatively the fat is similar to human milk fat but the actual fatty acids present in human milk and formula are not necessarily the same.

The introduction of vegetable fats with high polyunsaturated fatty acid content has further complicated formula manufacture. Higher levels of vitamin E are necessary for metabolism with high polyunsaturated fatty acid intakes. DHSS (1980) recommendations are that α-tocopherol (vitamin E) should be present in formulas in the proportion of 0.4 mg α-tocopherol to 1 g polyunsaturated fatty acids and vitamin E content in infant formula should not be less than 0.3 mg α-tocopherol/100 ml reconstituted feed.

Linoleic and linolenic acid are both essential fatty acids in infancy but the levels found in cows' milk fat (each about 1.5% total fatty acids) appear sufficient to prevent deficiencies in term human infants. The essential fatty acid content of human milk fat depends on maternal diet and varies widely. DHSS (1980) recommendations are that α-linolenic and linoleic acids together should provide not less than 1% of the total energy in the milk and should not exceed 20% of the total fatty acids.

Human milk has a slightly higher lactose content than cows' milk. Lactose is an expensive sugar and for practical reasons – as much as any other – manufacturers have tended to introduce carbohydrates other than lactose to formula milks. These are glucose, sucrose, maltose and maltodextrin (breakdown products of starch). Amylose is also used. All standard infant formulas will be poorly tolerated if infants develop lactose (or disaccharide) intolerance or cows' milk protein intolerance (*see* Chapter 15).

It must be clear that formula milks represent multiple modifications of cows' milk. Quantitative changes that make the milk appear closer in composition to human milk may not have equivalent qualitative effects or may unmask hitherto unrecognized nutritional needs or interrelations between nutrients. All formula changes must be followed carefully for adverse effects. Whether any of the differences between formulas and human milk have significant effects in adult life and for the prevention of the degenerative diseases of age has so far proved impossible either to demonstrate or disprove although associations have been drawn (Barker and Osmond, 1986). The possibility that methods of infant feeding may be relevant to later health and longevity should always be remembered (*see* Chapter 21).

Making up the formula

Powdered or freeze dried granular formula is usually sold with standard scoops. All standard formulas are now made up by the same method of mixing one flat, not packed, scoop of powder and 28 ml or 1 fl oz water. The powder dissolves readily. Pre-packed liquid feeds are available, but usually for hospital use only. Liquid feeds are unnecessarily bulky for home use, although they avoid the problems of sterilization of teats and bottles. Prepacked liquid feeds may contain some lactulose formed during processing and sterilization. Occasionally this causes soft, frequent stools and detectable reducing substances in the stools. Lactulose stools may be misdiagnosed as lactose intolerance (Hendrickse, Wooldridge and Russell, 1977).

How much is fed?

The milk requirements of young infants are usually stated as 150 ml/kg/day (105 kcal/kg/day). Most infants take less than this in the first days of life but can be expected to consume this amount by the end of the first week. This figure is only an average and some infants consume much more, once feeding is established. Intakes at 4–6 weeks of life may be greatly in excess of 'recommended' volumes (Wickes, 1952; Fomon, Owen and Thomas, 1964), but by the age of 3–4 months intake/kg/day has declined and total daily intake may remain more or less constant, despite increasing weight (Fomon, Owen and Thomas, 1964). Six feeds a day, on average, are required in the first days of life, but most infants settle to a five feed per day regimen, missing out one night feed, in the course of a few weeks. Infants under 3 kg with smaller stomachs and more rapid growth should be offered feeds three hourly initially since they may be unable to take requirements on a four hourly basis without dangerous gastric over-distension or risk of vomiting and inhalation.

Infant feeding regimens provide guidelines only. Variations in demand and need between individuals are enormous. The evidence for whether infants are receiving sufficient milk should be taken from their growth rates and general health and well-being and not from the absolute values for their milk intakes. The misinterpretation of growth charts and recommended allowances has led to a lot of confusion and misunderstanding about appropriate diets for young infants. We have discussed in the previous chapter how early infant growth is more rapid than indicated on most growth standards but slows by 4–6 months so that growth may settle back on to earlier centiles (Whitehead and Paul, 1984).

International Code of Marketing Breast-Milk Substitutes

In recent years there has been considerable international concern over the marketing of breast-milk substitutes. It was felt by many people concerned with the health of children that advertisements and pressure from salesmen acting for the infant formula manufacturers were encouraging women to change from traditional breast feeding to formula feeding. Advertisements even suggested that formula feeding was better and produced larger, healthier, infants. In affluent countries this was unfortunate. In developing countries it was disastrous (Puffer and Serrano, 1973). Mortality secondary to gastroenteritis and malnutrition in non-breast-fed infants in some developing countries is very high indeed. The topic of advertisement of breast-milk substitutes in the developing world was given a lot of media coverage. Emotions for both sides ran high and precipitated legal action.

Infant formula manufacturing is carried out by powerful 'multinationals' which provide financial support for many medical and paramedical projects. Scientific knowledge of infant nutrition has often advanced as a result of such funded projects. Thus the interactions between infant food manufacturing firms, nutritional scientists and clinicians are full of ethical complexities. WHO have tried to rationalize the situation through the International Code of Marketing Breast Milk Substitutes (WHO, 1981). This presents guidelines for acceptable formula marketing and is supported by many countries, particularly those of the Third World. The Code of Practice of Food Manufacturers' Federation (1983) is the UK manufacturers' answer to the WHO Code. At the very least these latter practices should be followed. In Britain, the WHO Code has not been ratified but there are moves within Europe to develop more stringent controls on the advertising and marketing of infant formulas.

Formula feeding and its advertisement may be undesirable in developing countries but the problem of what to feed young infants in these countries when a mother dies or is too sick to suckle or when breast milk secretion fails early in lactation (a situation which does occur occasionally) remains. Food mixes of a sloppy nature that can be fed by spoon using local staple, fortified with local protein sources such as egg or ground-nut sauce, can be tried, but they are slow to feed and recipes need careful design if energy and other nutrient intakes are to be adequate. These mixtures require thorough cooking and feeding from clean vessels if they are to be safe. Cooking may diminish the nutrient quality. Yet formula may be too expensive or supply unavailable in a rural society. Preparation of formula with contaminated water and utensils may be unavoidable. Reluctantly, it has to be accepted that many of these infants end up being fed cows' milk. Cows' milk obtained in these circumstances is likely to be contaminated by pathogenic organisms before sale and may even have been diluted in order to increase profits. To make neat cows' milk safer (but still hazardous) for young infants, milk should be diluted to four-fifths its volume with clean, boiled water to reduce the protein and electrolyte content, and 10 g sugar should be added to every 200 ml to bring the energy content back to an acceptable level. Infants should be offered extra boiled water after feeds especially if febrile, breathless or suffering diarrhoea.

Cows' milk

In circumstances such as those of developed countries where infant formulas are available, neat cows' milk should not be fed to young infants. DHSS (1988) policy in Britain has been to suggest that cows' milk is safe for infants greater than 6 months. However, low levels of vitamins and iron in cows' milk compared with modern formulas and the continuing, although reduced, risk of hypernatraemia in the second half of the first year, make it inadvisable to feed cows' milk until infants are on mixed diets and taking considerable volumes of non-milk fluids. A safe lower age limit for the introduction of cows' milk is 1 year rather than 6 months, in our view.

It is sometimes suggested (erroneously) that goats' milk is a more suitable milk for young infants than cows' milk. Goats' milk may have slightly less allergenic properties than cows' milk but in other respects it is as bad, or worse, than cows' milk. It too, has a high protein and electrolyte content and in addition it is deficient in folic acid. In Britain, regulations governing the conditions for keeping dairy herds and selling cows' milk do not currently apply to goats or the sale of goats' milk. The risks of milk-borne infection from goats' milk are thus higher than from cows' milk (Lawton, 1984).

Problems of cows' milk feeding (*Table 4.3*)

Several of these problems have already been mentioned briefly. Cows' milk presents the greatest risk to the youngest infants and the problems described have more or less vanished since modified milks became the only ones recommended in early infancy (DHSS, 1988).

Table 4.3 Problems with cows' milk feeding for young infants

Inspissated curd syndrome
Hypocalcaemia secondary to hyperphosphataemia
Hypernatraemia and hyperosmolar dehydration
Cows'-milk protein intolerance (CMPI)
Iron deficiency due to low iron content or blood loss due to CMPI
Vitamin deficiencies, especially C and D

Inspissated curd syndrome
Cows' milk has a higher proportion of casein protein than human milk and a higher total protein content. Young infants may have difficulty digesting the tough casein curds, and inspissated undigested curds can cause intestinal obstruction. Abdominal surgery may be necessary to exclude other causes of obstruction and to wash out the curds. This problem has become less common since the protein content of formulas has been decreased, but it still occurs occasionally in very young or immature infants fed feeds with predominantly casein protein.

Neonatal hypocalcaemia
Hypocalcaemia is common in infants in the first week of life. In the first few days it is particularly common in small, premature, sick infants (*see* Chapter 5) and those born with vitamin D deficiency. In the past, however, hypocalcaemia was also common in normal full-term infants who were thriving on unmodified cows' milk formulas. These infants developed hypocalcaemia around the end of the first week of life. The high phosphate content in cows' milk and unmodified cows' milk formula led to high absorption of phosphate. Calcium absorption from cows' milk is less efficient than phosphate absorption in infancy and the high plasma phosphate induced falls in plasma calcium due to alterations in the calcium-phosphate product. This caused hypocalcaemia with jitteriness, tetany and convulsions in

otherwise well-fed, thriving infants. Introduction of low phosphate feeds was effective treatment. Nowadays the problem is unusual in infants who are appropriately fed on modified formulas.

Hypertonic dehydration
Hypernatraemic, hypertonic dehydration was a relatively frequent and disastrous occurrence for infants fed formula milks high in protein, sodium and chloride. In Britain in the late 1960s and early 1970s, early weaning on to high-protein- and high-salt-containing solids from the age of a few weeks contributed to the prevalence of hypernatraemia.

The risk of hypertonic dehydration is one of the main reasons why it is inadvisable to introduce cows' milk to infants under 6 months of age. We recommend keeping infants on formula until about 1 year of age since hypernatraemic dehydration can present in infants in the second 6 months of life, although less frequently than in the first 6 months.

The renal solute load is those solutes derived from food in excess of metabolic requirements, or derived from normal tissue metabolism, which have to be excreted by the kidney. The kidneys of young infants are unable to excrete highly concentrated urine. Young infants fed unmodified cows' milk consequently have plasma sodium, urea and osmolality values in the high normal range following feeds (Davies, 1973). If fluid intake is reduced or extra renal fluid loss increased, the solute load presented to the kidneys may be in excess of the load the infant is capable of excreting in the volume of urine produced. Urine osmolality is maximal, plasma urea and sodium rise and intracellular osmolality also rises as water is drawn out of the cells into hypertonic extracellular fluid. The extracellular fluid compartment and particularly the vascular compartment are reduced in volume late in dehydration. Dehydration is not obvious until circulatory collapse occurs by which time there is severe intra- and extracellular dehydration. The correction of hypertonic dehydration in young infants is difficult since rapid replacement of fluids results in extracellular fluid moving into the intracellular compartment due to the intracellular hypertonicity. Cerebral oedema is a common sequel to treatment. Renal failure secondary to the severe circulatory collapse is also common.

The correction of hypertonic dehydration involves restoration of circulation with plasma and then slow rehydration with dextrose–saline solution (usually dextrose 5%, saline 0.45%) aiming to reduce the serum sodium by about 10 mmol/l/day. The mortality and morbidity of young infants with hypernatraemia in the early 1970s in Britain was high but since modified cows' milk formulas have been the only cows' milk based formulas available in Britain, the incidence of hypertonic dehydration has declined dramatically.

Vitamin deficiencies
In the recent past, deficiencies of vitamins C and D were associated with feeding unsupplemented cows' milk formulas to infants for prolonged periods without weaning or with inadequate exposure to sunlight. Modern infant formulas on sale in Britain have added vitamins A, B, C, D and K, and deficiencies of these in normal full-term infants receiving formula milk weaned at 4–6 months of age are rare. There should be no need to supplement normal full-term infants with extra vitamins so long as they continue to take supplemented formula milks. Once infants change to doorstep milk, vitamin supplementation is advisable. DHSS (1988) recommendations are that Children's Vitamins Drops (5 drops: vitamin A 200 µg;

vitamin C 20 mg; vitamin D 7 μg) should be given to all infants from 6 months (but from 1 month may be preferable) to 2 years, or preferably 5 years (DHSS, 1988).

An early modification of cows' milk based formula aimed to 'humanize' the fat content by increasing the proportion of polyunsaturated fatty acids (PUFA) to saturated fatty acids. Vegetable fats were substituted for the butter fat of cows' milk. Proportions of the essential fatty acids linoleic and linolenic acids were greatly increased. These essential fatty acids are readily oxidized within the body if fed in large amounts in the absence of sufficient vitamin E. Since they are constituents of red-cell membranes, oxidation has significant effects on red-cell survival. Vitamin E responsive haemolytic anaemia developed as a direct result of the fat substitution in at-risk infants (Hassan et al., 1966). Increased vitamin E content in high PUFA milks has removed, so far as mature healthy infants are concerned, vitamin E deficiency haemolytic anaemia. Vitamin E deficiency still occurs in immature infants.

Iron deficiency anaemia with cows' milk feeding
Cows' milk provides little iron, and the iron that is present is not readily absorbed. Cows' milk protein intolerance may cause a haemorrhagic colitis with insidious blood loss or overt gastrointestinal bleeding. Blood loss increases the need for iron in the cows' milk fed infant. Early introduction of cows' milk is not an uncommon precipitant of iron deficiency anaemia in the first year of life.

Soya based formulas

Soya based formulas are widely used in the United States as initial formula feeds for infants. In Britain they have tended to be used as an alternative to cows' milk based formulas when infants appear unable to tolerate cows' milk based formula. Examples are listed in *Table 4.4*. These milks are widely used in cases of cows' milk protein intolerance but it is inadvisable for infants to be changed to them from cows' milk formulas without causes for infants' symptoms being properly defined. Change to soya (not only cows' milk protein but usually lactose-free formula) may relieve symptoms of true milk intolerance but infants may still be offered other foods containing milk products, thus preventing complete resolution. If infants'

Table 4.4 Some soya protein based formulas suitable for infant feeding

Formula	Manufacturer	Protein source	Fat source	Carbohydrate source
Formula S	Cow & Gate	Soy protein isolate L-methionine	Vegetable oils	Glucose syrup solids
Isomil	Ross	Soy protein isolate L-methionine	Vegetable: soy and coconut oil	Corn syrup solids and sucrose
Prosobee	Mead Johnson	Soy protein isolate L-methionine	Vegetable: coconut and corn oil	Glucose syrup solids
Wysoy	Wyeth	Soy protein isolate L-methionine	Animal and vegetable: beef fat, coconut and soy oils	Sucrose and corn syrup solids

symptoms are not related to the formula, time will be wasted before infants present for further investigation.

Soya formulas contain protein from water-soluble soy isolates. Methionine is deficient in soy isolate protein and must be added to formulas to make them nutritionally safe (Hervada, 1984). Soya 'milk' bought at health food shops is unsuitable for infants and should *not* be fed. Because of the differences in amino acid content of the protein compared with human milk, the protein content of soya formula should exceed 1.6 g protein/100 kcal (420 kJ) (DHSS, 1980b). Soya formulas on sale in Britain do not contain lactose, which may account for some studies suggesting that mineral absorption from these milks is less good than from cows' milk based formulas. In the past, soya milks have been associated with development of goitre and iodine fortification of formulas is common. Vitamins and iron are also added as with cows' milk formulas (*see Table 4.1*).

Soya protein is probably no less allergenic than cows' milk protein. There seems little reason therefore to start infants on soya-based formulas rather than cows' milk based formulas with the aim of avoiding allergies. The main use of soya milks should be for nutrition of formula-fed ovo-lacto vegetarians who abjure dairy products and as one alternative to cows' milk formula for infants who are known to be intolerant to cows' milk protein. Since, however, the gastrointestinal damage resulting from cows' milk protein intolerance may make the gut more likely to be intolerant of other foreign proteins, soya formulas may not be the most appropriate for the immediate management of cows' milk protein intolerance.

'Follow-on' formulas

These are cows' milk based formulas designed to fit a theoretical gap between standard infant formulas and moving on to cows' milk and an adult diet. There is no particular reason why infants should not stay on standard formulas for the whole of the first year. 'Follow-on' formulas have higher protein and salt content than standard infant formulas but also contain added iron and vitamins in higher concentration than in cows' milk. The formulas are popular on the Continent, perhaps because milk is drunk less by children and not delivered to doorsteps as is the custom in Britain. There seems little need for these formulas in Britain, and there is concern that mothers may offer them to infants younger than 6 months and thus risk hypernatraemia. It is also unnecessary to encourage mothers to adopt these formulas when they offer no nutritional advantages over standard infant formulas. Understandably the greater prevalence of breast feeding has threatened infant-formula manufacturing firms and has stimulated diversification of products to develop new markets. Diversification may only confuse mothers.

References

BARKER, D. J. P. and OSMOND, C. (1986) Infant mortality, childhood nutrition and ischaemic heart disease in England and Wales. *Lancet*, **i,** 1077–1081

DAVIES, D. P. (1973) Plasma osmolality and feeding practices of healthy infants in the first three months of life. *British Medical Journal*, **ii,** 340–342

DEPARTMENT OF HEALTH AND SOCIAL SECURITY (1977) *The Composition of Mature Human Milk*. Report on Health and Social Subjects, No. 12. London: Her Majesty's Stationery Office

DEPARTMENT OF HEALTH AND SOCIAL SECURITY (1980) *Artificial Feeds for the Young Infant.* Report on Health and Social Subjects, No. 18. London: Her Majesty's Stationery Office

DEPARTMENT OF HEALTH AND SOCIAL SECURITY (1988) *Present Day Practice in Infant Feeding: Third Report.* Report on Health and Social Subjects, No. 32. London: Her Majesty's Stationery Office

FOMON, S. J. (1974) *Infant Nutrition,* 2nd edn. Philadelphia: W. B. Saunders Company

FOMON, S. J., OWEN, G. M. and THOMAS, L. M. (1964) Milk or formula volume ingested by infants fed *ad libitum. American Journal of Diseases of Children,* **108,** 601–604

FOOD MANUFACTUER'S FEDERATION (1983) *Code of Practice for Marketing of Infant Formulae in the United Kingdom and Schedule for a Code Monitoring Committee.* London: Food Manufacturer's Federation (Now Food and Drink Federation.)

HASSAN, H., HASHIM, S. A., VAN ITALLIE, J. B. and SEBRELL, W. H. (1966) Syndrome of premature infants associated with low plasma vitamin E levels and high polyunsaturated fatty acid diet. *American Journal of Clinical Nutrition,* **19,** 147–157

HENDRICKSE, R. G., WOOLDRIDGE, M. A. W. and RUSSELL, A. (1977) Lactulose in baby milks causing diarrhoea simulating lactose intolerance. *British Medical Journal,* **i,** 1194–1195

HERVADA, A. R. (1984) Soy bean formulas. In *Health Hazards of Milk,* edited by D. L. J. Freed, pp. 157–158. London: Baillière Tindall

LAWTON, R. (1984) Goats' milk. In *Health Hazards of Milk,* edited by D. L. J. Freed, pp. 150–156. London: Bailliére Tindall

LUCAS, A. (1986) Feeding the full-term infant. In *Textbook of Neonatology,* edited by N. R. C. Roberton, pp. 193–203. Edinburgh: Churchill-Livingstone

PUFFER, R. R. and SERRANO, C. V. (1973) *Patterns of Mortality in Childhood.* Scientific Publications No. 262, Pan American Health Organisation. Washington: World Health Organisation

RASSIN, D. K., STURMAN, J. A. and GAULL, G. E. (1978) Taurine and other free amino acids in milk of man and other mammals. *Early Human Development,* **2,** 1–13

WHITEHEAD, R. G. and PAUL, A. A. (1984) Growth charts and the assessment of infant feeding practices in the Western world and in developing countries. *Early Human Development,* **9,** 187–207

WICKES, I. G. (1952) Rate of gain and satiety in early infancy. *Archives of Disease in Childhood,* **27,** 449–456

WORLD HEALTH ORGANISATION (1981) *International Code of Marketing Breast Milk Substitutes.* Geneva: World Health Organisation

Chapter 5
Low-birthweight infants

Low-birthweight (LBW: <2.5 kg) infants have increased nutrient needs per unit body weight:

1. Increased heat and fluid losses due to large surface area to volume ratio and – in the very immature – relatively permeable skin.
2. Higher growth rates and greater nutrient requirements for deposition of new tissues.
3. Immature gastrointestinal and renal function leading to poor absorption and retention of nutrients.
4. Commonly, respiratory disease or other illness increasing physiological work and stressing metabolism.

The predominant and persisting needs for extra nutrients are for rapid growth. Premature (short gestation, SG: <37 weeks' gestation) infants must grow more rapidly than term infants in order to maintain expected intrauterine growth rates. Light, or small, for dates or small for gestational age (SFD: <tenth centile weight for gestational age) infants must have accelerated or 'catch-up' growth in order to achieve normal growth centiles for age.

The body composition of LBW infants, especially SG, differs from that of term infants (*Table 5.1*). Total body water, in particular extracellular water, is increased in SG infants and both SG and LFD infants have low body fat. Infants less than 34 weeks' gestation may be clinically oedematous at birth. SFD infants may be

Table 5.1 Approximate body composition related to gestational age*

Component (as % total body weight)	Total water	Extracellular fluid	Intracellular fluid	Fat
Gestation (weeks):				
12	90	70	20	0.5
26	86	62	24	1
30	85	60	25	2
33	80	55	26	6
36	77	50	27	7
40	72	40	32	14
1 year post term	65	25	40	24

* Data from Fomon, 1974; Widdowson, 1981; Friis-Hanson and Anderson, 1985.

marginally dehydrated at birth (Widdowson, 1981; Friis-Hansen and Anderson, 1985).

Term infants have sufficient liver glycogen, if unfed, to meet energy requirements for 8–12 hours and body fat to supply energy for 10 or more days – assuming normal requirements and normal ability to mobilize these reserves. Glycogen stores in the liver are built up in the last months of pregnancy so immature infants are likely to have much smaller reserves of rapidly available energy. Glycogen stores may only provide energy for 2–3 hours in very low birthweight (VLBW: <1.5 kg) infants (Heird *et al.*, 1972). Their body fat and consequently total energy reserves are low. Surface area is relatively large and heat loss rapid. Immature metabolism may result in delay in mobilizing fatty acids to meet energy needs since the newborn infant has to convert energy production from almost total glucose metabolism *in utero*, to metabolism of both glucose and fatty acids after birth. Respiratory quotients fall from 1.0 at birth to about 0.7 on the second day of life (Maniscalco and Warshaw, 1978). Both SG and LFD infants are particularly at risk of hypoglycaemia and hypothermia if not provided with readily metabolizable sources of energy early in life. Hypothermia and hypoglycaemia are particularly likely in those who are asphyxiated, anoxic, or stressed by cold, infection or respiratory distress.

The dilemma in feeding LBW infants lies in the clinical conflict between these infants' urgent needs for nutrition and the probability that they will be unable to tolerate the large volumes of milk or formula necessary to meet these needs. The problem increases with decreasing size and decreasing maturity of the infants. VLBW infants present many clinical problems other than those of feeding and nutrition, which exacerbate the problems of maintaining adequate nutrition.

Feeding LBW infants

Sucking and swallowing reflexes are present in the fetus from 18–20 weeks' gestation but under about 35 weeks' gestation these reflexes are poorly co-ordinated and infants may have insufficient strength to suck effectively from breast or bottle. Experienced nurses can often manoeuvre a teat against the palate of an immature infant so as to express milk into the back of the mouth from where it can be swallowed, but this is a rather different procedure from the normal forceful sucking of the mature infant. Thus a need for specialized feeding procedures is one of the main reasons why SG infants – and to a lesser extent SFD infants – require special care.

Methods of feeding LBW infants – enteral feeding

LBW infants – and other sick infants unable to suck from breast or bottle – can be fed either by gavage through a variety of enteral methods or parenterally. *Table 5.2* lists possible methods. All have advantages and disadvantages and it is not possible to state categorically how infants of a particular weight or gestation should be fed since so much depends on their clinical state, the facilities available and the experience of nursing and medical staff caring for them. Those involved in feeding LBW infants should be properly trained in the procedures (all nursing and medical procedures not just those relating to feeding) necessary for care of LBW and sick newborn. Units caring for sick newborn should also have equipment that both works and is appropriate for monitoring the clinical care of these infants.

Table 5.2 Possible methods of feeding LBW infants

Enterally:	
From breast or bottle	Usually only possible with healthy infants >35 weeks' gestation
By gavage:	
Nasogastrically	Feeds can be given as bolus or continuous drip feeds
Orogastrically	Bolus feeds only
Nasojejunally }	Continuous drip feeds only
Orojejunally }	
Parenterally:	
Into peripheral vein }	Risk of encouraging sepsis; should be accompanied by small enteral
Into central vein via }	feeds whenever they can be tolerated
long venous catheter }	

Where possible, mothers of infants on special care units should be encouraged to learn the simpler techniques such as tube feeding (usually once the tube is in place, although some may learn to pass tubes as well) so they can be involved in the care of their infants. This may help control the anxiety and frustration they have to endure during weeks or months of watching their infants. It also encourages the mother–child interaction important for the survival, normal growth and emotional development of LBW infants once they are discharged. Prolonged separation or lack of contact between mothers and their premature infants risks rejection of infants when they are at last well enough to be cared for at home (Budin, 1907; Klaus and Kennell, 1976; Boxall and Whitby, 1983).

Tube feeding: nasogastric
Here the feeding tube (usually a 5FG PVC tube) is passed through one nostril and into the stomach. The distance the tube needs to be inserted is measured before introduction against the nostril to left hypochondrium distance and the tube is marked or taped at the level of the nostril. The tube is then fed through the nostril to the level of the mark and lightly secured at the nostril. The tube is aspirated and, if it is in the stomach, acid secretions (pink change with litmus paper) are obtained. If the secretions are not acid or no secretions are obtained the tube may have curled up in the mouth or at the back of the nasopharynx. The tube should be withdrawn except for the last 1–2 cm and then passed again. Once correctly sited the tube can be secured firmly if it is planned to leave it in place between feeds. The position of the tube should always be checked prior to any feed by aspirating acid secretions. Tubes should be changed at least every 2–3 days since they stiffen with use and may become difficult to withdraw.

Feeds given nasogastrically can be given either as intermittent bolus feeds or as continuous drip feeds. For intermittent feeds, feed frequency depends largely on the state of the infant but in sick infants it is common to offer very small feeds hourly rather than larger feeds at longer intervals. Initially the stomach should be aspirated three hourly to determine whether the feeds are being digested and absorbed. If large volumes of aspirate are obtained (50% or more of the feed given since the previous aspiration) this suggests poor gastrointestinal motility and feeds should be stopped or reduced in volume for some hours. Drip feeds may be tolerated better than bolus feeds as stomach distension is kept to the minimum.

Drip feeds should be administered by continuous perfusor pumps to control infusion rates. Because a drip feed is relatively stagnant, loss of nutrients, particularly fats, by adhesion to the sides of the container may be significant and weight gain may be less by this method than by bolus feeding.

The advantages of nasogastric feeding are those gained in feeding infants with little disturbance since tubes need not be passed before each feed and the infants do not need to suck. It is easier to keep the tube in the stomach than by orogastric positioning. However, the main and important disadvantages of this method are obstruction to the airway by the tube in one nostril and increased respiratory difficulty or apnoea consequent upon stomach distension by food (Shivpuri et al., 1983). (This last is a problem that restricts any gavage feeding into the stomach in infants with significant respiratory distress or respiratory centre immaturity.) Prolonged use of nasogastric tubes may also lead to persistent deformity of the nostrils.

Orogastric feeding
This is an alternative to nasogastric feeding which does not have the complication of obstructing the airway. The tube is measured against the infant for mouth to left hypochondrium distance, and passed into the stomach through the mouth. It may be passed before each feed or secured between feeds by taping lightly against the middle of the bottom lip. Again, the position of a tube in the stomach must always be checked by obtaining acid secretions before feeding. Orogastric tubes are more difficult to keep in place than nasogastric tubes and are thus unsuitable for continuous drip feeding. Nevertheless intermittent orogastric feeding is now the method of choice in many units.

Transpyloric (naso-jejunal and oro-jejunal) feeding
Here the feeding tube is sited in the second part of the jejunum or beyond. This makes regurgitation less likely and this can be a useful method of feeding infants who are unable to tolerate – because of regurgitation or respiratory embarrassment – feeds placed in the stomach. The procedure has advantages but these are, in this author's opinion, largely outweighed by the disadvantages. The method is relatively little used since safer, more satisfactory parenteral feeding has largely superseded the use of transpyloric feeding. A long silicon rubber feeding tube is used and the length to be inserted determined by measuring mouth (or nose) to *ankle* distance on the tube and marking the tube at this level. With the infant lying on the right side, the tube is inserted into the stomach via nose or mouth. When the marked position on the tube has reached the level of the umbilicus the other end of the tube should be in the stomach and it should be possible to aspirate acid secretions. Water 1–2 ml passed down the tube at this stage may help its passage into the jejunum.

Alternatively a little air (1–2 ml) is pushed down a separate nasogastric tube to distend the stomach and encourage passage of the tube through the pylorus. The tube is advanced 1–2 cm every 5–10 minutes until the end of the tube is at the mouth, where it is taped in position. If water 1–2 ml passed down the transpyloric feeding tube cannot be aspirated through the intragastric tube, the transpyloric tube is almost certainly through the pylorus into the duodenum or jejunum. The site of the tube in the jejunum can be checked by straight abdominal X-ray. It is important that there is a tube into the stomach also. This is used to aspirate regurgitated feeds or accumulating secretions every 6 hours. These are replaced down the jejunal feeding tube. If much of the feed is found in the stomach it is likely that the jejunal tube has slipped back into the stomach. Feeds given down transpyloric tubes must be given by slow continuous drip feed via perfusor pump. Initially 1–2 ml of feed are given per hour but the volumes can be built up gradually to full volume feeds, provided that the infant tolerates them.

The problems of naso-jejunal feeding lie in the difficulty of getting the tube into the correct position in the first place and the need to provide isosmolar feeds. Correct siting of the tube may take over 24 hours. Meanwhile the infant must be fed by other means. Tubes left *in situ* for the duration of feeding may stiffen and become extremely difficult to remove. Infants fed transpylorically are more liable to necrotizing enterocolitis (*see below*) and frequently do not gain weight as well as those fed nasogastrically (Whitfield, 1982). Bypassing both mouth and stomach bypasses many of the normal gastrointestinal stimuli to hormone and enzyme secretion (Lucas, 1981). Lingual lipase stimulation and intragastric digestive activity are avoided. Fat and other nutrients may adhere to the container and perfusion set, thus reducing the nutrient content of the feed reaching the infant. Fat absorption and probably absorption of other nutrients is reduced. Reduced gastrointestinal hormone secretion due to lack of normal food stimuli in mouth and stomach could theoretically impair growth and maturation of the gastrointestinal system as well.

How much should be fed?

Once a feeding tube is in place enteral feeds should be introduced cautiously. Food in the stomach may embarrass respiration or induce apnoea (Shivpuri *et al.*, 1983). Small intestinal motility is less in immature infants and peristalsis poorly organized. Necrotizing enterocolitis (*see below*) develops easily in infants who are unwell, particularly if there is bowel distension due to large increases in feed volumes. High fluid intakes predispose to other complications, notably persistent patent ductus arteriosus (*see below*).

Most infants who are not overtly unwell at birth and who are over 1.3 kg body weight tolerate feeding by gavage a few hours after birth. Breast milk or formula should be fed within 2 or 3 hours of birth or intravenous dextrose solution 10% infused instead. Feeds should be offered on the first day at 40–60 ml/kg/day or in smaller quantities if the infant's ability to tolerate enteral feeding is in doubt. Feeds are usually given as small bolus feeds although very slow continuous drip feeds from perfusor pumps may be better tolerated in those who are only just coping with enteral feeding. Infants under 2 kg should be fed one or two hourly initially if fed bolus feeds, although the heavier of these infants will tolerate three hourly feeding fairly rapidly. Feed volumes can be increased by 10–20 ml/kg/day (provided the infants tolerate this) until full volumes of 200 ml/kg/day are reached. Infants nursed under radiant heaters or phototherapy have increased insensible water loss and, with phototherapy, decreased intestinal water absorption. Fluid intakes should reflect these needs.

Infants below 1.3 kg birth weight, even when well, are often managed by 'nil by mouth' for the first 24 hours of life or even longer. Hydration and normoglycaemia are maintained with intravenous dextrose solution 10% (40–60 ml/kg/day on the first day of life). Sick infants of any gestation should not be fed enterally until their condition has stabilized. The postnatal age at which sick and VLBW infants are given enteral feeds depends on their clinical state although transpyloric feeding may enable them to be fed enterally earlier than by gastric feeding. When feeds are being introduced, the stomach should be aspirated every 3 hours, just before a feed, to check that excessive pooling of feed in the stomach is not occurring. Aspirates equivalent to 50% or more of the volume fed in the previous 3 hours indicate significant gastrointestinal stasis. Enteral feeding should cease temporarily.

Common complications resulting from enteral feeds in LBW infants

Increasing respiratory distress and apnoea
Splinting of the diaphragm by a distended stomach increases respiratory problems in infants who may have decreased lung compliance due to hyaline membrane disease (idiopathic respiratory distress syndrome) or primary atelectasis. Apnoea is one response to the increasing effort of respiration (Wilkinson and Yu, 1974). It is also a reflex response to stomach distension. Neonates with respiratory distress due to any cause should not be fed orally until their condition is showing signs of improvement.

Gastro-oesophageal reflux and aspiration of feed
Infants reflux stomach contents to oesophagus readily. This is particularly likely if food is fed into the stomach, if the stomach is over-full, or if the infant is distressed by respiratory difficulty. Aspiration of stomach contents can cause aspiration pneumonia or severe acute apnoea. Nursing infants after feeds in the prone 'knee–chest) position reduces pressure on the gastro-oesophageal junction and diminishes the risks of reflux as well as discouraging aspiration of refluxed feed (*Figure 5.1*).

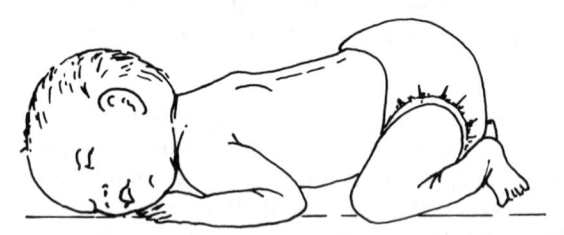

Figure 5.1 Knee–chest position for nursing LBW infants postprandially.

Necrotizing enterocolitis
This is a curious condition of uncertain aetiology. Particular organisms such as *Clostridia* spp. or *Klebsiella* spp. may be responsible, but the condition is more probably the result of a combination of adverse circumstances including relative anoxia to the bowel wall and the presence of intestinal gas-forming bacteria capable of invading the ischaemic wall. The condition sometimes occurs in small epidemics on (usually overcrowded) neonatal special care units.

Many aspects of feeding contribute to the development of necrotizing enterocolitis. It is rare in infants who have received no food enterally and it is less common in infants fed their own unprocessed mother's milk. It is common in sick enterally fed infants. It is also common in infants introduced to large volumes of feed rapidly. It sometimes occurs in mature infants with severe cyanotic congenital heart disease. Rapid distension of the neonatal bowel, particularly in the presence of anoxia or hypotension, may cause ischaemia of the bowel and provide the opportunity for bacterial invasion. Infants present with abdominal distension, vomiting, bloody stools, paralytic ileus or evidence of obstruction, peritonitis, circulatory collapse and septicaemia. The characteristic X-ray appearances are of loops of distended bowel with the double wall or 'tramlining' appearance of air within the bowel wall due to gas-forming bacteria invading the bowel wall. Treatment involves stopping enteral feeds for 7–10 days and aspirating the stomach regularly to relieve gastrointestinal distension. Antibiotics, including those active against anaerobic bacteria, are also given. Parenteral feeding is necessary.

Patent ductus arteriosus
This is a common problem of both enterally and parenterally fed LBW infants but particularly those who have severe respiratory problems in the newborn period. It can be considered a potential complication of feeding since high fluid loads early in life encourage the ductus to stay patent (Stevenson, 1977; Bell *et al.*, 1980). The presence of full pulses and/or audible murmur in the pulmonary area or second intercostal space suggests that the ductus is still functioning. Feed or intravenous fluid volumes should be reduced by 20% for a few days and then volumes increased again very gradually. This policy must be pursued with circumspection. Indomethacin therapy is sometimes effective in closing the ductus but some ducti require surgical management. It is unwise to persist with low feed levels to the extent that the infant is inadequately hydrated or nourished if it is obvious that reducing feed volumes has not been effective in closing the ductus.

What should be fed?

The choice of feeds for LBW infants is between the infants' own mothers' milk, expressed or banked; other banked breast milk; fortified human milk (own mother's or banked); and standard infant formula or preterm infant formula. As explained earlier, these infants have greater needs for energy, protein and other nutrients than full-term, normal-weight infants if they are to attain the rapid growth rates they would have pursued *in utero* or which they need for 'catch-up' growth. If they are to obtain an increased nutrient intake/kg body weight, they will have to consume either larger volumes/kg/day of the feeds received by term infants or more nutrient dense feeds. What are the relative advantages and disadvantages of the feeds available for LBW infants?

Human milk
The advantages for the human infant of own mother's milk are better absorption, particularly of fats, and some protection against infection for LBW infants who have increased susceptibility to infection. In extremely immature infants it may be the only enteral feed tolerated in early life (Lucas, 1987). The composition of milk from mothers delivering preterm is variable but usually richer in protein, sodium and energy than milk of mothers delivering at term (Gross *et al.*, 1980; Schanler and Oh, 1980). This may be a reflection only of the small volume of milk that these mothers produce. Increased output with suckling tends to lower concentration (Lucas and Hudson, 1984).

Infants over 2 kg, if relatively well, can often tolerate the high volumes of milk (200 ml/kg/day) necessary to achieve energy intakes of 630 kJ (150 kcal)/kg/day within about 10 days of birth. Expressed own mother's milk can probably meet their nutrient requirements. LBW infants under 2 kg birth weight require feeds of even greater nutrient density since feed volumes may need to be kept low for a prolonged period to avoid fluid overload. Milk from the infants' own mothers may not achieve adequate nutrient concentration to fulfil their requirements, particularly for energy, protein, sodium and phosphate.

If own mother's milk can be fed directly to infants through gavage immediately after expression from mother, little nutrient or antibacterial quality is lost. The advantages of better nutrient absorption and some protection against infection together with the emotional satisfaction for the mother may outweigh the disadvantage of difficulty in achieving adequate total nutrient intake except by large volume feeding, in the heavier, stronger infants. However, some fat will be lost by adherence to the sides of the tube, especially if the feed is given by continuous gavage (Brooke and Barley, 1978). There will also be some loss of cells by adherence to collecting and administering vessels. With storage, pasteurization or deep freezing the anti-bacterial, hormonal and enzymatic actions of the milk are diminished and the unique qualities of own mother's milk are reduced. The particular advantages for LBW infants are likely to be so diminished as to make it unlikely that unsupplemented banked human milk has any significant advantage for unsupplemented long-term feeding of LBW infants.

Pooled breast milk of mothers delivering at term and in well-established lactation and 'drip' breast milk are not suitable for VLBW infants as nutrient quantity is inadequate and anti-infective properties minimal. But some units now fortify banked milk and even own mother's milk fed to LBW infants using either skim and cream components derived from mature human donor milk (Schanler, Garza and Nichols, 1985) or energy from glucose polymer or medium-chain triglycerides, whey protein, sodium, calcium and phosphate supplements. This may improve rates of weight gain but the composition and particular properties of the milk are altered substantially. This may be nutritionally important (Lucas, 1986). For example, fortification of human milk with calcium reduces the efficiency of fat absorption (Chappell *et al.*, 1986).

Table 5.3 Some LBW formulas available in Britain and USA

Formula	Manufacturers
Osterprem	Boots/Farley
Nenatal	Cow & Gate
Prematalac	Cow & Gate
SMA low birthweight formula	Wyeth
Pre Aptamil	Milupa
Enfamil premature	Mead Johnson
Similac 24 LBW	Ross Abbott
Alprem	Nestlé

LBW formula
Recent years have seen the development of formulas (*Table 5.3*) which aim to provide greater nutrient density thus providing for the increased nutrient needs/kg of LBW infants without the necessity to feed large volumes. Energy, protein, mineral and vitamin content of the formulas are increased and other nutrients such

as carnitine also added. The formulas available vary quite widely in composition (*Table 5.4*) but none has been shown to have definite advantages over others. These preterm formulas are available only in liquid form and are intended for infants under 2 kg body weight. Bulk, due to their liquid preparation, prevents them being used outside hospital.

Studies of LBW infants fed LBW infant formulas suggest that not only are growth rates improved but fewer nutritional problems occur (Brooke, Wood and Barley, 1982; Gross, 1983; Lucas *et al.*, 1984; Cooper *et al.*, 1985).

In one large multicentre study of LBW infants fed either banked human milk, expressed breast milk fortified with banked human milk, expressed breast milk fortified with preterm formula or preterm formula in early life, weight gain was maintained closer to expected centiles in the infants fed preterm formula. Length and skull circumference also appeared to increase more rapidly in this group. Hyponatraemia, hyperbilirubinaemia, hypophosphataemia and bone disease of prematurity were all less prevalent in the infants on the preterm formula. Nitrogen retention was also greater in these infants (Lucas *et al.*, 1984; Roberts and Lucas, 1985).

Modern preterm formulas have advantages over other enteral feeds for LBW infants which suggest they are the feeds most likely to encourage optimum growth in early life. This would seem likely to encourage both resistance to infection and normal brain development so as to minimize the morbidity and handicap that might result from inadequate nutrition in very early life. It is possible, particularly perhaps for the VLBW infant who is being introduced to enteral feeds, that fresh expressed own mother's milk may have advantages in protection against infection and facilitated nutrient absorption which outweigh its questionable nutrient adequacy for the infant (Lucas, 1987). However, long-term very *frequent* expression by mothers in order to provide the fresh expressed breast milk these infants require is not usually practical. And once human milk has to be stored or pasteurized its unique advantages are lost.

Thus where mothers of VLBW infants plan to breast feed once their infants are able to suck vigorously, the infants can be fed own mother's expressed breast milk supplemented with preterm formula to tolerance. In this way mothers can express breast milk at home regularly and bring their refrigerated milk collections up to the Special Care Unit once or twice a day for feeding their infants.

Parenteral feeding

This is now the method of choice for VLBW infants with major respiratory or gastrointestinal problems. Yet parenteral nutrition should not be undertaken lightly. It is a discipline that requires intensive care and close clinical and biochemical monitoring. Those practising parenteral nutrition must be familiar with procedures for preparation, setting up, infusing and monitoring both the intravenous line and the infusion. Thus parenteral feeding should be practised only:

1. In units where there are facilities to make up intravenous solutions under sterile conditions.
2. Where there is biochemical and microbiological support.
3. Where there is suitable equipment for the delivery of intravenous infusions, including intravenous constant infusion pumps.

Table 5.4 Approximate composition (unites/l) of LBW formulas commonly used in Britain* (manufacturers' data)

Milk:	Human (term)	Osterprem (Boots/Farley)	Nenatal (Cow & Gate)	Prematalac (Cow & Gate)	SMA LBW Formula (Wyeth)	Pre Aptamil† (Milupa)
Energy:						
MJ	2.94	3.34	3.18	3.30	3.34	3.08
kcal	700	800	760	790	800	740
Protein (g)	11	20	18	24	20	21
Fat (g)	42	49	45	50	44	36
Saturated and unsaturated	50:50	40:60	48:52	48:52	49:51	48:52
Carbohydrate (g)	74	70	70	66	82	83
Sodium (mmol)	7	20	9‡	26‡	14	15
Calcium (mmol)	9	18	25‡	17	19	15
Phosphorus (mmol)	5	11	16	17	13	15
Potential renal solute load (mosmol)	79	132	107	169‡	128	132
Osmolality (mosmol)	290	300	340	342	268	350

* Composition of formulas changes frequently. Consult recent manufacturers' data for exact values.
† Low zinc content compared with other LBW formula.
‡ Nutrients marked indicate considerable deviation from other formula values.

4. Above all, where staff are trained and experienced in changing drip sets and infusion liquids under aseptic conditions and aware of how complications of intravenous feeding may present in these infants.

Infection is a major problem in intravenous nutrition, particularly for LBW infants, but can be reduced by:
1. Scrupulous attention to aseptic techniques.
2. The use of bacterial filters on intravenous lines.
3. Daily changes of infusion sets.
4. Frequent changes of infusion sites when these are peripheral.

The site at which the catheter enters the body must be observed constantly. If there is any suggestion of infection or extravasation, the infusion must be stopped. The hypertonic glucose solutions and calcium-containing solutions used in intravenous feeding are very likely to cause skin sloughing after extravasation, leaving unsightly scars.

Parenteral feeding can be given through a short 22 or 24G peripheral venous cannula extending 2–3 cm into a peripheral vein. Ten percent glucose is the maximum glucose concentration that can be given into a peripheral vein without frequent venous thrombosis and this may limit the usefulness of peripheral veins in these small infants with high energy requirements but often low tolerance of fluid volumes. Alternatively, parenteral feeding can be given through a long venous line usually inserted into a vein in the antecubital fossa or the long saphenous vein at the ankle, and introduced up to the superior or inferior vena cava. A 19G butterfly needle, with the catheter section removed, is introduced into the peripheral vein and a thin Broviac silastic catheter threaded up this. The distance the catheter needs to be inserted is measured against the infant's body prior to introduction. The final position of the catheter should be checked by X-ray (if necessary a small quantity of radio-opaque dye is introduced to mark the position of the catheter tip). The whole procedure must take place under strict aseptic technique. The site of insertion of the catheter must be inspected frequently for evidence of thrombosis, tissue necrosis, obstruction or sepsis. Catheters and cannulae used for intravenous feeding should not be used to give or take blood nor for the administration of drugs other than the intravenous feeding mixtures. The infusion sets should be changed daily under strict aseptic techniques. Management of sepsis should include removal of the cannula or catheter and culture of the cannula or catheter tip.

Parenteral feeding can be total or partial, that is it provides all the infant's nutrition or it supplements oral feeds in order to achieve nutritional requirements. If possible, intravenous feeding should be combined with some oral feeding. This often removes the necessity to give fat emulsions intravenously as a source of essential fatty acids and also means that vitamins can be given orally. More importantly, however, the process of oral feeding may be very important for normal growth and maturation of the infant gut. The stimulus to gastrointestinal hormones produced by even small feeds and, if fresh breast milk is fed, the effect of the enzymes and hormones in the milk may be important in the development of gastrointestinal function so that when the infant can tolerate enteral feeding without respiratory embarrassment, it can also digest and absorb adequately. Infants fed some oral feed appear to grow better than those receiving no feed enterally. Many units now feed 1–2 ml expressed breast milk to otherwise totally parenterally fed infants with the intention of stimulating maturation of gut function.

62 Low-birthweight infants

Parenteral feeding is discussed in Chapter 16, but *Table 5.5* presents a possible programme for full intravenous nutrition in an infant taking nothing by mouth. The rates at which the feeding is 'built-up' depends on how well it is tolerated.

Table 5.5 Possible plan for total intravenous feeding (IVF) of LBW infants (adapted from Tripp and Candy, 1985)

	Day 1* (per kg/day)	Day 5 (per kg/day)
Fluid (ml)	60	150†
Amino acids (g)	0.5	2.5
Glucose (g)	8	15
Fat (g)	–	3‡
Sodium (mmol)	3	3
Potassium (mmol)	2.5	2.5

Volumes of solutions meeting these and other basic needs:

	ml/kg/day	ml/kg/day
Vamin 7% Dextrose 10% (KabiVitrum)	7	36
10% Dextrose	40	80
10% Intralipid (KabiVitrum)	–	30‡
Vitlipid (KabiVitrum)	1.0	1.0
Solivito (KabiVitrum)	0.5	0.5
Ped-El (KabiVitrum)	2	2

* Complications in infant's progress or response to IVF may necessitate slower build-up to this nutrient intake level.
† Increased volumes needed with radiant heaters and/or phototherapy.
‡ Avoid fat if infant infected, acidosed, jaundiced and start after first 24 hours. Build up slowly and always check for triglyceride clearing (under 2.7 mmol/l (250 mg/100 ml) 4–6 hours after stopping Intralipid infusion).

The need is to provide energy, protein, vitamins and minerals, sufficient to meet requirements. This may be as difficult in small sick immature infants as providing enteral nutrients adequately, since the fluid volumes needed to provide the nutrients may be greater than those which the infants can tolerate without overload. Because maturity and state of health influence fluid requirements greatly and because the process of intravenous feeding may influence metabolic rate and thus heat and fluid loss, volumes of fluid/kg/day need to be judged on an individual basis after observing the clinical and biochemical effects of a particular volume. However, full-volume intravenous feeding should not be given initially. Both amino acid and glucose loads must be increased gradually in order to allow opportunity for metabolism to adapt. Units using intravenous nutrition regularly have usually developed their own regimens and in many cases have computers programmed to calculate the composition of the daily infusate for individual infants, taking into account weight, age, day of infusion, fluid and electrolyte losses and blood biochemistry. This makes it easier for pharmacy departments to make up supplies of intravenous solutions and may minimize metabolic derangement in the infants (MacMahon, 1984).

The risks of intravenous feeding for LBW and other neonates are:

1. Infection
2. Cholestatic jaundice.
3. Hyperglycaemia.

4. Hyperammonaemia.
5. Hyperaminoacidaemia.
6. Essential fatty acid deficiency.
7. Trace element deficiency.

These are discussed further in Chapter 16.

Nutritional problems in LBW infants

Some of the nutritional complications of LBW infants are common in all LBW infants however they are fed. Others are more likely as a result of particular methods of feeding or the composition of feeds (*Table 5.6*).

Table 5.6 Nutritional complications of different methods of feeding LBW infants

Enteral feeding:	
Human milk	Failure to thrive, hyponatraemia, bone disease of prematurity, copper deficiency
Standard formula	As above; also taurine deficiency, carnitine deficiency
Preterm formula	Possibly fewer complications; bone disease of prematurity still quite common
Parenteral feeding	Failure to thrive; essential fatty acid deficiency (if Intralipid not given); carnitine deficiency; copper deficiency; bone disease of prematurity

Hyponatraemia
Normal levels of plasma sodium are 135–145 mmol/l in infancy. With sodium levels below 130 mol/l infants are particularly likely to be apathetic, intolerant of feeds (owing to reduced gastrointestinal motility) and hypotensive. They may even convulse. Hyponatraemia is common particularly in VLBW infants and those who have been asphyxiated since renal function may be compromised by anoxia. Frusemide, given perhaps for fluid retention due to patent ductus arteriosus, also predisposes to hyponatraemia from excess renal sodium excretion.

The infant kidney has limited capacity to vary sodium excretion to meet requirements. Sodium chloride infusions may induce oedema, and low sodium intakes may result in hyponatraemia. Renal function is affected by hypoxia, shock, immaturity and sepsis so hyponatraemia is particularly likely in *sick* LBW infants fed standard formula or breast milk – or neither (breast milk and standard formula have very low sodium content). High fluid intakes increase sodium excretion but fluid restriction increases resorption and helps resolve hyponatraemia. The sodium requirement of LBW infants is usually 2–3 mmol/kg/day. Deficit can be calculated and administered orally with feeds, using sodium chloride solution 1 mmol/ml strength.

Hypocalcaemia

Hypocalcaemia is also common in LBW and sick neonates. It usually occurs in the first few days of life and reflects metabolic difficulties in maintaining normal calcium levels in early infancy rather than the difficulty in absorbing calcium to meet requirements, even though this is a problem with long-term effects (*see below*) in LBW infants. Calcium levels in the cord blood are high in the fetus owing to active transport from mother to fetus. Adaptation to extra-uterine life without this vigorous influx of calcium takes time, particularly in immature and sick infants. Hypocalcaemia seems to result from the relative insensitivity of tissue to parathormone although albumin levels are low so protein-bound calcium is at low levels also. Infants present with jitteriness, irritability, convulsions or oedema, usually in the first few days of life. Serum calcium levels under 1.7 mmol/l should be considered significant and calcium gluconate given, either by mouth 0.5–1.1 mmol (200–500 mg)/kg/day or intravenously 1–2 ml 10% solution given slowly and *carefully* intravenously – subcutaneous extravasations of calcium solutions are very liable to cause skin sloughing. Some cases of hypocalcaemia are secondary to hypomagnesaemia (more common with intravenous feeding) and will not resolve until magnesium levels are corrected.

Bone disease of LBW infants ('rickets of prematurity')

This is a problem seen in VLBW infants, particularly those who have had significant periods of IVF or who have received breast milk or standard (not LBW) infant formula. It is easy to overlook the condition since presentation with florid 'rickets' is comparatively rare and the condition may not present clinically until 6–8 weeks of age by which time infants may be at home. Radiographic changes without clinical signs or symptoms are common (Callenbach *et al.*, 1981). The infants present around 2 months of age with:

1. Swollen ends of the shafts of long bones.
2. Rickety rosary with swelling of the ends of the bony ribs.
3. Soft bossed skull with more obvious side-to-side flattening than usually seen in LBW infants.
4. Large anterior fontanelle due to poor skull bone development.
5. Fractures of ribs or long bones.

Bony X-rays show:

1. Gross osteoporosis of all bones.
2. Flaring of the ends of the metaphyses.
3. Lack of definition to the ends of the metaphyses; or
4. Early healing with development of the provisional line of calcification.

Epiphyseal development is commonly delayed. Blood biochemistry shows a greatly raised alkaline phosphatase value (>800 International Units/l), low plasma phosphate and low or normal plasma calcium values. Since the X-ray appearances take time to develop and only indicate severe disease, the earliest indication of bone disease of prematurity may be a persistently raised alkaline phosphatase activity without other explanation such as cholestasis.

The explanation for 'rickets' of prematurity is not clear but it seems likely that most cases are not due to vitamin D deficiency nor to immature metabolism of vitamin D but to deficiency of bone mineral substrate (Brooke and Lucas, 1985). Inadequate intakes of protein, copper and calcium have been blamed for some

Table 5.7 Factors contributing to bone disease ('rickets') of prematurity

Deficiency of bone substrate:	
Inadequate intake:	calcium, phosphate, protein, copper
Increased substrate loss:	hypercalcuria in acidosis, hypercalcuria with diuretics (especially frusemide)
Inadequate active hormones for bone mineralization:	
Vitamin D:	low content in breast milk, poor absorption if relative steatorrhoea, diminished synthesis of 1–25 $(OH)_2$ vitamin D in VLBW
Parathormone:	relative peripheral unresponsiveness of VLBW

cases of bone disease but phosphate deficiency seems the commonest cause (*Table 5.7*). Hypercalcaemia secondary to inability to utilize calcium due to gross phosphate deficiency can occur.

The fetus accrues about 7.5 mmol (300 mg) calcium and 5 mmol (150 mg) phosphate daily from the maternal circulation in the last trimester of pregnancy. It is virtually impossible for VLBW infants to ingest or receive this amount of calcium and phosphate by enteral or parenteral feeding and thus a deficiency of mineral for deposition in bone develops. Low birthweight formulas with higher phosphate content are associated with greater percentage absorption of calcium and phosphate than breast milk and less evidence of bone disease. A calcium:phosphate ratio near two with about 1.3–2.0 mmol (50–80 mg) calcium/100 ml feed and 1–1.5 mmol (20–45 mg) phosphorus/100 ml feed has been recommended for LBW formulas (Lucas, 1986).

The usual management of bone disease is to increase the bone mineral intake of these infants by supplementing 0.3–0.5 mmol (10–15 mg) neutral phosphate per 100 ml feed or increasing (if possible) the phosphate in the intravenous feeding infusate. Infants with falling serum phosphate values and rising alkaline phosphatase activity (>800 International Units) should be supplemented before clinical bone disease develops. VLBW infants fed breast milk should probably be supplemented routinely from early life. Calcium supplementation may also be advisable with 0.5–1.0 mmol (20–40 mg) calcium per 100 ml feed.

Carnitine deficiency
Carnitine (β-hydroxy-trimethyl-gamma-aminobutyric acid) is necessary for transfer of free fatty acids across inner mitochondrial membranes prior to oxidation. It is therefore important for normal lipolysis, thermogenesis, ketogenesis and perhaps also regulation of nitrogen balance. Normally carnitine is synthesized in the body from lysine and methionine. The neonate's ability to synthesize carnitine is less than that of older individuals. Thus the carnitine in breast milk and cows' milk based formulas may be important in maintaining normal lipid metabolism. Levels of carnitine rise slowly after birth. LBW infants may have low carnitine levels due to relatively increased carnitine requirements, and failure to thrive has occasionally been attributed to carnitine deficiency. Carnitine is now added to many LBW formula feeds so deficiency in enterally fed infants may cease to be important. Carnitine deficiency is still likely in those infants who have had prolonged intravenous feeding when it may present as delayed lipid clearance from the plasma.

Essential fatty acid (EFA) deficiency

EFA deficiency has been described in intravenously fed neonates, particularly when there is associated carnitine deficiency. It is also described in enterally fed neonates with cholestasis. These infants present after some weeks of intravenous feeding with poor growth, dry scaly skin and mucocutaneous ulceration. The intravenous feeding solutions will not have contained EFA and giving occasional infusions of Intralipid (KabiVitrum) prevents the complication. Infusions of fresh plasma once weekly may reduce the need for other sources of EFA. Alternatively small oral feeds of preterm formula or breast milk can probably provide sufficient EFA to prevent deficiency. Formula milks should contain linoleic acid to the level of at least 1% of total energy intake to prevent EFA deficiency (Hansen et al., 1963).

Taurine deficiency

Taurine is present in higher concentration in human milk than in cows' milk and, until recently, all infant formulas. The need for this high taurine value has not been clear since bile acids can be conjugated with glycine rather than taurine by even the immature neonate. In kittens taurine deficiency has been associated with abnormalities in retinal development but no such association has been shown for man. However, there is now evidence that taurine supplementation can reduce fatty acid loss in cystic fibrosis (Darling et al., 1985) and the fat malabsorption of the LBW infant is reduced by taurine supplementation (Galeano et al., 1987). Taurine 'deficiency' does not seem to lead to clinical features (even failure to thrive) but taurine supplementation of LBW formulas may have resulted in subtle improvements in growth and development through more normal fatty acid composition of the tissues.

Copper deficiency (see also Chapter 9)

There have been a number of reports of clinical conditions associated with very low serum copper in VLBW infants which have responded to copper supplementation of the diet. These infants have usually been totally parenterally fed or fed breast milk or low copper content formula. Since about 1984 the copper content of most infant formulas in Britain has increased although copper content is very variable.

Infants with copper deficiency fail to thrive and are often anaemic, severely neutropenic with oedema and gross osteoporosis (Sutton et al., 1985). Some have decreased skin pigmentation. Diagnosis of clinical deficiency from serum copper levels is not easy since low levels are common in asymptomatic LBW infants. Activity of erythrocyte superoxide dismutase, a copper-dependent enzyme, is low.

Copper requirements in LBW infants are uncertain but levels of 1 μmol/kg/day have been suggested (Sutton et al., 1985). Most LBW infants do not achieve these intakes yet do not show evidence of deficiency.

Vitamin E deficiency

The place of vitamin E in the management of LBW infants is controversial. Levels of vitamin E are low in the newborn. They rise rapidly in full-term infants but stay low for longer periods in LBW infants. There is evidence that vitamin E protects against intra-ventricular haemorrhage in SG infants (Chiswick et al., 1984). Thus vitamin E should probably be administered from birth to VLBW infants. Vitamin E may also protect against retinopathy of prematurity (Hittner et al., 1981). However, enthusiastic therapy with vitamin E has been incriminated in the development of necrotizing enterocolitis and infection (Finer et al., 1984).

When infant formulas containing high unsaturated fatty acid content were first introduced, there was an outbreak of vitamin E dependent haemolytic anaemia in infants on these formulas. Addition of vitamin E to the milks has prevented this. A similar haemolytic anaemia responding to water-soluble α-tocopherol acetate 10 mg daily has been described in LBW infants after about 2 weeks of life. Falling haemoglobins and high reticulocyte counts in premature infants may be an indication for vitamin E supplementation.

Since longstanding deficiency of vitamin E is now recognized as causing neurological degeneration in chronic fat malabsorption states, vitamin E may be more important than previously recognized for brain structure and function. Whilst vitamin E deficiency in LBW infants has not been shown to correlate with later neurological damage (not related to intraventricular haemorrhage) it would seem wise to avoid significant deficiency during the period of rapid brain growth and development.

Anaemia
Anaemia is common in all LBW infants irrespective of method of feeding. The haemoglobin level of SG infants is not as high as in full-term infants (14.5 g/dl at 28 weeks; 17.0 g/dl at term) and drops to lower levels than in term infants because of:

1. More rapid growth rates leading to greater dilution of available red cells and greater difficulty of bone marrow in maintaining red-cell production to meet needs of growth.
2. Bone marrow suppression following comparatively high oxygen tensions in blood at birth compared with *in utero*.
3. Low blood volume (80 ml/kg) and loss of blood iatrogenically for investigations (blood gases, electrolytes, etc.).
4. Slightly shorter half life of immature red cells (70 days in term infants; 40 days in 28 weeks' gestation infants).
5. Deficiency of vitamin E or folic acid in early weeks of life.
6. Infection.

These are reasons for anaemia developing around 4–8 weeks after birth. Later in the first year, once birth weight has doubled, rapid growth and poor initial iron stores make LBW infants particularly at risk of iron-deficiency anaemia.

Vitamin E deficiency and folate deficiency (*see below*) can be avoided by supplementation. Anaemia due to growth, venesection and infection in early life may require small 'top-up' transfusions with partially packed cells. Those dealing with LBW infants must be constantly aware of the need to keep blood investigations to a minimum in these children because of the small total blood volume.

LBW infants fed infant formula should be given iron from 1 month of age (or from weaning if they are breast fed) for the first year of life to prevent iron deficiency anaemia. Before 1 month of age, iron is unnecessary and may affect resistance to infection. Low levels of vitamin E allow damage to red-cell membranes by free radicals, including iron, and thus encourage haemolysis. In breast-fed infants, iron orally could interfere with the anti-infective properties of lactoferrin. Thus it is more appropriate to give totally breast-fed infants iron supplements only if they show evidence of significant iron deficiency or at weaning.

What levels of haemoglobin are acceptable in LBW infants in the first months of life? Levels over 10 g/dl should not cause concern (unless they have developed rapidly due to haemorrhage or haemolysis) and should be symptom free for otherwise normal LBW infants. With levels below this, symptoms such as difficulty with feeding, breathlessness, cardiac failure and signs of reopened ductus arteriosus are common. Symptomatic anaemia requires 'top up' transfusion. It may be advisable to 'top up' all those LBW infants with haemoglobin below 8 g/dl as the chances of this becoming symptomatic are very high. Reticulocyte counts above 5% total red cells may indicate resolution with spontaneous improvement of haemoglobin levels in the course of a few days. Anaemia and high reticulocyte count may also indicate either haemolysis if haemoglobin is not rising *or* excessive blood letting for haematological investigations.

Folic acid deficiency
Occasionally megaloblastic anaemia and/or folate dependent poor growth have been demonstrated in LBW infants in the first months of life. The rapid growth of LBW infants requires more folate than is contained in the small volumes of milk these infants may be consuming and deficiency develops (Strelling, Blackledge and Goodall, 1979). Treatment is with folic acid 2.5 mg daily. A similar dose on a weekly basis is sufficient to prevent folate deficiency.

Other vitamin deficiencies
Premature infants are more prone to vitamin K deficiency than full-term infants particularly if they are breast fed, intravenously fed or given antibiotics. We recommend vitamin K 1 mg by month, intramuscularly or intravenously for ALL infants at birth. This is usually adequate to prevent vitamin K deficiency developing except in infants on parenteral feeding where the injection should be repeated weekly. Any infant, particularly the LBW infant, developing unexplained bleeding in the first month of life should be given a second injection of vitamin K as a precaution.

The small size and small intakes of milk or formula by LBW infants mean that vitamin intakes may not meet requirements. Vitamin deficiencies are a greater potential risk in LBW than term infants. Policies regarding vitamin and iron supplementation vary between units, but we believe it is important to supplement all infants below 2 kg birth weight and very important to supplement VLBW infants. Our regimen is outlined. It has the virtue of being relatively cheap and palatable. Once started, the regimen should continue until infants are 1 year old at least, since it is when the infant is weaned that the combination of exhaustion of prenatally acquired stores and relatively low dietary intakes reaches a critical state. It is often late in the first year before LBW infants are established on satisfactory mixed diets with adequate intakes of vitamins and iron.

Programme for vitamin supplementation in LBW infants

> From 2 weeks old (all LBW infants) – Children's vitamin drops (BNF): 7 drops daily (providing vitamin A 300 µg (1000 units), vitamin C 30 mg, vitamin D 10 µg (400 units). Folic acid syrup (Lexpec; R. P. Drugs): 2.5 mg in 5 ml once weekly.

> From 1 month old (all except wholly breast milk fed infants) – Sodium edetate elixir (Sytron; Parke-Davis): 1 ml daily (containing 100 µmol (5.5 mg) iron/ml).

> Infants less than 1.5 kg at birth – Vitamin E (water-soluble α-tocopherol acetate): 10 mg daily.

This regimen has one potential problem. The vitamin supplement supplies no B vitamins. Lucas and Bates (1984) have demonstrated transient biochemical evidence of riboflavin deficiency in the second week of life in LBW infants. This was prevented by feeding preterm formula which has a higher riboflavin content than human milk (human milk, 0.82 µmol/l, 310 µg/l; preterm formula, 4.76 µmol/l, 1.8 mg/l), or even by complementing human milk with some preterm formula. Thus B vitamin supplementation should perhaps be considered for LBW infants whilst they are wholly fed on expressed breast milk.

Iron is unnecessary in the first month of life and may encourage haemolysis (especially if there is vitamin E deficiency) through free radical effects on red-cell membranes. It may also encourage infection through saturation of transferrin in the blood. In breast-fed infants it interferes with the anti-infective effects of lactoferrin and should be avoided before weaning except when there is symptomatic iron deficiency anaemia.

Failure to thrive
Failure to thrive is discussed more extensively in Chapter 7. It is common for LBW infants to fail to gain weight for prolonged periods over the first weeks or months of life. The reasons are varied. SG infants are usually slower to start to gain weight than normal full-term infants. SFD infants, if well and fairly mature, may show very little initial weight loss and rapid catch-up growth.

1. SG infants have greater extracellular fluid volume than term infants so initial weight loss involves a greater proportion of body weight.
2. SG infants often have feeding difficulties. Early intakes may be inadequate to sustain growth.
3. When fed human milk or standard formula, the energy, protein, vitamin and mineral content of the feed may be inadequate for SG infants despite apparently adequate volumes.
4. Infants with severe respiratory distress and persistent tachypnoea or significant patent ductus arteriosus use extra energy for respiratory and cardiac work. This prevents energy being available for growth. LBW infants with respiratory problems show delayed onset of weight gain compared with those without respiratory problems (Davies, 1981).
5. Infection is common in SG infants and is often difficult to diagnose. Acidosis and poor weight gain may be the only clinical signs of infection.
6. Infants may be inadequately warmed so that energy is wasted in thermogenesis rather than used for growth.
7. If infants have been fed intravenously for prolonged periods, persisting trace nutrient (mineral or essential fatty acid) deficiency could inhibit growth.

Catch-up growth in LBW infants

If LBW infants are not to remain small all their lives they must show accelerated growth rates in order to catch up with other infants – both term and appropriate for dates. Once weight gain is established, the minimum acceptable rate should be over 1.5% body weight per day (>15 g/kg/day). The problems of SG infants often result in delayed onset of weight gain. However, by term, most SG infants are achieving a growth curve between the tenth and fiftieth centiles for gestational age. Weight and length accelerate across the growth centiles after the expected date of delivery

(Davies, 1981). LBW formulas enable acceleration to take place earlier. Rapid skull circumference growth may occur before rapid weight gain but the side-to-side flattening of the skull common in SG infants as they grow makes this measurement difficult to interpret.

The outlook for SFD infants is less certain. The aetiology of the growth retardation is significant to prognosis. Infants with disproportionate growth retardation (discussed in Chapter 2) with relatively normal intrauterine skull growth are expected to show more or less complete catch-up growth as the period of 'malnutrition' *in utero* has been short. Infants with proportionate growth retardation and without marked wasting have less predictable catch-up – possibly because so many of them pass from a less than satisfactory environment *in utero* to a less than satisfactory environment *ex utero*. Amongst these proportionate SFD infants will be those with intrauterine TORCH (toxoplasmosis, rubella, cytomegalovirus, herpes simplex) infections or chromosomal or other major abnormality. These infants are likely to remain small and show little catch-up. However, since most infant growth charts underrate the rapid growth of many normal infants in the first 6–8 weeks of life, some of these SFD infants may appear to be catching up with their peers shortly after birth if growth is reviewed against gestationally matched centiles, only to appear to fail to thrive at 3–4 months and to end the first year in much the same weight centile position as at birth. Early reassurance on the extent of catch-up should be guarded but as with so many aspects of child rearing, good nutrition and a stimulating, loving home environment are likely to minimize the effect of the antenatal growth insult.

References

BELL, E. F., WARBURTON, D., STONESTREET, B. S. and OH, W. (1980) Effect of fluid administration on the development of symptomatic patent ductus arteriosus and congestive heart failure in premature infants. *New England Journal of Medicine*, **302**, 598–603

BOXALL, J. and WHITBY, C. (1983) The role of the nurse in mother–baby interaction. In *Parent–Baby Attachment in Premature Infants*, edited by J. A. Davis, M. P. M. Richards and N. R. C. Roberton, pp. 129–138. London: Croom Helm

BROOKE, O. G. and LUCAS, A., (1985) Metabolic bone disease in preterm infants. *Archives of Disease in Childhood*, **60**, 682–683

BROOKE, O. G. and BARLEY, J. (1978) Loss of energy during continuous infusions of breast milk. *Archives of Disease in Childhood*, **53**, 344–345

BROOKE, O. G., WOOD, C. and BARLEY, J. (1982) Energy balance, nitrogen balance and growth in preterm fed expressed breast milk, a premature infant formula and two low-solute adapted formulae. *Archives of Disease in Childhood*, **57**, 898–904

BUDIN, P. (1907) *The Nursling*. London: Caxton Publishing

CALLENBACH, J. C., SHEEHAN, M. B., ABRAMSON, S. J. and HALL, R. T. (1981) Etiologic factors in rickets of very low birth weight infants. *Journal of Pediatrics*, **98**, 800–805

CHAPPELL, J. E., CLANDININ, M. T., KEARNEY-VOLPE, C., RETCHMAN, B. and SWYER, P. W. (1986) Fatty acid balance studies in premature infants fed human milk or formula: effect of calcium supplementation. *Journal of Pediatrics*, **108**, 439–447

CHISWICK, M. L., JOHNSTON, M., WOODHALL, C. et al. (1984) Protective effect of vitamin E on intraventricular haemorrhage in the newborn. In *Biology of Vitamin E*, edited by R. Porter and J. Whelan. Ciba Foundation Symposium number 101, pp. 186–200. Tunbridge Wells: Pitman Medical

COOPER, P. A., ROTHBERG, A. D., DAVIES, V. A. and ARGENT, A. C. (1985) COMPARATIVE GROWTH AND BIOCHEMICAL RESPONSE OF VERY LOW BIRTHWEIGHT INFANTS FED OWN MOTHER'S MILK, A PREMATURE INFANT FORMULA, OR ONE OF TWO STANDARD FORMULAS. *Journal of Pediatric Gastroenterology and Nutrition*, **4**, 786–794

References

DARLING, P. B., LEPAGE, G., LEROY, C. and ROY, C. C. (1985) Effect of taurine supplements on fat absorption in cystic fibrosis. *Pediatric Research*, **19**, 578–582

DAVIES, D. P. (1981) Physical growth from fetus to early childhood. In *Scientific Foundations of Paediatrics*, 2nd edn., edited by J. A. Davis and J. Dobbing, pp. 303–330. London: William Heinemann Medical Books

FRIIS-HANSEN, B. and ANDERSEN, G. E. (1985) Water – the major nutrient. In *Pediatric Nutrition*, edited by G. C. Arneil and J. Metcoff, pp. 109–126. London: Butterworths

FINER, N. N., PETERS, K. L., HAYEK, Z. and MERKEL, C. L. (1984) Vitamin E and necrotising colitis. *Pediatrics*, **73**, 387–393

FOMON, S. J. (1974) *Infant Nutrition*, p. 69. Philadelphia: W. B. Saunders

GALEANO, N. F., DARLING, P., LEPAGE, G., LEROY, C., COLLET, S., GIGVERE, R. and ROY, C. C. (1987) Taurine supplementation of a preterm formula improves fat absorption in preterm infants. *Pediatric Research*, **22**, 67–71

GROSS, S. J. (1983) Growth and biochemical response of preterm infants fed human milk or modified infant formula. *New England Journal of Medicine*, **308**, 237–241

GROSS, S. J., DAVID, R. J., BAUMAN, L. and TOMARELLI, R. M. (1980) Nutritional composition of milk produced by mothers delivering preterm. *Journal of Pediatrics*, **96**, 641–644

HANSEN, A. E., WIESE, H. F., BOELSCHE, A. N., HAGGARD, M. E., ADAM, D. J. D. and DAVIS, H. (1963) Role of linoleic acid in infant nutrition. *Pediatrics*, **31**, 171–192

HEIRD, W. C., DRISCOLL, J. M. Jr., SCHILLINGER, J. M., GREBIN, B. and WINTERS, R. W. (1972) Intravenous alimentation in pediatric patients. *Journal of Pediatrics*, **80**, 351–372

HITTNER, H. M., GODIO, L. B., RUDOLPH, A. J., *et al.* (1981) Retrolental fibroplasia: efficacy of vitamin E in a double-blind clinical study of preterm infants. *New England Journal of Medicine*, **305**, 1365–1371

KLAUS, M. H. and KENNELL, J. H. (1976) *Maternal–Infant Bonding*. St. Louis: C. V. Mosby

LUCAS, A. (1981) Gut hormones and infant feeding. In *Scientific Foundations of Paediatrics*, 2nd edn., edited by J. A. Davis and J. Dobbing, pp. 87–91. London: William Heinemann Medical Books

LUCAS, A. (1986) Feeding low birth weight infants. In *Textbook of Neonatology*, edited by N. R. C. Roberton, pp. 204–210. Edinburgh: Churchill-Livingstone

LUCAS, A. (1987) AIDS and human milk bank closures. *Lancet*, **i**, 1092–1093

LUCAS, A. and BATES, C. (1984) Transient riboflavin depletion in pre-term infants. *Archives of Disease in Childhood*, **59**, 837–841

LUCAS, A. and HUDSON, G. J. (1984) Preterm milk as a source of protein for low birthweight infants. *Archives of Disease in Childhood*, **59**, 831–836

LUCAS, A., GORE, S. M., COLE, T. J., *et al.* (1984) Multicentre trial on feeding LBW infants: effects of diet on early growth. *Archives of Disease in Childhood*, **59**, 722–730

MacMAHON, P. (1984) Prescribing and formulating intravenous feeding solutions by microcomputer. *Archives of Disease in Childhood*, **59**, 548–552

MANISCALCO, W. M. and WARSHAW, J. B. (1978) Cellular energy metabolism during fetal and perinatal development. In *Temperature Regulation and Energy Metabolism in the Newborn*, edited by J. C. Sinclair, pp. 1–37. New York: Grune and Stratton

ROBERTS, S. B. and LUCAS, A. (1985) Effects of two extremes of dietary intake on protein accretion in preterm infants. *Early Human Development*, **12**, 301–307

SCHANLER, R. J. and OH, W. (1980) Composition of breast milk obtained from mothers of premature infants as compared to breast milk obtained from donors. *Journal of Pediatrics*, **96**, 679–681

SCHANLER, R. J., GARZA, C. and NICHOLS, B. L. (1985) Fortified mothers' milk for very low birth weight infants: Results of growth and nutrient balance studies. *Journal of Pediatrics*, **107**, 437–445

SHIVPURI, C. R., MARTIN, R. J., CARLO, W. A. and FANAROFF, A. A. (1983) Decreased ventilation in preterm infants during oral feeding. *Journal of Pediatrics*, **103**, 285–289

STEVENSON, J. G. (1977) Fluid administration in the association of patent ductus arteriosus complicating respiratory distress syndrome. *Journal of Pediatrics*, **90**, 257–261

STRELLING, M. K., BLACKLEDGE, D. G. and GOODALL, H. B. (1979) Diagnosis and management of folate deficiency in low birth weight infants. *Archives of Disease in Childhood*, **54**, 271–277

SUTTON, A. M., HARVIE, A., COCKBURN, F., FARQUHARSON, J. and LOGAN, R. W. (1985) Copper deficiency in the preterm infant of very low birth weight. *Archives of Disease in Childhood*, **60**, 644–651

TRIPP, J. H. and CANDY, D. C. A. (1985) *Manual of Paediatric Gastroenterology*. Edinburgh: Churchill Livingstone

WHITEFIELD, M. F. (1982) Poor weight gain of the low birth weight infant fed nasojejunally. *Archives of Disease in Childhood*, **57**, 597–601

WIDDOWSON, E. M. (1981) Changes in body proportions and composition during growth. *Scientific Foundations of Paediatrics*, 2nd edn., edited by J. A. Davies and J. Dobbing, pp. 330–342. London: William Heinemann Medical Books

WILKINSON, A. R. and YU, V. Y. H. (1974) Immediate effects of feeding on blood gases and some cardiorespiratory functions in ill newborn infants. *Lancet*, **i**, 1083–1085

Chapter 6
Weaning

Weaning has had many definitions – changing feeding from breast to cup; from breast to bottle; from bottle to cup; from milk to solids. The definition most widely used today is 'the process of introducing any non-milk food into the infant diet, irrespective of whether or not breast or bottle feeding continues'.

When?

When should weaning occur? This again has undergone change. In Britain in the past, and in many developing countries today, weaning is an event late in the first year of the infant's life or even in the second year. In Western Europe and North America in the late 1960s it was an event often taking place in the first week or month of life. Recent studies have tried to demonstrate the optimal time for weaning, by determining when breast-milk intake ceases to maintain optimum growth (Waterlow and Thomson, 1979; Whitehead, Paul and Rowland, 1980; Whitehead and Paul, 1984). Deciding this from studies of infant growth is more difficult than might be thought.

A need for energy is the main factor determining the time at which foods other than milk should be introduced to infants' diets. When does this need arise? A study of infant growth rates in relation to milk intakes might be expected to give some indication of when milk intake ceases to meet requirements. However, normal growth is usually assessed in relation to reference standards, of which the most widely used are either the WHO (World Health Organisation, 1983) or the NCHS standards (Hamill, 1977), although many countries have developed growth standards of their own (Tanner, Whitehouse and Takaishi, 1966; van Wieringen, 1972). Growth standards only indicate average growth for the group from which the standards are derived. Deviation from the mean of one set of standards does not necessarily indicate abnormality if those children reviewed have different racial origins, environments and nutritional customs.

This is particularly true in early infancy when many groups of infants follow very different growth curves from those indicated by the standards (Whitehead and Paul, 1984) and yet appear well and adequately nourished (*see* Chapter 1). This is partly because standards refer to populations studied cross-sectionally rather than longitudinally. Growth is so rapid that very frequent longitudinal measurements on populations of infants are necessary to produce growth curves that represent growth velocity changes accurately. Current British standards underestimate rates of growth of most healthy infants in the first 2–3 months of life (Wickes, 1952; Whitehead, Paul and Rowland, 1980).

The milk intakes of breast-fed infants should give the best indication of the needs of infants. The need to wean would then be indicated by the age at which the energy intake of breast milk alone can no longer support normal rates of growth. However, we have already suggested that it is difficult to assess the limits of *normal* infant growth, and the measurement of energy intake from breast milk is inaccurate and tedious. Moreover, the volumes of milk mothers produce are enormously variable. Many factors other than infants' needs affect the volumes of breast milk produced. Studies of the intakes of formula-fed infants are easier and indicate the maximum quantities of milk that infants can ingest comfortably at any age, thus providing evidence for when weaning is essential. Such studies still do not indicate optimum age for weaning.

Fomon, Owen and Thomas (1964) showed that bottle-fed infants increased their total daily intakes rapidly in the first months of life, even though intake/kg/day tended to drop from an averge of 199 ml (563 kJ, 134 kcal)/kg/day at 8–30 days to 150 ml (420 kJ, 100 kcal)/kg/day at 3–5 months. Once the infants achieved weights of about 5 kg, further daily volume increments were small. Thus intake/kg/day fell between weights of 5 and 7 kg although infants continued to grow satisfactorily. More recently, Whitehead, Paul and Cole (1981) have demonstrated that infants' energy requirements are higher than previously thought soon after birth, but drop rapidly to levels of 357–378 kJ (85–90 kcal)/kg/day at 4–5 months and then rise again towards the end of the year. Such a demonstration explains both the previously anticipated inadequacy of breast feeding to meet the needs of infants from 3 months onwards and the satisfactory growth of many breast-fed infants despite apparently inappropriately low milk intakes.

Why?

If weaning is not necessarily indicated before 4 months of age, there seem good reasons to begin to wean most infants between 4 and 6 months, so that a considerable energy intake from foods other than milk has been established early in the second half of the first year. It is at about 6 months that the volumes of milk needed to sustain adequate growth become difficult for infants to tolerate. Deficiencies of iron and vitamins may also begin to develop after 6 months in wholly breast-fed infants. Infants of 5 months onwards start putting objects in their mouths. It is appropriate that some of these objects should be edible. At this age also, teeth begin to erupt and infants develop the ability to chew. Delay in feeding chewable food may result in delayed development of chewing.

The aims of weaning

Although growth has slowed considerably by the age of 6 months when compared with the rate immediately after birth, about 7% of total energy intake is still needed for growth. Tissue deposition requires a more varied diet than body maintenance with greater needs for amino acids, fatty acids, vitamins and minerals and high requirements for energy. Thus weaning diets need to be varied in content so as to cover the vitamin and mineral needs. Infants who continue high milk or formula intakes as well as taking solids will receive a high proportion of protein requirements from the milk and thus they have no great need for protein-rich solids. It is particularly important to introduce iron, zinc and vitamins C and D into the diet early, since deficiencies of these nutrients occur readily.

Currently there is a lot of concern about the effects of foreign protein on inducing allergic states in young infants (*see* Chapter 14) particularly for infants with strong family predisposition to eczema and asthma. If ingested allergens are a problem, they present maximum risk in very young infants. The permeability and sensitivity of the intestinal tract to 'foreign' proteins has diminished by the age of 4 months when first weaning solids are likely to be introduced. Nevertheless, it is probably wise to reduce the allergenic load to young infants by avoiding proteins known to precipitate allergic responses as long as nutritionally practical.

The most well-defined foreign substance that affects some, presumably genetically sensitive, infants adversely is gluten. Historically British infants have been weaned on to wheat products first. Gluten is present in wheat, rye, oats and barley but not rice or maize. Although wheat-containing weaning foods are still very popular, rice-based cereals have increased in popularity and are, on *theoretical* grounds, more appropriate as first cereal food. Transient gluten intolerance occurs occasionally in young infants after gastrointestinal infection. Other precautions include allowing egg yolk, but not the more allergenic and less digestible egg albumen, to infants aged less than 6 months. Infants with a family history of allergy and atopy may benefit from weaning after 6 months, although the evidence that this really protects against eczema or asthma is not conclusive.

How?

The protein needs of a 1-year-old child can be met by the protein in about 750 ml cow's milk or about 1 litre formula. About 1500 ml cows' milk or formula are needed to meet the energy needs of a child of the same age. If weanling infants continue on – for example – three '8 ounce' (240 ml) bottles of milk or formula a day plus a little milk with cereal, their protein requirements from other foods will be relatively small. Thus initial weaning foods are usually energy- and vitamin-B providing cereals, vitamin-C containing fruit juice, and puréed fruits and vegetables to provide a variety of minerals and vitamins. It is important, whether using home-prepared or manufactured infant foods, to present variety to infants since this avoids deficiency of trace nutrients which may not be present in all foods. Further, infants are basically conservative and resist change. It is possibly important for later appetite and diet that they learn to accept variety in tastes and, as they grow and learn to chew, variety in textures.

First weaning foods are usually semi-sloppy in nature and must be well mashed, strained or homogenized (*Table 6.1*). As children begin to make chewing efforts, lumpy solids which soften readily in the mouth can be introduced as well as rusks and chewable, suckable solids. Gradually infants learn effective chewing movements. Manufactured foods are commonly presented to mothers as 'baby', 'infant' or 'junior' foods depending on their relative lumpiness. These foods have great advantages to the modern mother from the point of view of convenience, hygiene and nutritional variety. Their protein and mineral content have been reduced since the problems experienced in the early 1970s from hypernatraemia secondary to cows' milk feeding and early weaning with protein- and salt-rich solids. The energy content of tinned infant foods is usually less than 420 kJ/100 g (100 kcal/100 g) and commonly only 210–290 kJ/100 g (50–70 kcal/100 g). This is

Table 6.1 Outline for weaning (foods listed roughly according to likely order of introduction)

Introduce small volumes of vitamin C containing fruit juices (preferably sugar free)
Introduce cereal softened with milk or water: soft rusks or rice preparations
Introduce increasing amounts of powdered infant cereals or 'strained' foods, both 'puddings' and 'dinners'
Home-prepared foods include:
  Slightly sweetened puréed stewed apple and other fruits
  Banana mashed with milk
  Mashed potato (mashed with a little milk and margarine) and gravy
  Mashed spinach and egg yolk
  Puréed carrots, turnips and other vegetables
  Minced meat
  Hard rusks to be sucked and chewed
  Bread and butter 'soldiers' (thin fingers of bread; no crusts)

---

frequently less energy dense than many home-produced weaning foods or even milk and formula, although the volume of food for the same energy content may be less than with formula.

The sodium content of weaning foods is important. Hypernatraemia is still seen occasionally in infants secondary to high salt intakes, often associated with early weaning and early change to unmodified cows' milk. For this reason alone, it would be sufficient to discourage the addition of salt to weaning foods. In addition, there are suggestions that in adults the development of hypertension may be related to sensitivity of some individuals to salt. Populations where the mean daily salt intake is low generally have a low prevalence of hypertension. Hypertension is very prevalent amongst some high salt consuming populations. Genetic factors predisposing to hypertension may be dependent or independent of sodium sensitivity. A modest intake of sodium seems advisable and might discourage young children from liking their foods 'salty'. The proof of the risks of a high salt intake are, however, not totally convincing (*see* Chapter 21).

Another aspect of weaning on to a wholesome mixed diet is the educative effect it may have on the infant. Infants, although reluctant to take solids initially, seem to develop likes and dislikes to some extent determined by how they are fed. It is important to establish habits, such as taking food without added salt or sugar, which encourage good dietary practices continuing into childhood and adult life. Current views on adverse nutritional habits would suggest that foods should not be sweetened unnecessarily since this may encourage dental caries and a craving for sweet foods. High-fibre, whole foods should be encouraged, although it may be inappropriate to present them to very young infants who have limited abilities to chew, since fibre tends to lend a coarse texture to the food. Moreover the relatively low energy density of some high-fibre foods risks the infants receiving inadequate energy intakes despite satiety. Wholemeal cereals and whole but well-mashed fruit and vegetables should be introduced as soon as posible. Animal fats should form only a modest part of the energy intake, and fried foods should be discouraged.

Table 6.2 lists problems that may arise secondary to weaning. Many of the problems of weaning in affluent societies are behavioural rather than nutritional. Mothers often attribute nutritional knowledge to their infants suggesting that foods initially rejected by infants are rejected because infants 'do not need', 'want', or 'like' that food, or that the food does not 'suit' them. More often infants appear to reject foods initially in order to express unfamiliarity with a food. Once a new taste is familiar, acceptance is likely. The consequence of accepting as food refusal the

Table 6.2 Problems that may arise secondary to weaning

Gastrointestinal infection secondary to contaminated foodstuffs or utensils
Inadequate intake of energy, protein, vitamins or minerals due to ignorance of infants' needs or too ready acceptance of food refusal
Overfeeding due to continuation of full milk intake with substantial solid intake
Malnutrition (protein-energy, vitamins, minerals) due to deficiencies of essential nutrients in diet
Allergic responses to foods
Presentation of specific nutritional disorders:
   Gluten-sensitive enteropathy
   Fructose intolerance
   Acrodermatitis enteropathica

---

natural reluctance by infants to take new foods is that children may develop strong food likes and dislikes, particularly if mothers tends to feed them bland, mashed foods because they have rejected stronger tastes and textures. This view is speculative but seems logical. Reluctant weaners may become faddy toddlers who are also reluctant to chew meat, vegetables and fruit and who live off juice, chips, crisps, sweets and biscuits. If nutrition education is to be effective, it should begin by example in infancy.

Weaning in developing countries

Weaning is a time of much greater concern for infants in underdeveloped societies than in affluent situations. The conflict of needs and problems created by the need for non-milk food sources – despite the risks of infection and nutritional deficiency from contaminated and low-nutrient developing-country diets – has been labelled the 'weanling dilemma' (*Figure 6.1*). The need to introduce non-milk food sources introduces the risks of gastrointestinal infection and parasitic infestation because of the heavy contamination of foodstuffs with infecting organisms. Local diets may be energy poor, monotonous staple fed once or twice a day. Meals are not specially prepared for infants and young children. Young children partake of the family meal. Small infants need feeding four or more times a day with energy-dense foods if they are to tolerate sufficient food to meet their needs.

Thus the sheer bulkiness of the diet together with the infrequent meals may prevent adequate energy intakes by infants in developing countries. Monotony and limited nutrient content of the staples may also prevent infants receiving the variety of minerals and vitamins necessary for rapid growth. A staple low in one essential amino acid requires mixing with other complementary proteins (perhaps in sauces, vegetables or stews) in order to provide for protein needs. Superimposed infection may affect appetite and precipitate a vicious cycle of deteriorating nutrition and increasing infection.

What should be offered as weaning foods in developing countries? There are various possibilities. Food mixes (Cameron and Hofvander, 1983) containing various local foods with relatively high energy and varied nutrient content may be cooked along with the family staple in covered tins within the same cooking pots as the staple. Or the child may be fed the traditional staple, but with a larger proportion of the sauce than generally received by adults. Sauces are usually prepared from ground-nuts, beans, meat or other nutritious, but less available than the staple, food. They provide protein and/or vitamin and mineral sources. Some

78 Weaning

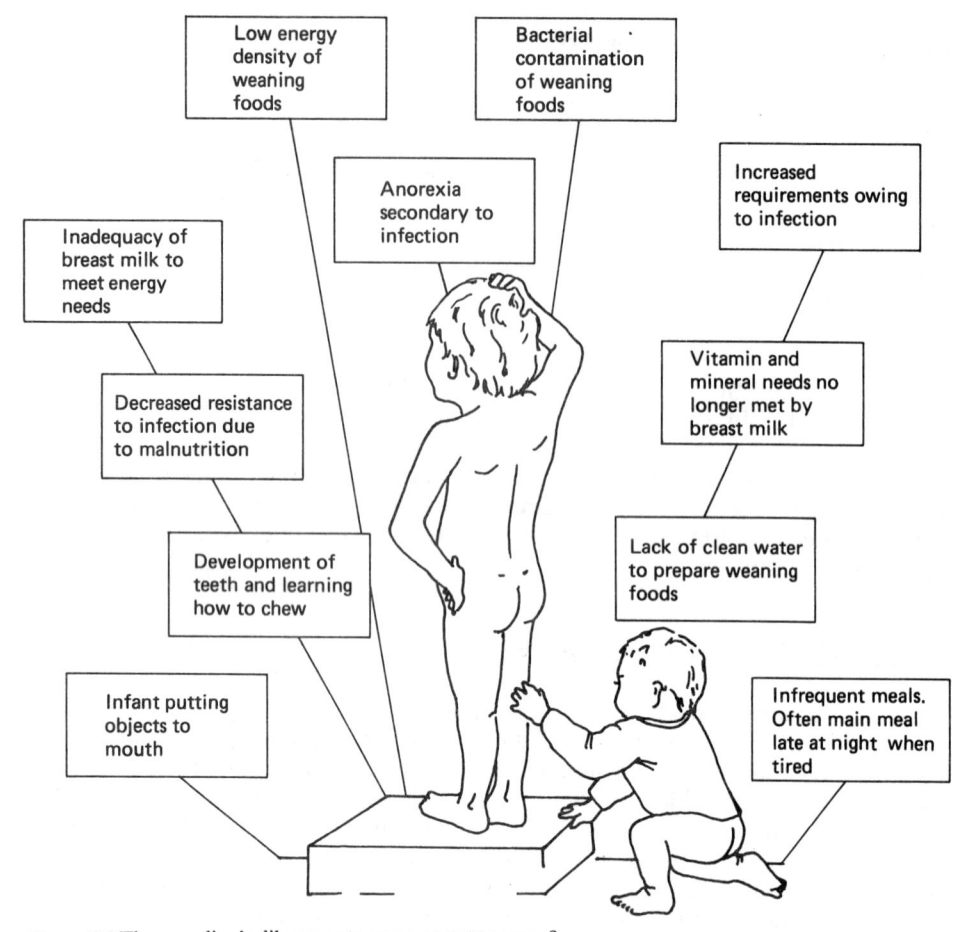

Figure 6.1 The weanling's dilemma: to wean or not to wean?

Labels around the figure:
- Low energy density of weaning foods
- Bacterial contamination of weaning foods
- Increased requirements owing to infection
- Anorexia secondary to infection
- Inadequacy of breast milk to meet energy needs
- Vitamin and mineral needs no longer met by breast milk
- Decreased resistance to infection due to malnutrition
- Development of teeth and learning how to chew
- Lack of clean water to prepare weaning foods
- Infant putting objects to mouth
- Infrequent meals. Often main meal late at night when tired

traditional diets need to be supplemented with vitamin sources in the form of fruit or dark green vegetables and protein sources such as milk powder cooked in the food or added at serving (*not* made up into milk with dirty water) before adequate nutrient density is achieved. In theory, prepared baby foods from tins or jars provide satisfactory weaning foods and have the great advantage of being initially more hygienic than home-prepared foods. In practice, the cost of manufactured foods is generally prohibitive and discourages them being given to infants in adequate quantities. Infants should continue dietary supplementation from regular breast feeds for as long as possible since breast milk will contribute considerable protein to the daily diet.

The following principles should be followed when weaning children in developing countries in particular. They are applicable (and generally practised) in developed countries as well:

1. Continue breast feeding as long as possible during the weaning process.
2. Feed children at least four times a day.
3. Mix foods: choose foods from protein, energy and vitamin sources at each meal.

4. Introduce new foods gradually and accept that infants may take solids reluctantly initially. Persist with the weaning process.
5. Boil all water used in cooking and scour utensils with boiling water.
6. Avoid large volumes of fluid in between meals, since these will detract from infants' appetites for food. Offer drinks towards the end of meals.
7. Feed the children. Use spoons if there are liquid sauces or gravies, otherwise essential nutrients may be lost.

Children in developing countries are often weaned on to vegetarian, or predominantly vegetarian, diets. Even in the Western World vegetarian diets may have hazards for children in the weaning period. These are discussed further in Chapter 11.

References

CAMERON, M. and HOFVANDER, Y. (1983) *Manual on Feeding Infants and Young Children*. Oxford: Oxford University Press

FOMON, S. J., OWEN, G. M. and THOMAS, L. M. (1964) Milk or formula volume ingested by infants fed *ad libitum*. *American Journal of Diseases of Children*, **108**, 601–604

HAMILL, P. V. V. (1977) *NCHS Growth Curves for Children*. US Department of Health Education Welfare Publication No. PHS 7B-1650. Hyattsville: National Center for Health Statistics

TANNER, J. M., WHITEHOUSE, R. M. and TAKAISHI, M. (1966) Standards from birth to maturity for height, weight, height velocity and weight velocity. British Children 1965. *Archives of Disease in Childhood*, **41**, 454–471, 613–675

WATERLOW, J. C. and THOMSON, A. M. (1979) Observations on the adequacy of breast feeding. *Lancet*. **ii**, 238–242

WHITEHEAD, R. G. and PAUL, A. A. (1984) Growth charts and the assessment of infant feeding practices in the Western world and in developing countries. *Early Human Development*, **9**, 187–207

WHITEHEAD, R. G., PAUL, A. A. and ROWLAND, M. G. M. (1980) Lactation in Cambridge and in the Gambia. In Nutrition in Childhood. *Topics in Paediatrics*, Vol. **2**, edited by B. A. Wharton, pp. 22–23. Bath: Pitman Press

WHITEHEAD, R. G., PAUL, A. A. and COLE, T. J. (1981) A critical analysis of measured food intakes during infancy and early childhood in comparison with current international recommendations. *Journal of Human Nutrition*, **35**, 339–348

WICKES, I. G. (1952) Rate of gain and satiety in early infancy. *Archives of Disease in Childhood*, **27**, 449–457

Van WIERINGEN, J. C. (1972) *Seculaire Groeiverschuving*. Leiden: Nederlands Instituut voor Preventieve Geneeskunde

WORLD HEALTH ORGANISATION (1983) *Measuring Change in Nutritional Status*. Geneva: World Health Organisation

Chapter 7
Failure to thrive

Failure to thrive is failure to gain in height and weight at the expected rate. As the problem is common in infancy – an age when accurate length measurements are not easy to obtain – height/length measurements are often overlooked and failure to thrive interpreted as failure to gain in *weight* at the expected rate.

Failure to thrive should be a three-dimensional diagnosis over time. Healthy infants and children grow so rapidly that even when sick or inadequately nourished, some weight gain may still occur. The *rate* of growth is therefore more important in diagnosis of failure to thrive than absolute size or the presence of growth. Some children may be small overall but nevertheless growing at normal rates and thus thriving within their own growth pattern (*Figure 7.1*). Children found on one occasion to be below the third centile for weight are often described as showing failure to thrive, but evidence that they have abnormally slow growth over a period of time is necessary to confirm true failure to thrive rather than constitutional small size.

The clinical diagnosis of failure to thrive

The symptoms and signs of failure to thrive are those of its causes. Possible causes are numerous but the vast majority of children with failure to thrive have either a readily recognizable cause or failure to thrive determined by their nurturing environment and which will not be diagnosed by clinical investigative procedures. Differential diagnosis demands thorough history and examination. Particular attention should be given to details of dietary intake; problems with feeding or gastrointestinal function; the psychosocial background of the family; and the home environment.

Many causes of failure to thrive in young infants are conditions that also affect neurological development. Poor nutrition in early life may, if severe and prolonged, influence brain growth and possibly contribute to developmental delay. Sick, poorly nourished children learn more slowly through apathy, physical weakness or failure to stimulate attention and interest from their carers. Developmental assessment of young infants who are failing to thrive is an important part of the clinical assessment although it may be difficult at presentation to decide whether developmental delay is a feature of the cause of failure to thrive, or whether it is secondary to the consequent poor nutrition.

The clinical diagnosis of failure to thrive 81

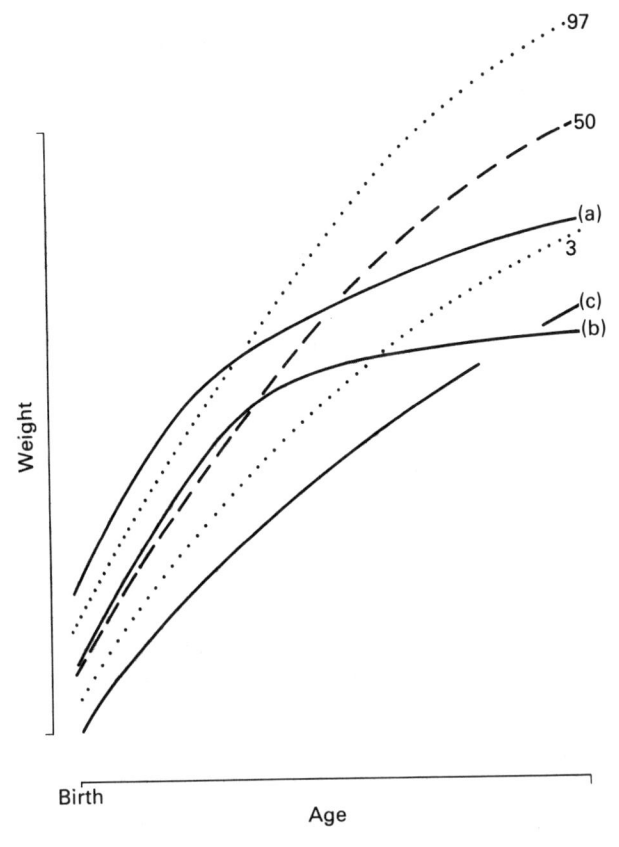

Figure 7.1 Diagrammatic representation of weight gain in failure to thrive (*a,b*) compared with that of constitutionally small normal (*c*) and with 3, 50 and 97 centiles for age.

The following are particular points relevant to clinical assessment of the child presenting with failure to thrive:

1. *History:* Appetite and feeding – detailed dietary history of all meals and snacks, specifying food refusal or vomiting; feeding difficulties, problems with swallowing or chewing.
   Bowel function – frequency of stools; nature of stools – consistency, colour, odour.
   Details of past history – pregnancy, birth history, birth weight; postnatal growth problems; frequency of infections, especially diarrhoea and respiratory infections.
   Developmental history – assess motor and social aspects separately if possible.
2. *Family history:* Family illnesses. Social circumstances – home, persons/room, where, and with whom the child sleeps.
3. *Clinical examination:*
   Observe parent–child interaction.
   Observe general state of care – cleanliness, clothing, etc.
   Look for evidence of wasting of muscles, loss of fat.

82 Failure to thrive

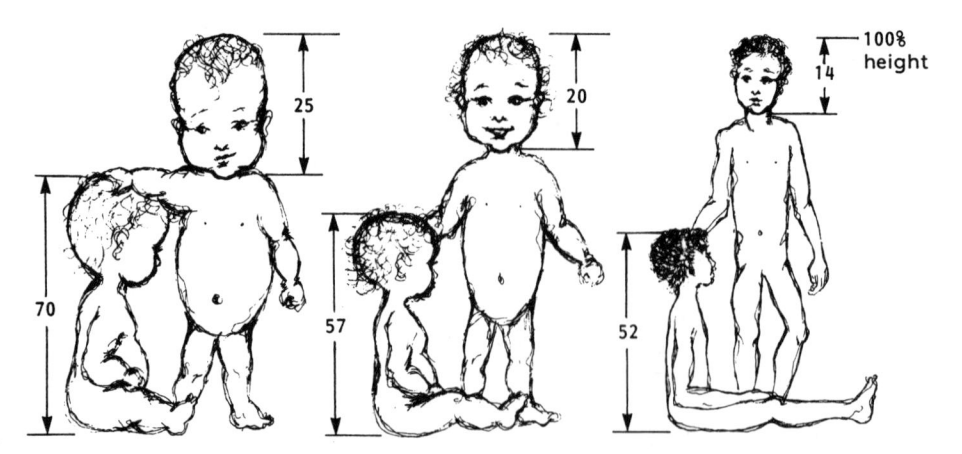

Figure 7.2 Changes in relative head size and sitting to standing height at birth, 2½ years and adolescence (menarche in girls, age 15 in boys). Rest of child not drawn in proportion!

Measure weight, length, skull circumference and plot them on growth charts.
Measure body proportions: upper segment to lower segment (*Figure 7.2*).
Assess developmental progress and responsiveness.
Watch the child feed.

The likely causes of failure to thrive are influenced by age although no age group is exclusive of other conditions. The following are likely causes according to age:

1. *Premature infant:* Congenital disorders, metabolic problems, nutrition inadequacy, infection – acute and acquired *in utero* – chronic lung disease, cardiac failure (patent ductus arteriosus).
2. *Term neonates:* Congenital abnormalities, infection, inborn errors of metabolism, minor feeding problems.
3. *Post-neonatal infants:* *Infections – recurrent, acute, and chronic.
   Congenital heart disease.
   Inborn errors of metabolism.
   Endocrine problems – hypothyroidism.
   Renal problems.
   *Gastrointestinal:
     pyloric stenosis,
     gastro-oesophageal reflux;
     malabsorption.
   *Inadequate intake.
   *Psychosocial deprivation.
4. *Toddler:* Inadequate or inappropriate diet with feeding and behavioural problems; infections due to poor environmental hygiene; malabsorption syndromes.
5. *Older child:* Psychosocial deprivation; causes of short stature presenting as poor weight gain; malabsorption syndromes.

* Most frequently encountered causes in general paediatric practice.

Failure to thrive can be classified according to the types of situation that precipitate failure to thrive:

1. Too little in.
2. Too much out.
3. Failure to absorb.
4. Failure to utilize.
5. Increased requirements.

Specific causes often act through several of these general causes but the classification provides a useful approach to investigation of the underlying disorder. This approach to the classification of causes of failure to thrive can be used for classification of other nutrient deficiencies (*see*, for example, iron deficiency, Chapter 9).

Too little in: Inadequate intake (*Table 7.1*)

Energy intakes may be low because of poverty, ignorance or neglect. Children are simply fed too little. Infrequent meals of bulky food of low energy density make it difficult for small children with poor appetites and perhaps poor skills at feeding themselves to ingest sufficient food at each meal to meet requirements. This is often the case in developing countries where children may receive only two meals per day of bulky, energy-poor, staple. In this country, children remaining on a wholly milk diet beyond 6 months may also have difficulty in ingesting the large volumes required to meet energy needs unless fed very frequently. Toddlers allowed to drink fruit squash and 'pop' (aerated drinks, Pepsi, Coca-Cola, lemonade) *ad libitum* may sate their appetites with fluid yet ingest inadequate energy and other nutrients.

Table 7.1 Causes of inadequate energy intake

Inadequate offered:	poverty, ignorance, deliberate neglect; infrequent feeding; low energy density, bulky diet
Anorexia:	infection; chronic illness; unhappiness or fear; psychological disturbance; deficiency of other nutrients (iron, zinc); coeliac disease
Feeding difficulty:	wrong-shaped teat; too small or too large a hole in teat in bottle feeding; abnormality of palate or lips; bulbar palsy; extreme breathlessness; blocked nose in infants who are obligate nose breathers when sucking; inappropriate management of feeding
Vomiting:	pyloric stenosis; hiatus hernia and reflux oesophagitis; general illness (e.g. urinary tract infection); raised intracranial pressure; emotional disorders

The child – usually a toddler – who will not eat as parents expect is a major worry for parents and a frequent presentation in clinics. Often these are children whose birth weight and parental size are such that their growth expectations are below average anyway. They may not need to eat much to grow at their expected rate, particularly in the toddler years when growth rates are much slower than in infancy. They quickly learn to manipulate their parents by not eating. All too often they receive adequate energy intakes but as drinks and snacks in between meals. Dietary history may indicate clearly why these children have no appetite for meals!

These healthy, sometimes underweight, finicky children require firm management. If children do not eat their meals, drinks and snacks in between meals should be stopped. Drinks can easily reduce appetite for meals without providing alternative nutrition. Parents should try to reduce their own anxiety over the child (who usually provides evidence of adequate intake by vigorous activity and displays of temperament).

Small children resist being forced to eat. They should be allowed to join in family meals so they see others eating around them but left to eat at their own pace (often slow and episodic). The less attention paid to whether they are eating or not, the more likely they are to get on with the meal. Fussing and forcing is usually ineffective. These children require dietary management, not investigation. However, any suggestion from clinical examination that there is genuine anorexia, significant growth faltering or malaise should precipitate investigation for urinary tract infection, coeliac disease or other causes of anorexia and failure to thrive. Faddy eaters are often iron deficient and may present with anaemia and misery. Correction of iron deficiency may improve appetite and temperament thus helping parental management.

Anorexia and difficulty with feeding are other problems leading to inadequate intake. Vomiting will result in inadequate intake since food vomited back can be regarded as failed ingestion rather than failed absorption. The variety of conditions leading to anorexia or vomiting is great but in childhood infection is a very common explanation.

Table 7.2 Conditions leading to failure to thrive through malabsorption

Congenital:
    Cystic fibrosis
    Schwachman syndrome
    Abetalipoproteinaemia
    Glucose–galactose malabsorption
    Biliary atresia

Genetic predisposition:
    Gluten-sensitive enteropathy (coeliac disease)
    Lactose intolerance

Acquired:
    Lactose and disaccharide intolerance
    Transient gluten-sensitive enteropathy
    Infestations, e.g. giardiasis, ascariasis
    Anatomical lesions, e.g. blind loop syndrome, short gut syndrome
    Crohn's disease
    Cirrhosis

Failure to absorb

Table 7.2 lists the main malabsorption syndromes of childhood. Cystic fibrosis is likely to present as a hungry, wasted child with bulky, particularly foul smelling (because they contain undigested protein as well as undigested fat), stools present since birth. Rectal prolapse is common and respiratory symptoms may be the dominant complaint. There may be a family history (*see* Chapter 15).

Coeliac disease only occurs in children who have been weaned on to gluten-containing solids (wheat, rye, oats, barley). Children may present soon after weaning, or at any age throughout life thereafter. Iron deficiency is common and short stature may be marked in older children (*see* Chapter 15).

Lactose and other disaccharide intolerances affect children secondary to gastrointestinal infection, particularly with pathogenic *E. coli* and rotavirus, but also affect non-Caucasians in later childhood due to genetic tendencies to lose lactase activity. *Giardia* infestation seems particularly common amongst infants and toddlers attending day nurseries. It may be difficult to diagnose since the cysts and parasites are not always found in stools. Diagnosis may be made coincidentally with jejunal biopsy, when *Giardia* are seen in the jejunal juice or attached to the mucosa.

Too much out: Increased losses (*Table 7.3*)

Tissue loss in severe eczema, burns, or exfoliative dermatitis may be considerable.

Maintenance of increased energy and protein intakes is important for management. In treatment of burns this may necessitate intravenous feeding. Folate deficiency readily arises when there is tissue loss.

Table 7.3 Sites of increased nutrient losses causing failure to thrive

Skin:
  Generalized tissue loss – eczema
  Exfoliative dermatitis
  Burns

Gastrointestinal tract:
  Protein losing enteropathy
  Protein and iron: gastrointestinal bleeding

Renal tract:
  Protein – nephrotic syndrome
  Glucose – diabetes mellitus, renal tubular disorders

Other sites:
  Protein loss from tapping pleural or pericardial effusions
  Protein loss in peritoneal dialysis
  Protein loss in pus from empyema or osteomyelitis
  Protein loss in major haemorrhage

The development of diabetes in childhood is usually so acute that weight loss is rarely sufficiently prolonged to be diagnosed as failure to thrive. Inadequate control of diabetic children may cause sufficient sugar loss in the urine to precipitate energy deficiency and failure to thrive (*see* Chapter 18). Wasting or failure to thrive secondary to renal protein loss is also marked in the nephrotic syndrome although the actual tissue loss is not apparent until remission, because of masking oedema (*see* Chapter 17).

Failure to utilize (*Table 7.4*)

This is a nebulous but most important aetiological class leading to failure to thrive. Children with a wide variety of conditions, often with severe metabolic impact, may eat adequately and yet fail to thrive. Children with uncontrolled inborn errors of

Table 7.4 Examples of conditions without clear nutritional explanation for failure to thrive ('failure to utilize' group)

Congenital and antenatal:
  Slow growth both *in utero* and *ex utero*
  Genetic – both non-specific and specific syndromes
  Chromosomal – Down's syndrome, etc.
  Severe congenital abnormalities
  Intrauterine infections
  Maternal 'toxins' – cigarettes, alcohol, anti-convulsant drugs
  Other intrauterine growth retardation, e.g. Russell–Silver 'dwarfism'

Postnatal:
  Metabolic – inborn errors of metabolism, hypothyroidism in infancy
  'Toxic' – infection, uraemia
  Specific nutrient deficiency – zinc deficiency, iron deficiency, rickets
  Congenital heart disease
  Severe mental handicap
  Psychosocial deprivation

metabolism, uraemia and severe infection may fail to thrive despite reasonable intakes. Children with intrauterine growth retardation or severe congenital abnormality may eat adequately and yet fail to thrive. Sometimes such children grow at a normal rate but fail to achieve catch-up and thus remain small. Isolated nutrient deficiency leads to failure to utilize the energy available for normal growth. The child with vitamin D deficiency, for example, fails to thrive as part of the clinical picture of rickets. Zinc and trace element deficiencies are associated with poor growth in otherwise adequately nourished children (*see* Chapter 9). Amongst this group also are those children who fail to thrive, despite adequate intake, because of their unsatisfactory nurture (*see below*).

Increased requirements (*Table 7.5*)

The classic example of failure to thrive or weight loss secondary to increased requirements must be thyrotoxicosis. Here basal metabolic rate is increased in association with high circulating thyroid hormones. Thyrotoxicosis in older children

Table 7.5 Conditions leading to increased nutrient requirements

Prematurity
Catch-up growth
Thyrotoxicosis
Cerebral palsy: choreoathetoid, spastic
Severe chronic asthma
Congenital heart disease
Pyrexia

is associated with wasting, restlessness, anxiety, large appetite or anorexia and vomiting. It is uncommon in young children and infants except as congenital thyrotoxicosis secondary to elevated maternal long-acting thyroid stimulators. Usually mother has a history of thyrotoxicosis which has resolved with treatment.

Infants are thin, restless, tachycardic and at risk of congestive heart failure. They are hungry and yet fail to thrive. The condition resolves gradually as maternal immunoglobulins are metabolized over the first few months of life. Propranolol, carbimazole and/or potassium iodide may be necessary to control the condition meanwhile.

Premature or small for gestational age infants need extra food for accelerated growth and will fail to thrive if their increased energy needs are not recognized. Children with increased cardiorespiratory workload secondary to congestive heart failure or respiratory disease such as chronic asthma fail to thrive due to the need for extra energy for increased respiratory work.

Failure to thrive in specific conditions

Several common causes of failure to thrive will now be discussed in the hope that an understanding of the reasons for failure to thrive will help management or prevention.

Infection

Infection precipitates failure to thrive through the following mechanisms.

Inadequate intake
Anorexia and vomiting are important features of many infections and form a major contributing factor to wasting in even fairly trivial infections. Children who are ill with infection should be offered good quality palatable foods to reduce the inadequate intake. Convalescent diets should include extra food for catch-up growth.

Increased losses
Certain infections (*see* diarrhoea below) induce protein loss through the formation of pus or through protein-losing enteropathy (measles, for example) even though the disease is not primarily a gastroenteritis (Sarker *et al.*, 1986).

Malabsorption
This is particularly a feature of diarrhoea (*see below*) but pyrexia inhibits absorption of iron by the gastrointestinal tract (Beresford, Neale and Brooke, 1971), and other nutrient absorption may be similarly affected.

Failure to utilize
The 'toxicity' of infection and pyrexia remain largely unexplained. It has been suggested that infection uncouples oxidative metabolism, thus misdirecting energy released from metabolism to form heat. Independent of all the other effects of infection on energy balance, there does seem to be an effect at the intracellular level contributing to energy wastage.

Increased requirements
Pyrexia is an important cause of increased requirements in infection. A 1°C rise in body temperature increases basal metabolic rate by 13%. Infection stimulates accelerated production of leucocytes and extra protein synthesis for antibody

formation. The need to provide increased requirements is greatest in the convalescent period. When weight loss has occurred children must have accelerated growth rates to make up the growth deficits during the period of illness. If increased requirements are *not* provided during this period, growth may continue at normal rates for age – but along lower centiles (*Figure 7.3*).

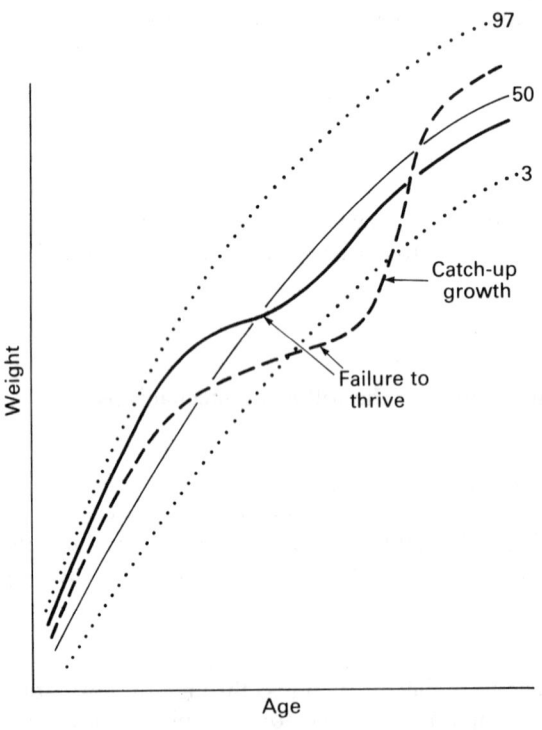

Figure 7.3 Diagrammatic representation of failure in thrive with total catch-up growth (- - - -) and no catch-up growth despite resolution of failure to thrive (——) plotted against weight centiles.

Diarrhoea

Most diarrhoea in childhood originates with infections, as discussed above. However, diarrhoea is such an important cause for failure to thrive that I shall discuss it separately. Hopefully, a clearer analysis of why diarrhoea causes failure to thrive and sometimes severe protein-energy malnutrition will encourage vigorous management of diarrhoea so as to reduce its growth-damaging effects.

World-wide, acute diarrhoeal infections are probably the most important cause of failure to thrive. Persisting diarrhoea due to infections such as rotavirus, pathogenic *Escherichia coli*, *Campylobacter*, *Cryptosporidia* or recurrent episodes of acute diarrhoea are common amongst infants, even in well-developed countries. In the developing world, where weaning foods provide inadequate nutrition and are likely to be heavily contaminated with enteric organisms, the interaction of diarrhoeal infection and lowered host resistance due to malnutrition presents a formidable problem (Mata, 1985).

Undoubtedly, a major part of the malnutrition due to diarrhoea is secondary to poor intake (Molla, Molla and Rahaman, 1986). Either the child is deprived of normal diet and fed on energy-poor, sloppy foods, or all food is stopped and oral rehydration solution proferred instead (*see* Chapter 15). Energy deficiency for a short period (24 hours) in a well-nourished child can be made up rapidly in convalescence. But if the diarrhoea persists or recurs and oral rehydration without food becomes recurrent, the energy deficiency accumulates and wasting follows.

In addition to anorexia and reduced intake, diarrhoea causes impaired absorption of nutrients – an effect that may persist for several weeks even when the infection seems to have resolved. There may be reduced absorption of protein, fat and carbohydrate secondary to mucosal damage from bacterial adhesions to the mucosa; release of enterotoxins; and hydrolysis of bile acids and carbohydrates by bacterial overgrowth in the small intestine (Molla *et al.*, 1983). In some infections there may even be a protein-losing enteropathy secondary to damage to the mucosa (Sarker *et al.*, 1986). Losses of electrolytes, and probably other nutrients, occur as part of the secretory diarrhoea which may follow damage to intestinal epithelial cells by bacterial toxins. Infectious diarrhoea may also precipitate more specific enteropathies such as lactose intolerance or transient gluten sensitivity. Associated pyrexia may increase metabolism and thus energy requirements.

Prevention of failure to thrive resulting from infection or diarrhoea involves:

1. Educating families in hygiene so as to reduce the prevalence of infection.
2. Provision of clean accessible water supplies.
3. Reducing the period of oral rehydration to the minimum practical in diarrhoea.
4. If possible, reintroducing full-strength milk without regrading (*see* Chapter 15).
5. Continuing breast feeding with oral rehydration in weanling diarrhoea.
6. Providing appetizing, easily swallowed, small, frequent, meals during illness and infection.
7. Providing frequent, nutrient-dense, meals in convalescence.

Congenital heart disease

Failure to thrive is common in congenital heart disease. Usually the failure to thrive develops in the first 2 years of life and affects particularly those infants with cyanotic congenital heart disease or pulmonary hypertension and congestive cardiac failure. The potential causes of failure to thrive in congenital heart disease are multiple:

1. Inadequate intake due to breathlessness and anorexia:
   (a) Child fails to thrive.
   (b) Child is fed for actual weight rather than expected weight for age.
   (c) Child receives inadequate food for catch-up growth.
2. Malabsorption:
   (a) Secondary to poor nutrition, anoxia or congestion of intestinal wall.
   (b) Due to increased prevalence of gluten-sensitive enteropathy in congenital heart disease (Congdon *et al.*, 1982).
3. Failure to utilize food due to severe anoxia, acidosis or poor perfusion of tissues.
4. High energy requirements (in cardiac failure and pulmonary hypertension particularly); inadequate intakes thus become even further from requirements.

Sondheimer and Hamilton (1978) have demonstrated malabsorption in association with congenital heart disease. Others have shown an increased incidence of enteropathy (presumed gluten sensitivity) in children with congenital heart disease (Congdon et al., 1982). In our experience, however, the main problem is that the intakes of these children may be adequate for their small size but inadequate for the catch-up growth necessary or for the increased requirements shown by some children (Menon and Poskitt, 1985).

Measurement of oxygen consumption in infants with congenital heart disease shows increased oxygen consumption/kg/min in infants with congestive failure or pulmonary hypertension (e.g. large ventricular septal defect), or both. This is presumably similar to the raised metabolic rate seen in cardiac cachexia in adults (Pittman and Cohen, 1964) and is probably related to increased cardiac and respiratory work with relatively inefficient cardiorespiratory function.

If resting metabolism in infants with congenital heart disease is high, management of these infants should include encouraging high energy intakes to anticipate failure to thrive secondary to increased needs. All too often the volumes of feed these infants can ingest are insufficient for their needs. We have had only limited success so far in improving energy intakes and growth rates by attempts to increase energy intakes without increasing feed volumes. Methods for doing this include introducing energy-dense solids as substitute for milk feeds in infants of 2 months or over – monitoring fluid and electrolyte balance closely – and increasing the energy density of feeds with carbohydrate or fat sources (see *Tables 15.10* and *15.11*). The electrolyte content of substances used to increase energy density is important since sodium intakes may affect fluid retention. Many of these infants are receiving intensive diuretic therapy and may even be sodium deficient.

Bougle et al. (1986) have improved growth rates in infants with congenital heart disease through continuous enteral feeding. This offers another method of increasing energy intake in these children.

Although the prospects for successful surgery or bypass are increased if cardiac infants are larger and heavier and better nourished, the benefits of getting these infants to grow better may be less than anticipated. If cardiac function is inadequate in a small body, will it be any more adequate in a larger body or will increase in body size result in irretrievable cardiac failure? This we do not know.

Children with congenital heart disease should be given fluoride drops or tablets, starting before tooth eruption to help prevent dental caries. Subacute bacterial endocarditis is a severe problem, easily developing unnoticed in the early stages, and often precipitated by treatment of caries.

Neurological handicap

It is not unusual for children with severe spastic cerebral palsy or mental retardation to fail to thrive. Again, the causes of this are multiple.

Failure to thrive in severe neurological handicap may be consequent upon:

1. Inadequate intake due to difficulties with chewing and with co-ordinating swallowing.
2. Inadequate intake due to being fed sloppy foods in order to overcome feeding/swallowing difficulties.
3. Specific nutrient deficiencies (e.g. vitamin C) due to poor intake from a sloppy diet or effect of drugs (e.g. anti-convulsant induced vitamin D deficiency).

4. High energy requirements due to continuous neuromuscular activity in choreoathetosis or the extra work required to counteract muscle spasm in spastic cerebral palsy.
5. Deprivation syndrome (*see below*) in some rejected handicapped children.
6. Neurologically induced growth failure in some severely brain damaged children (mechanism not understood). Rarely hypopituitarism is contributing to growth failure.

Again it is important that these children are fed diets that are nutritionally adequate. Children who are unable to consume normal diet for their age on nutrient dense but non-bulky diets even in liquidized form, should be referred for paediatric dietetic advice. Growth failure due to inadequate dietary intake or specific nutrient deficiency can easily be overlooked by attributing it to the primary cerebral damage.

Children with severe neurological handicap are particularly prone to caries. Poor nutrition in early life may contribute to poor dental enamel. High-carbohydrate diets, often given because diets need to be soft and sloppy rather than chewable, encourage cariogenic bacteria in the mouth. Teeth grinding by handicapped children probably contributes to damage. Cleaning the teeth is not an easy exercise in these children. Since unnoticed dental abscesses cause unnecessary ill health, fluoride drops should be introduced from an early age (*see* Chapter 12).

Psychosocial deprivation

The concept that unhappy, unwanted or rejected children are small, and yet hungry, is one that reaches out beyond the medical literature (*see* Dickens: *Oliver Twist*). It is easy to connect many of these children with starvation secondary to their uncaring environment. However, poor growth may occur in the presence of plenty if the environment is inappropriately harsh. In a classic study of children in German orphanages, Widdowson (1951) showed how the effects of nutritional supplementation may be insufficient to overcome the growth-retarding effects of an unkind carer.

McCarthy (1974) has commented that 'in deprivation there is nothing. Feeling has gone and attachments do not exist, except on a very superficial level and of a kind which are not worth the child's preserving'. Sometimes the child is subject to physical abuse, sometimes simply emotional abuse. The effect may be that the child is deprived of food through deliberate callousness or oversight. The child may be offered food but be too miserable or unhappy to eat. Or the child may eat – and even eat excessively – and yet not grow. With the first two possibilities the failure to thrive is understandable. With the third possibility the failure to thrive is mysterious and still inadequately explained.

The child with failure to thrive due to deprivation (emotional or psychosocial deprivation; maternal rejection; failure to thrive syndrome; psychosocial dwarfism) is often from a home with an obvious background of disturbance, violence or neglect. Occasionally the rejection is more subtle and may occur in a well-to-do home. Only one child may be affected either because this particular child is disliked by a parent for some, not necessarily acknowledged, cause or perhaps because this child has a personality or constitution that reacts to rejection this way. For reasons that could be genetic, other children in the same family may respond differently to the environmental stress.

92   Failure to thrive

Clinically these children are diagnosed on specific features rather than by exclusion of other causes of failure to thrive (*Table 7.6*). Young children are usually quiet, apathetic and may assume catatonic (fixed) postures yet practise eye avoidance whilst remaining alert and watchful (radar gaze). Older children may present with behaviour problems with bizarre, aggressive, destructive behaviour and uncontrollable appetites. It is often the large appetite with poor growth which draws attention to the child's problems.

Table 7.6 Clinical features of emotional deprivation syndrome

History:	appetite may be large or even abnormal (e.g. stealing food, eating leftovers from school plates), behaviour quiet and apathetic or aggressive and attention seeking
Clinical signs:	short; often underweight for height; passive, unresponsive; avoid eye contact; radar gaze or frozen watchfulness; abdominal distension; cold, reddish-blue hands, feet and nose (acrocyanosis); chilblains

Rapid development, growth and emotional awakening with tender, loving, care but without significant change in diet

The proof of the diagnosis of deprivation syndrome is in the effect of change of environment. When placed in an emotionally warm, caring and stimulating environment these children grow very rapidly despite no change in nutritional intake. Moreover, they 'blossom'. The quiet, apathetic children assume a more

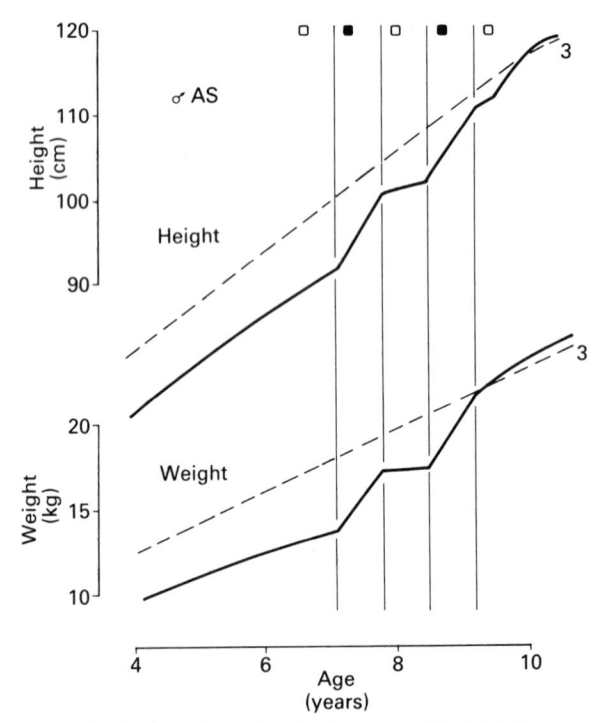

Figure 7.4 Growth of emotionally deprived child with failure to thrive (———) plotted against third centiles for height and weight (- - - -) during periods at home ☐ and foster care ■.

alert, responsive affect. The aggressive children usually become more co-operative. When placed back at home, unless there have been significant changes, growth may slow once more (*Figure 7.4*).

We assume that one of the effects of emotional insult in children with deprivation syndrome is that the higher centres of the brain act on areas such as the hypothalamus to interfere with the normal hormonal and neurological controls of appetite and growth. Growth studies of children at the time of removal from the adverse envrinment have demonstrated depressed growth hormone (Rayner and Rudd, 1973) and adrenocorticotrophic hormone responses to stimulation tests. After a few days of 'tender, loving care' these responses return to normal. Cerebral function may also affect catecholamine production. Stress may induce a state of semi-permanent anxiety and increased catecholamine secretion, thus increasing metabolism and causing failure to thrive despite high energy intakes. This has not been demonstrated convincingly. Catecholamines are not easily measured, and study of these children necessitates altering the environment responsible for their abnormalities – and thus altering the abnormal responses.

The management of emotional deprivation is not nutritional, but social and psychological, help for the family. Place of Safety Orders and Care Proceedings may be necessary in severe cases. However, it is important to provide a diet of high energy and good nutrient quality so as to optimize growth in a caring environment. This diminishes any developmental delay that may accompany poor nurturing and makes the child happier, rounder and potentially more 'cuddly'. If mother is having difficulty bonding with her child, she is more likely to bond with a cheerful, well-nourished, even rotund, infant than a whingey, skinny one.

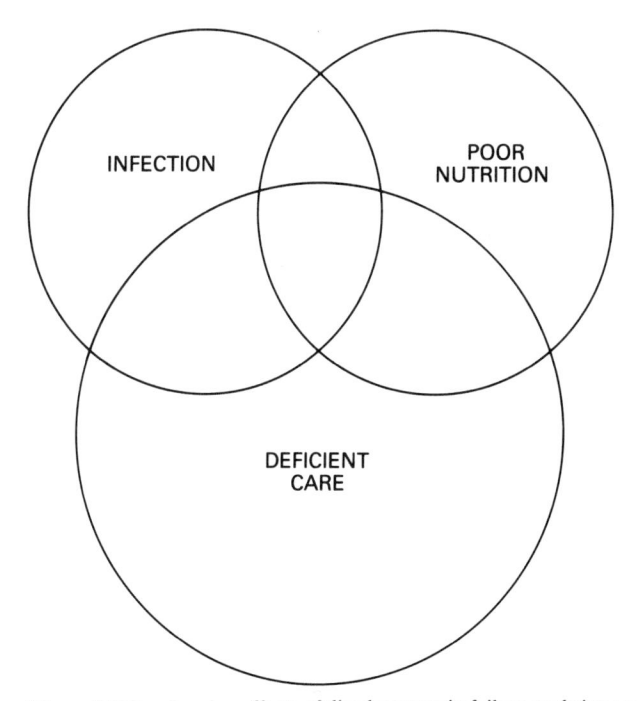

Figure 7.5 Overlapping effects of disadvantage in failure to thrive amongst children from poor environments.

94 Failure to thrive

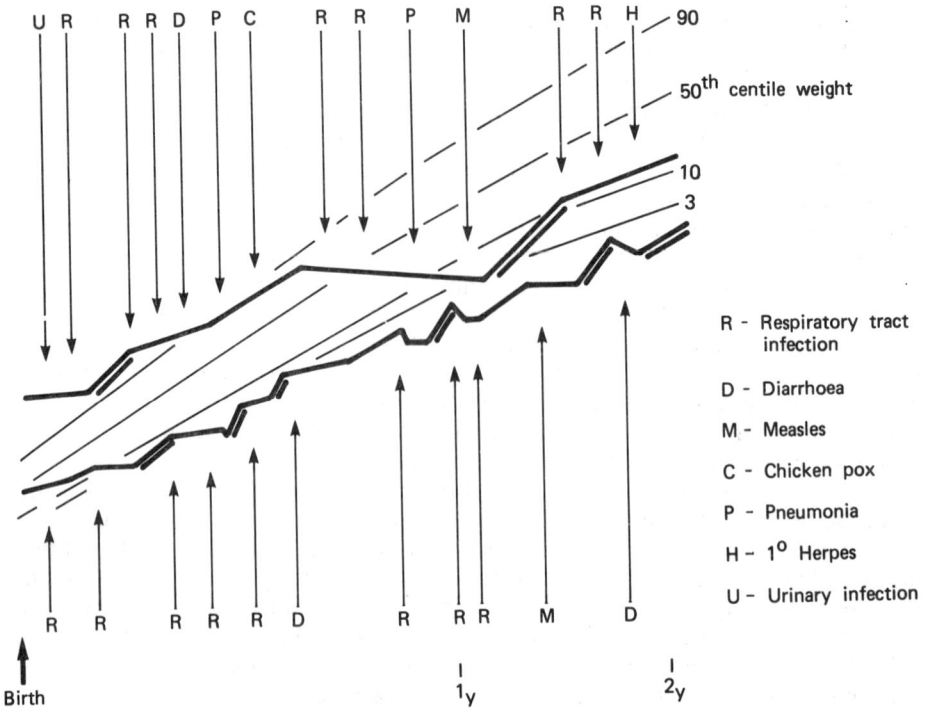

Figure 7.6 Weights of two British children in first 2 years of life showing failure to thrive secondary to repeated infection associated with deprived urban environments. Periods of catch-up growth indicated by double lines.

R - Respiratory tract infection
D - Diarrhoea
M - Measles
C - Chicken pox
P - Pneumonia
H - 1° Herpes
U - Urinary infection

It is often stated that the majority of children who have failure to thrive without obvious clinical cause have psychosocial deprivation. The majority of children with unexplained failure to thrive that we see come from poor environments, often with a background of family strife. Many of these families have poor standards of hygiene and live in overcrowded households. The prevalence of infection – chronic or repeated acute infection – in poor urban environments probably contributes as much to failure to thrive as the emotional deprivation (*Figure 7.5*). Certainly, short stature and underweight are much commoner in children from poor environments although their dietary intake may actually be more than that of children from better environments (Nelson and Paul, 1981; Donnet *et al.*, 1982). For whatever reason growth is affected – whether due to repeated infections (*Figure 7.6*), the nutritional environment, or the emotional environment – children in poor social environments appear to need more food to achieve the same growth as children from more affluent environments (Donnet *et al.*, 1982). This is yet another indication of how difficult it is to predict the nutritional needs of any individual!

References

BERESFORD, C. H., NEALE, R. J. and BROOKE, O. G. (1971) Iron absorption and pyrexia. *Lancet*, **i**, 568–572

BOUGLE, D., ISELIN, M., KAHYAT, A. and DUHAMEL, J-F. (1976) Nutritional treatment of congenital heart disease. *Archives of Disease in Childhood*, **61**, 799–801

CONGDON, P. J., FIDDLER, G. I., LITTLEWOOD, J. M. and SCOTT, O. (1982) Coeliac disease associated with congenital heart disease. *Archives of Disease in Childhood*, **57**, 78–79

DONNET, M. L., COLE, T. J., SCOTT, T. M. and STANFIELD, J. P. (1982) Diet, growth and health of infants in a disadvantaged inner city environment in Glasgow. In *Nutrition and Health*, edited by M. R. Turner, pp. 183–195. Lancaster: MTP Press

McCARTHY, D. (1974) Effects of emotional disturbance and deprivation (maternal rejection) on somatic growth. In *Scientific Foundations of Paediatrics*, edited by J. A. Davis and J. Dobbing, pp. 56–67. London: William Heinemann Medical Books

MATA, L. (1985) Global importance of diarrhoeal disease and malnutrition. In *Diarrhoeal Disease and Malnutrition*, edited by M. Gracey, pp. 1–14. Edinburgh: Churchill Livingstone

MENON, G. and POSKITT, E. M. E. (1985) Why does congenital heart disease cause failure to thrive? *Archives of Disease in Childhood*, **60**, 1134–1139

MOLLA, A., MOLLA, A. M., SARKER, S. A., KHATOON, M. and RAHAMAN, M. M. (1983) Effect of acute diarrhoea on absorption of macro nutrients during disease and after recovery. In *Diarrhoea and Malnutrition*, edited by L. C. Chen and M. S. Scrimshaw, pp. 143–154. New York: Plenum Publishing

MOLLA, A. M., MOLLA, A. and RAHAMAN, M. M. (1986) The impact of acute diarrhoea of different aetiologies on food intake in children. In *Diarrhoea and Malnutrition in Childhood*, edited by J. A. Walker-Smith and A. S. McNeish, pp. 14–18. London: Butterworths

NELSON, M. and PAUL, A. A. (1981) Socioeconomic influences of nutrient intake in children. In *Preventive Nutrition and Society*, edited by M. R. Turner, pp. 121–130. Lancaster: MTP Press

PITTMAN, J. G. and COHEN, P. (1964) The pathogenesis of cardiac cachexia. Part I. *New England Journal of Medicine*, **271**, 403–409

RAYNER, P. H. W. and RUDD, B. T. (1973) Emotional deprivation in three siblings associated with functional growth hormone deficiency. *Australian Paediatric Journal*, **9**, 79–84

SARKER, S. A., WAHED, M. A., RAHAMAN, M. M., ALAM, A. N., ISLAM, A. and JAHAN, F. (1986) Persistent protein losing enteropathy in post measles diarrhoea. *Archives of Disease in Childhood*, **61**, 739–743

SONDHEIMER, J. M. and HAMILTON, J. R. (1978) Intestinal function in infants with severe congenital heart disease. *Journal of Pediatrics*, **92**, 572–578

WIDDOWSON, E. M. (1951) Mental contentment and physical growth. *Lancet*, **i**, 1316–1318

Chapter 8
Protein-energy malnutrition

Protein-energy malnutrition (PEM) is the term most frequently used to embrace the severe forms of malnutrition seen in childhood – marasmus and kwashiorkor – and the nutritionally determined growth failure that precedes these clinical syndromes. There has been enormous research into these conditions. Much has been written about their definition, recognition and interrelation, but much remains to be understood.

Classification of PEM

It is easy to recognize gross abnormality in the severe forms of PEM. It is much more difficult to decide the boundary between mild malnutrition and normal light weight or short stature. Making distinctions between normality and malnutrition provides an area of great controversy and an opportunity for a variety of classifications, none of which is entirely satisfactory. An early classification is that of Gomez et al. (1956) (*Table 8.1*) which uses deficit in weight for age to define mild, moderate and severe PEM. The Wellcome Working Party (Anon, 1970)

Table 8.1 Gomez classification of PEM*

First-degree malnutrition:	10–24% below expected weight for age†
Second-degree malnutrition:	25–39% below expected weight for age
Third-degree malnutrition:	>39% below expected weight for age and/or oedema

* Gomez et al. (1956).
† Standards not specified.

provided a simple clinical classification of the severe forms of PEM (*Table 8.2*). Waterlow (1972) has suggested that two classifications are necessary: one to assess the prevalence of mild to severe malnutrition in a community; one, for example the Wellcome Working Party definition, to differentiate the severe forms of clinical malnutrition. Waterlow and Rutishauser (1974) stress the importance of height deficit as indication of the duration of the malnutrition and, perhaps, evidence of adaptation to the adverse environment.

In both the Gomez and the Wellcome Working Party classifications the child's age is needed to relate weight to expected weight for age. Age – accurate even to a

Table 8.2 Wellcome Trust Working Party classification of malnutrition*

	Oedema	
	Absent	Present
60–80% expected weight for age†	Underweight	Kwashiorkor
<60% expected weight for age	Marasmus	Marasmic kwashiorkor

* Anon, 1970.
† Standards used are those of Stuart and Stevenson (1964).

year – is often not known in areas where malnutrition abounds. Attempts to make age-independent classifications of malnutrition usually involve relating weight to height. WHO (1983) tables include centiles for weight by height. Below two standard deviations or less than the 10th centile weight by height should be regarded as abnormal. The normal range of values for such ratios is still influenced by age and neither this, nor the Gomez and Wellcome classifications, include height for age (Rao, 1985). A child may be normal weight for height but grossly underweight for age, if he or she is significantly stunted. There are many causes for short stature but the child who grows slowly in an adverse environment and retains normal weight for height may be showing adaptation to the adverse environment. A child with gross wasting or oedema has not adapted successfully. Any classification that looks only at weight and height can also be misleading in kwashiorkor-inducing situations since the presence of oedema artificially increases weight.

Another problem for anthropometrical assessment of malnutrition is deciding which 'normal standards' should be used. The Wellcome Trust Working Party (Anon, 1970) classification used Harvard standards or the 'Boston boys' (Stuart and Stevenson, 1964). The Gomez classification (Gomez et al., 1956) does not state particular standards. In the future it may be appropriate that all except very local anthropometric studies relate data to the common standard of the WHO standards (WHO, 1983). This will take no account of racial differences in growth. However, Habicht et al. (1974) have shown that differences in weight and height for preschool children of the same racial origin but of different social classes are greater than differences in weight and height of children of different racial origins but of the most affluent social groups. Relating weight and height of young children to international standards gives a better representation of absolute nutritional state for the child population under study.

Other methods of assessing nutritional status without the need for accurate age or great technological skill (hence, suitable for quickly trained field workers) utilize the relative constancy of mid upper arm circumference between the ages of 1 and 5 years, and the relative constancy of mid upper arm circumference to height over the same period.

Shakir tape

A special tape is used to measure the mid upper arm circumference (on the left side) midway between the acromion and the olecranon with the arm hanging loosely by the side. A measuring point and coloured zones are indicated on the tape. When the tape is wrapped around the arm, the measuring point overlaps one of the coloured zones towards the other end of the tape: green (>13.5 cm) indicates normal or acceptable nutrition; yellow (>12.5–13.5 cm) indicates borderline nutrition; red (<12.5 cm) indicates malnutrition. The tape is useful in screening programmes but does not distinguish between loss of fat and loss of muscle and – more importantly – may be misleading with children with severe kwashiorkor and oedematous upper arms. (Such children should be easily recognizable as unwell and abnormal, without resort to the tape.)

QUAC stick

This is another field tool which uses the relative constancy of the mid upper arm circumference:height ratio of young children to screen out malnourished individuals (Arnhold, 1969). The height-measuring stick is marked off in arm circumference measurements (80% and 85% of normal) against appropriate height measurements.

Whichever classification of malnutrition is used, assessment of the nutritional state of individual children suspected of PEM must include thorough physical examination. *Table 8.3* outlines the particular clinical signs of PEM and the distinguishing features of marasmus and kwashiorkor.

Table 8.3 Symptoms and signs of marasmus and kwashiorkor

	Marasmus	*Kwashiorkor*
Symptoms:		
Affect	Miserable but alert	Apathetic, drowsy
Appetite	Hungry	Anorexic
Activity	Diminished	Grossly diminished
Diarrhoea	++	+
Hypothermia	++	++
Associated infections	+	++
Signs:		
*Oedema	No	Yes
†Hair changes:		
Thinning	±	0–++
Depigmentation	±	0–++
*Painless pluckability	–	+–++
Loss of curl	±	0–++
†Skin changes:		
Patchy depigmentation	±	0–++
Cracking, ulceration	±	0–++
Angular stomatitis	±	+
Facial features	Wizened, obvious buccal fat pads	Puffy eyes, moon face, pallor
Hepatomegaly	–	0–+++
Anaemia	±	+–++
Weight deficit	+++	+
Height deficit	0–+++	±
Muscle wasting	+++	++
Fat loss	+++	0–++

* The distinguishing feature.
† Very variable and less likely in cases developing acutely.

The majority of undernourished children from regions where marasmus and/or kwashiorkor are prevalent cannot be classified as suffering from either marasmus or kwashiorkor (Frank, 1985). They show evidence of sub-optimal nutrition with poor growth in weight and often stunting, wasting, reduced activity, and susceptibility to infection. National statistics reflect the overall poor state of nutrition through high early childhood mortality from infections such as gastroenteritis, measles and respiratory tract infections, thus reflecting the predisposition of marginally malnourished children to succumb to infection (Puffer and Serrano, 1973).

Malnutrition and the resistance to infection

Many abnormalities of immunology have been described in association with malnutrition, both in children and in experimental animals. The susceptibility of malnourished children to severe infection has a complex multifactorial aetiology. *Table 8.4* indicates some of the many immunological abnormalities detected in children with PEM.

Table 8.4 Immunological changes associated with PEM*

Reduced resistance at mucosal barriers	Lungs, gastrointestinal tract	Increased permeability, reduced repair, reduced mucus and lysozyme secretion, low intragastric pH	May respond to vitamins A, C, niacin and zinc
Suppression of immunological system	Lymph glands, bone marrow, spleen, thymus	Atrophy lymphoid tissue, reduced humoral and cellular immune responses	
Specific effects on cell lines	Phagocytes	Reduced cell migration, reduced opsonizing capacity, reduced bacteriocidal activity	
	Lymphocytes	Reduced T-cell-mediated immunity, reduced numbers of T cells, increased non-T, non-B cells, diminished production of humoral mediators	Due to low zinc, iron, vitamins
Other factors		Reduced complement factors; complement cascade inhibitors present in serum in PEM; reduced antibody production to some antigens; low serum IgA	

* Farthing and Keusch, 1985.

The effects of infection in children from malnourishing environments exacerbate the effects of the poor nutrition since infection leads to anorexia, pyrexia with increased metabolic rate, toxicity affecting metabolic reactions and often tissue loss due to diarrhoea (Mata, Urrutia and Garcia, 1967; Poskitt, 1972; Rowland, Cole and Whitehead, 1977; Duggan, Alwar and Milner, 1986). Nutrition deteriorates in these children during infection and is insufficient in between episodes of infection to allow complete catch-up growth (*Figure 8.1*). Increased susceptibility to infection resulting from poor nutrition leads to further deterioration in nutritional status. This interaction between nutrition and infection is epitomized by the 'weanling's dilemma' (*see also* Chapter 6). Prolonged breast feeding without weaning solids by malnourished mothers may fail to provide for children's

100 Protein-energy malnutrition

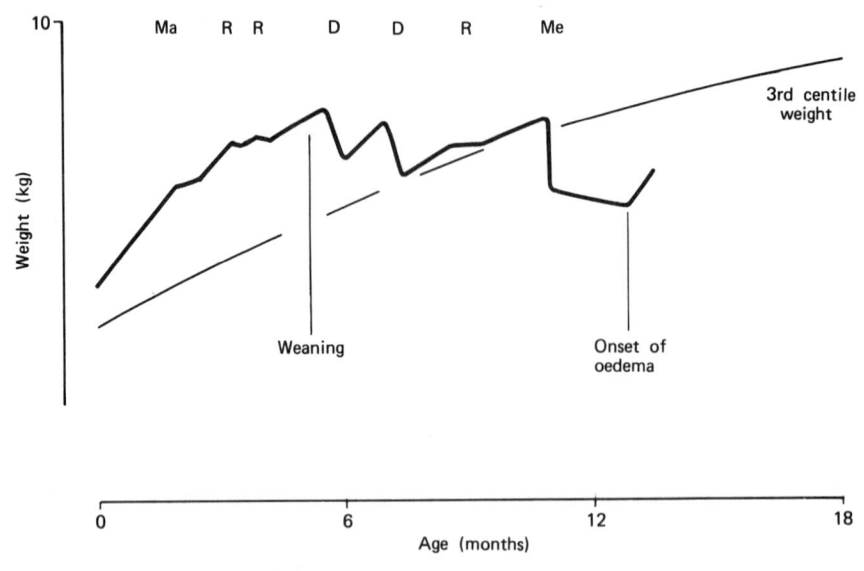

Figure 8.1 Weight faltering with infection progressing to kwashiorkor. Ma, malaria; R, respiratory tract infection; D, diarrhoea; Me, measles.

nutritional needs. By contrast, weaning introduces the child to a diet of low energy density, which is frequently deficient in specific nutrients and heavily contaminated with pathogenic organisms (*see Figure 6.1*).

All this occurs at an age when the children have lost passive immunity acquired from their mothers *in utero* and are beginning to move around more, put foreign bodies in their mouths, and contact respiratory and – particularly – gastrointestinal infections and infestations (Beisel, 1982). Reduction in the prevalence of infectious disease by improving water supplies, sanitation and by immunization (particularly against measles: Poskitt, 1971; Duggan, Alwar and Milner, 1986) should improve the nutritional status of populations of young children without change in the food supply. Nutritional supplementation might also reduce susceptibility to severe infection and thus avoid further deterioration in nutritional status with infection. In practice, however, it is usually easier to sink boreholes and latrines and to provide piped water to a community than to ensure that nutritional supplements reach the groups at risk. The former measures will also be effective for more than one generation of children. Too often the need for emergency feeding programmes diverts funds from more long-term community health measures.

We have discussed PEM in general terms. Let us now look at the specific disease entities.

Marasmus

Marasmus is severe undernutrition with weight less than 60% of that expected for age. In developed countries many children are described as clinically marasmic when they are severely wasted, even though their degree of underweight may not be as extreme as that defined above.

In developed countries where underweight is due to a wide variety of factors other than undernutrition, it is important to distinguish children whose predominant problem is primarily short stature with associated low weight, from those who are significantly underweight for their (low) height. The aetiology of the two conditions is distinct, and the former situation may have little to do with nutrition. In many developing countries, inadequate nutrition is so frequent that its prevalence overwhelms all other causes of underweight. Nevertheless, distinction between those who are short for age and underweight, and those who are normal stature for age but severely underweight, is important since those who are short are likely to have suffered more prolonged malnutrition or may conceivably have other causes for their poor growth. Failure to thrive, which only in its extreme form is marasmus, has been discussed in Chapter 7. Causes of primary short stature are discussed in most paediatric textbooks and will not be described further here.

Marasmus is the usual clinical presentation of severe childhood malnutrition during famine or as a result of starvation from – for example – breast feeding failure. It frequently follows prolonged or repeated gastroenteritis. Children are thin with loss of fat and muscle. Wasting is obvious and in young children the buccal fat pad may be apparent in an otherwise wizened face (*Figure 8.2*). Typically these children are miserable, but hungry and often feed well when food is offered. They

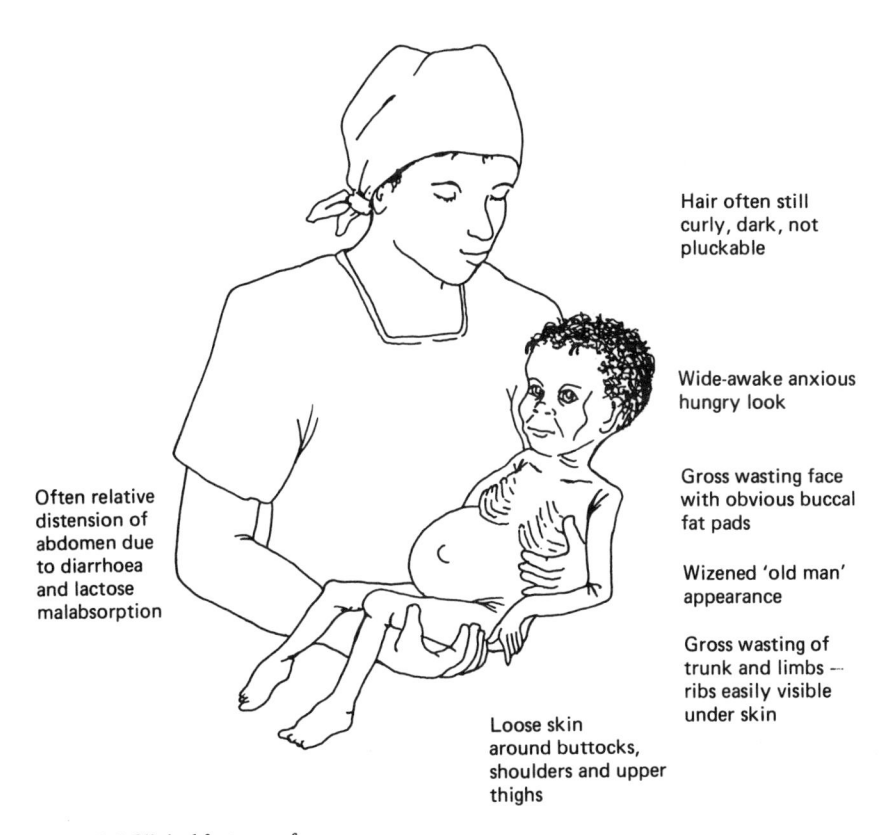

Figure 8.2 Clinical features of marasmus.

may have distended abdomens secondary to poor muscle tone, abdominal muscle wasting and/or disaccharide intolerance with excessive intestinal gas formation. They are commonly hypothermic and hypoglycaemic but haemoglobin (in the absence of parasitic infestations or severe iron deficiency) is within the normal range. Serum albumin and electrolytes are also usually normal although serum potassium may be low when there is severe diarrhoea. Total body potassium is depleted (Waterlow, Golden and Patrick, 1978). Hypothermia and hypoglycaemia are common, and even in hot climates these children may have difficulty maintaining normal body temperature particularly at night. Body temperature control may be achieved most easily by lying children under the same blankets as their mothers, next to their mothers' warm bodies – assuming that the mothers are themselves well and reasonably well nourished. Marasmic children should be screened for associated infections and vitamin deficiencies, both of which are very common complicating conditions.

Kwashiorkor

Kwashiorkor is oedematous malnutrition, but other features such as hair and skin changes and hepatomegaly due to fatty liver are characteristic (Williams, 1933) (*Table 8.3*, and *Figure 8.3*). The prevalence of features other than oedema and fatty

Sparse, straight, readily pluckable hair

Puffy eyes, mooned face

Apathy, misery, anorexia, anaemia

Wasting upper arms and upper trunk

Hepatomegaly

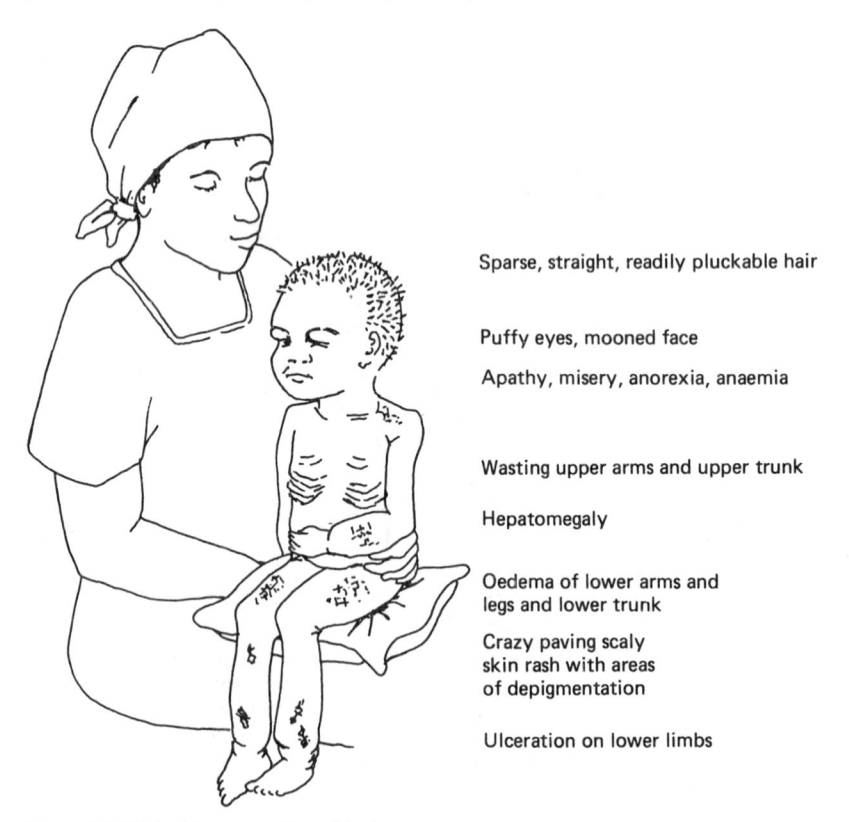

Oedema of lower arms and legs and lower trunk

Crazy paving scaly skin rash with areas of depigmentation

Ulceration on lower limbs

Figure 8.3 Clinical features of kwashiorkor.

liver vary with the area of origin of the children. In Uganda, for example, anaemia, cardiac failure and severe skin lesions are very common associations of kwashiorkor (Wharton, Howells and McCance, 1967). In the West Indies hypokalaemia and relative preservation of subcutaneous fat are more frequently seen. The age group affected by kwashiorkor also varies. Children in the West Indies tend to be younger than those in East Africa.

The derivation of the word kwashiorkor is from the Ga language of West Africa and refers to the 'supplanted one'. Typically, kwashiorkor children have recently been weaned, often because the mother finds she is pregnant. Since weaning may also include sending the child to live with grandmother, an element of emotional deprivation may contribute to the pathophysiology.

Kwashiorkor is associated with plasma protein levels below 25 g/l. The prevalence of oedema increases as albumin levels fall, but correlations between plasma albumin levels and the presence or severity of oedema are not close (Whitehead, Frood and Poskitt, 1971). Oedema often disappears at lower levels of serum albumin than those associated with gross oedema before treatment.

Why some children develop low serum protein values and oedematous malnutrition and others show only marasmus is not known. It is too simple (and incorrect) to explain the differences as due to less protein in the diets of children with kwashiorkor. It is difficult to demonstrate consistent differences in progress to severe PEM for the two conditions. Marasmus is extreme undernutrition usually precipitated by several conditions contributing to inadequate nutrient retention. Kwashiorkor is a more complex multifactorial condition with more severe metabolic and biochemical disturbance (*Table 8.5*). Jackson (1986) has discussed

Table 8.5 Biochemical blood abnormalities associated with kwashiorkor

Low haemoglobin

Low proteins:
    Low albumin
    High non-essential/essential amino acid ratio
    High alanine/valine ratio
    Low transferrin
    Low retinol binding protein
    Low thyroxine binding pre-albumin

Hormonal:
    Low thyroid hormone
    Low insulin
    Normal or high growth hormone
    Normal or high cortisol

Low glucose

Low cholesterol especially low density lipoprotein cholesterol

Low triglycerides

how marginal diets combined with noxious insults might lead to development of kwashiorkor rather than marasmus, possibly through the final common pathway of oxidant (free radical) damage to cells. Certainly it seems that severe PEM is the sad end point of a combination of adverse circumstances, no one of which appears to be a prime cause, but all of which may be aggravating factors (Golden, 1985) (*Figure 8.4*).

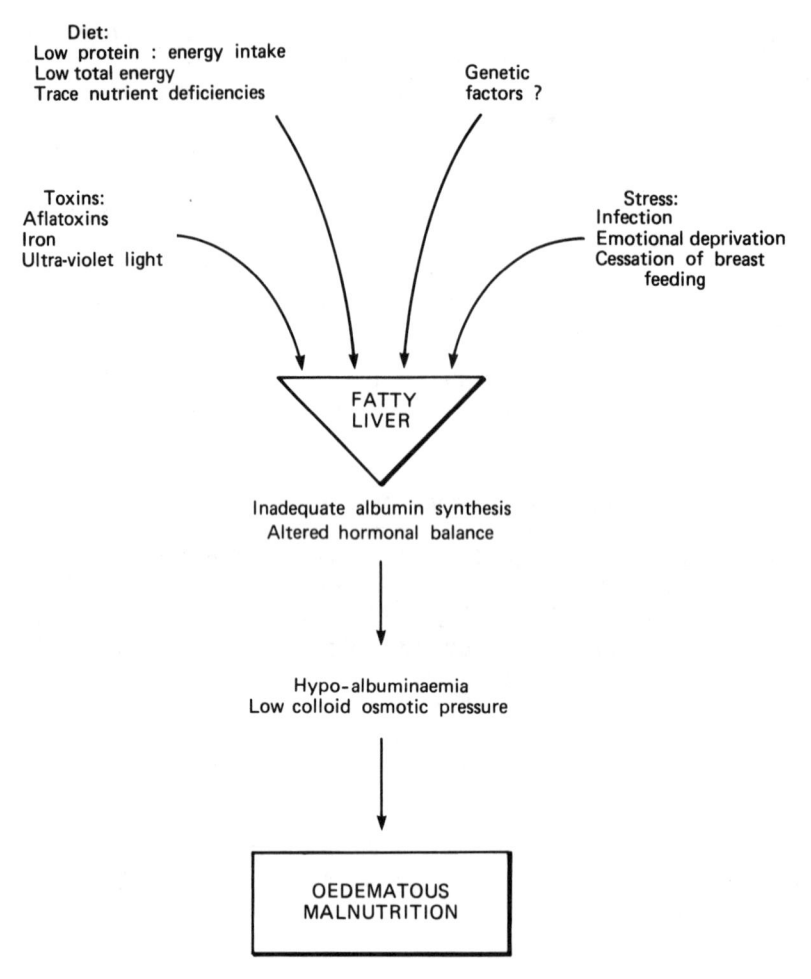

Figure 8.4 Diagrammatic representation of possible pathophysiological progress to kwashiorkor.

The progress to severe PEM may be much as follows:

1. The children are young and need high nutrient requirements for rapid growth.
2. The diet is staple of low energy density and poor quality protein, low in some essential amino acids. Recent weaning means the child is unaccustomed to the diet and takes with difficulty, reluctance or both.
3. The monotony of the diet leads to deficiencies of vitamins and minerals. Infrequent feeding encourages overall low nutrient intake.
4. The environment is unhygienic with prevalent bacterial and parasitic infections, particularly gastrointestinal pathogens.
5. The food and eating utensils are heavily contaminated with intestinal pathogens. The food itself is damaged by storage and contamination with fungi such as *Aspergillus*.
6. The child is of an age when immunity derived from mother *in utero* has been lost and natural immunity is only beginning to develop.

7. The child succumbs to repeated infection and appetite is diminished. The immune response is impaired by deteriorating nutritional state. Protein is lost in gastrointestinal infection and energy wasted as pyrexia.
8. Weight progress falters, trips or falls.
9. Specific nutrient deficiencies, food toxins or infections affect tissues already stressed metabolically by poor nutrition. Liver metabolism is affected, leading to development of fatty liver, reduced albumin synthesis, low serum albumin and altered hormonal balance.
10. Oedema develops as a result of some final insult on this clinical progression: infection; hormonal imbalance; toxins, especially aflatoxins (Hendrickse et al., 1982); specific nutrient deficiency; free radical damage, etc.

This progression may be halted or reversed at any stage by measures that improve general health and nutrition. Alternatively – and all too commonly – the progression is halted by overwhelming infection and death.

Management of severe PEM

Management depends largely on the severity of the illness and the facilities available for investigation and treatment. Unfortunately severe PEM is commonly found in areas where investigative and therapeutic facilities are very limited, and management may be dependent on feeding the children locally available foods prepared so as to provide optimum nutritional benefit. Where possible, three aspects of investigation should be considered in these children:

1. A search for infection.
2. Assessment of biochemical – especially electrolyte – abnormalities.
3. Assessment of anaemia, and cardiovascular state.

Treatment should be initiated even without definite results from investigations and should initially aim at treating infection and vitamin, electrolyte and water imbalance (*Table 8.6*).

Table 8.6 Management of severe PEM*

History and clinical examination
Assess hydration
Treat for infections, infestations and for malarial suppression
100 000 International Units water miscible vitamin A intramuscularly (under 1 year: half dose)
Repeat vitamin A dose orally on day 2
Where haemoglobin <3 g/dl slow, careful blood transfusion of packed cells
Folic acid 5 mg daily
Multivitamin drops or Ketovite (Paines & Byrne) liquid and tablets
Correct water, sodium, potassium and magnesium deficits orally if possible
When electrolyte–water imbalance corrected introduce ¼-strength formula (*see Table 8.7*)

* Adapted from Cameron and Hofvander, 1983.

The majority of children will have some, or all, of the following: malaria, measles, hookworm, ascariasis, gastroenteritis, pneumonia, septicaemia, skin sepsis, urinary tract infection. Screening for and treating infection is an essential part of the management of severe malnutrition. Where there are no facilities to do this, treatment of the parasitic infestations common in the locality in which the child lives, most notably helminthic and malarial infections, and immediate vigorous treatment with antibiotics when children appear toxic or pyrexial, are advisable.

Infection may not be obvious in poorly nourished children. Hypothermia, apathy, failure to respond to diet, low white blood cell count and falling haemoglobin levels are as suggestive of infection as the usual clinical features of pyrexia, toxicity and increased white blood cell count (Phillips and Wharton, 1968).

Antibiotic regimens are likely to be determined by the drugs available in the region. Bactericidal drugs should be used where possible. However, combinations of penicillin and chloramphenicol (watch dose carefully, particularly in young infants; preferably only one course) are cheap, usually available and effective against the *Pneumococci* and *Salmonellae* which so often overwhelm these children. Drugs should be used with caution in malnutrition since drug metabolism may be affected by poor nutrition (Poskitt, 1974).

Children with severe PEM have low total body potassium values although serum potassium level may be within normal limits. Total body water and total body sodium values are high (even in marasmus) although serum sodium level may be low. Total body magnesium level is low. Thus it is important to correct electrolyte imbalances which may not be apparent from routine biochemistry. It is advisable to concentrate on correcting hydration and biochemical deficits early in management and to introduce food only gradually.

Children may be dehydrated and hypovolaemic even though oedematous. Intravenous therapy is hazardous (although sometimes essential) in kwashiorkor children. Intravenous lines may be difficult to insert and it is easy to induce fluid overload and precipitate cardiac failure. Plasma, or normal saline, 20 ml/kg, may be helpful where there is circulatory failure secondary to hypovolaemia and dehydration. Where possible oral rehydration should be instituted (*see* Chapter 15). Frequent (one to two hourly) small feeds or even slow continuous nasogastric gavage feeding may be tolerated when less frequent larger volume feeds cause vomiting. Provided the child is passing urine, potassium 4–8 mmol/kg/day should be given routinely. Magnesium supplements (1–2 mmol/kg/day) are also advisable. Acute magnesium deficiency presents as irritability, convulsions, rigidity of the limbs or athetotic movements. Treatment of the acute reaction is with intramuscular 25% magnesium sulphate 0.5 ml/kg body weight (Waterlow, Golden and Patrick, 1978).

When the child is tolerating small amounts of oral fluid, food can be introduced in the form of diluted formula. Formula is gradually built up to full strength over 5–7 days or more slowly if the child is unable to tolerate full-strength milk.

Most units that treat PEM have developed their own therapeutic formulas which are more energy dense but have less protein than cows' milk (*Table 8.7*). Energy can be provided thus reducing the risks of hypoglycaemia (and accompanying hypothermia) without overloading the child with fluid or protein. The composition of these formulas depends on the local problems commonly associated with PEM and on locally available carbohydrate and oil sources. Most provide sugars other than lactose since lactose intolerance is common in these children (Dean, 1952).

The basic formula should be fed in sufficient quantities to provide 420 kJ/kg/day (100 kcal/kg/day). Since it is advisable to keep the volume of intake down to minimize vomiting and to avoid exacerbating heart failure and oedema, formulas are usually milk fortified with oil or carbohydrate source to an energy density of 420 kJ/100 ml (100 kcal/100 ml) or a combination of casein, or soy protein with

Table 8.7 Composition of formula for initial treatment of severe PEM*

	\multicolumn{3}{c}{*Type of 'milk' powder*}
	Whole milk	Dried skimmed milk	K-Mix 2†
'Milk' powder‡ (g)	150	75	100
Sugar (g)	50	50	0
Oil (g)	10	60	70
Water (ml)	to 1000	to 1000	to 1000

* Adapted from Cameron and Hofvander, 1983. Composition approximately 4.2 kJ (1 kcal)/ml.
† Distributed by UNICEF; calcium caseinate, dried skimmed milk, sucrose and vitamin A.
‡ Mix ingredients to a smooth paste with a little water and then gradually mix in remaining water.

added methionine, and energy sources. Provided feeds are tolerated orally or by intermittent or continuous nasogastric gavage, protein and energy strength can be gradually built up until children are receiving 3–4 g protein/kg/day and at least 500 kJ/kg/day (120 kcal/kg/day). Once children regain their appetites, energy intakes above 420 kJ/kg/day can be obtained through introduction of local staples. It is not unusual for children to consume over 850 kJ/kg/day (200 kcal/kg/day) during catch-up growth and recovery. An expected rate of weight gain is over 70 g/day.

Signs of deteriorating clinical state that indicate less intense re-feeding are:

1. Increasing drowsiness suggesting severe hypokalaemia, hepatic failure and protein intolerance, or infection.
2. Increasing weight (in oedematous children) suggesting either cardiac failure or grossly disturbed metabolism unable to tolerate the rate of re-feeding.
3. Profuse diarrhoea, secondary either to gastrointestinal infection and responsive to a short period of oral rehydration therapy (*see* Chapter 15) or to food intolerance, in which case a change of formula, usually to non-disaccharide version, is necessary.

Anaemia is common in kwashiorkor and usually resolves as nutritional state improves. Severe anaemia is not uncommon in both marasmus and kwashiorkor, often secondary to malaria or hookworm. Anaemia may precipitate cardiac failure, increased fluid retention and death (Wharton, Howells and McCance, 1967). Treatment with iron to overcome hookworm anaemia may reduce resistance to infection (*see below*). If possible, anaemia should be managed by treatment of the cause (antimalarials; antihelminthics). Where anaemia is severe and there is heart failure, very slow blood transfuion of packed red cells is indicated; but, in view of the ever-present danger of fluid overload, this procedure should not be undertaken lightly and the child should be closely observed for deteriorating cardiorespiratory status.

Complications of PEM that may develop during initiation of treatment are listed in *Table 8.8*.

Children with severe PEM are likely to be deprived of other nutrients than protein and energy. Vitamins should be given either as double the daily dose of standard vitamin preparations or as Ketovite liquid 5 ml daily and Ketovite tablets (one, three times daily) (Paines & Byrne) if available. Folic acid should be given as well as other vitamins in a dose of 5 mg daily. Folate deficiency is a common accompaniment of severe PEM since there is a metabolic block in the conversion of dihydrofolate to tetrahydrofolate which resolves with refeeding and which is – to some extent – overcome by high folate intakes. Trace minerals (Metabolic Mineral Mixture; Scientific Hospital Supplies) are advisable also.

Table 8.8 Complications of management of severe PEM

Hypothermia

Hypoglycaemia

Infection

Liver failure:
   Hypoglycaemia
   Hyperbilirubinaemia
   Increasing drowsiness

Cardiac failure:
   Breathlessness
   Increasing liver size
   Increasing weight and oedema

The role of iron therapy in the management of severe PEM is controversial. Many children present with severe anaemia as part of a clinical picture exacerbated by hookworm or other infestations. Plasma transferrin and iron binding capacity are low (Masawe and Rwabwogo-Atenyi, 1973). Plasma ferritin levels are often high indicating high iron stores. Unbound iron causes free radical damage, and it has been suggested that the features of kwashiorkor are a reflection of uncontrolled free radical damage due to the presence of – amongst other radicals – free iron. Certainly some children, and adults with malnutrition, deteriorate and develop overt infection in association with treatment following iron therapy (Murray *et al.*, 1975). This is particularly true when iron is provided parenterally. Either the presence of unbound iron in plasma encourages bacterial multiplication or iron causes free radical damage and prevents the normal antibacterial processes. It would seem advisable to avoid routine iron therapy early in the management of severe malnutrition. If anaemia requires urgent treatment, slow transfusion of packed red cells should be given. In the convalescent stage when the risks of acute infection in very sick children have diminished, iron therapy is advisable since requirements will be high for catch-up growth.

The first signs of response to treatment in malnutrition are usually increased interest and awareness in the child and some return of appetite in kwashiorkor when appetite is poor. In marasmus there is usually no weight loss. In kwashiorkor weight loss is often the first objective sign of improvement as oedema begins to resolve. Weight gain may not occur until 10 days or longer after initiation of treatment since the loss of oedema masks any increase in muscle or tissue mass. The child with kwashiorkor who has lost oedema but not regained significant weight often looks extremely thin (particularly in marasmic kwashiorkor) with little muscle mass and usually little subcutaneous fat. Once the children begin to show appetite, local staple should be added to the meals of formula to provide an extra source of energy. Minimum energy intake for a reasonable rate of catch-up growth and recovery is 630 kJ/kg/day (150 kcal/kg/day).

The outlook for children with the severe forms of PEM is variable and is influenced by the type of PEM; the area from which the children come; the facilities available to treat them; and other conditions affecting the children. Thus it is difficult to provide prognoses for the various forms of severe malnutrition. If the only problem is marasmus due to underfeeding (failure of breast feeding, for example) the outlook is good if food can be provided without undue delay. Children with kwashiorkor present more severe metabolic problems, and mortality rates are 10–25% for severe cases. Children with marasmic kwashiorkor generally fare worse than those with either marasmus or kwashiorkor alone since there are often associated problems. The precipitation of marasmus into kwashiorkor may represent the end point of nutritional stress where adaptation to stress has been extreme but has finally failed.

Nutrition Rehabilitation Units

It is not possible to treat all cases of childhood malnutrition with the special care and supervision suggested above. Such management must be reserved for centres where investigative and therapeutic facilities are available and for the more severe cases, since in many developing countries the numbers of affected children are too great for all children to be treated intensively when medical resources are severely limited. Moreover, there is little gain if children are cured only to go back to the environments that precipitated the malnutrition. They will be subjected to the same unsatisfactory dietary practices and poor domestic hygiene and may present again with PEM or die of overwhelming infection. The management of severe PEM should therefore be accompanied by education for the families of children with PEM so that they can care for their children more appropriately once the recovered children return home.

In Nutrition Rehabilitation Units (NRU) the policy is to feed moderately to severely malnourished children selected local food mixes in such proportions and quantities that they recover from malnutrition without recourse to more expensive or more refined therapeutic diets. It may be necessary initially to supplement local foods with formula milks or with dried milk powder to initiate recovery, and it may also be necessary to tube-feed children initially with fortified milk formulas. Such measures should be regarded as having negative educative effects and should be introduced only when they are clearly necessary.

In NRUs, nutrition education for the mothers is combined with instruction in dealing with simple illnesses such as fever, malaria and gastroenteritis; hygiene; contraception; literacy; simple agricultural techniques; simple income generating activities and budgeting. What is taught in these Units must be derived from the known or perceived problems, needs and sophistication of the local women. Unfortunately such Units have limited use in the arid areas or in urban slums where lack of water or lack of land and lack of money make it impossible for mothers to grow or buy sufficient food for their children, irrespective of how skilled their agriculture or budgeting. Under such circumstances, efforts may be better directed at mobilizing the political will to finance the construction of boreholes and irrigation systems, or to support minimum wage levels that enable the lowest paid – whether men or women – to buy adequate food for their families.

Prevention of severe PEM

The prevention of malnutrition is more likely to be achieved through political and economic solutions than through medical or nutritional ones. NRUs can be used as a forum for educating the public through teaching attendees to teach others and through inviting visitors to observe the work of the NRU or take part in the instruction. They must educate local people in better nutrition, hygiene and health care and better use of scarce resources. Critical to the prevention of PEM is the management of weaning (Rowland, Goh Rowland and Dunn, 1986).

Weaning education

In many areas severe malnutrition develops in young children despite available food. It develops from inappropriate weaning practices exacerbated by prevalent infections (Rowland, 1986). Mothers attending NRUs, and mothers and potential mothers at home, should be educated to use the local foods to make weaning diets more suitable in order to reduce malnutrition. The principles of weaning infants satisfactorily on to traditional low-energy dense monotonous diets have been discussed in Chapter 6. Children are frequently fed weaning diet only once or twice a day, and they may be expected to feed themselves with their hands – in many cultures with right hand only. Infants of 1–2 years may have considerable difficulty mopping up protein-containing sauces and stews with the staple by hand. Often they are fed late at night when they may be too tired or hungry to make the effort to feed. Thus food must be specially prepared or presented for weanlings and they must be helped to eat. When fed with spoons, the juices which may have higher nutrient quality than the staple, are not lost. Weanlings should be fed at least four times a day.

Table 8.9 outlines the food grouping method of designing food mixes which are suitable as weanling diets and constructed from likely local foods. Further examples

Table 8.9 Food grouping method of designing multi-mix weaning meals*

	Food group†		
Staple‡	*Protein source*	*Vitamin source*	*Additional energy source§*
Plantain (banana)	Ground-nuts	Dark green leafy vegetables	Local plant oils: ground-nut, red palm
Grains: rice, maize, millet, etc.	Legumes	Coloured vegetables: tomatoes, peppers, pumpkin, carrots	
	Fish	Fruits, especially citrus	Sesame seeds
Sweet potato	Meat	Red palm oil	Butter, margarine, ghee
Potato	Eggs		
	Dried skimmed milk		Sugar

* *See* Cameron and Hofvander (1983) for much greater detail.
† Plan meals to include foods from all groups at each meal. Staple forms greatest bulk of meal. Varying groupings and varying staple improves overall quality of diets (*see* Chapter 11).
‡ Parboiling and fermentation of grains may improve digestibility and nutrient quality (Rowland, 1986).
§ If more than 25% total energy from oils, food may become unpleasantly greasy.

are given in Cameron and Hofvander (1983). These mixes may be prepared separately; concocted after the various foods have been cooked; or cooked in a small tin put inside the main cooking pot. Which of these procedures is followed will depend on local customs. Little is usually achieved by turning traditional cooking methods upside down!

Recent tragedies in the Horn of Africa and the Sahel and other areas have shown what can be achieved by emergency feeding of populations. It would be churlish in the extreme to decry and diminish the magnificent human response in terms of aid that has greeted recognition of these disasters. Nevertheless, the emergency procedures met by this response have limited value as long-term solutions to the problems of famine since they tend to encourage dependency on outside aid, disrupt normal agricultural processes and worsen already low production and maldistribution of food. However, by grouping malnourished people together, education for survival is facilitated through, for example, setting up smallholdings within the confines of the emergency feeding centres and using these as demonstration areas. Sadly, it is often difficult for malnourished, displaced, demoralized and despondent adults to translate what they learn in demonstration centres to their own circumstances at home.

The long-term effects of PEM

There has been much argument over the effects of PEM in early childhood on late growth and intellectual development. This is a politically sensitive subject for understandable reasons. The difficulty in elucidating the long-term effects of PEM is the difficulty of isolating the effects of PEM from those of the PEM-inducing environment. Growth and development and intellectual achievement are – on average – less in children from deprived home environments even without severe PEM. Children from good environments who may have brief periods of severe undernutrition (such as infants with pyloric stenosis) do not usually show long-term sequelae in growth retardation or intellectual achievement. On the other hand, children who have had prolonged poor nutrition in early life are often, but not invariably, shorter than average as adults and may show poorer skills in general reasoning and spatial perceptual abilities with short-term memory and learning ability less affected. However, these differences are rarely marked (Alleyne et al., 1977).

The explanation for intellectual restriction as a result of PEM may relate more to the period of prolonged poor nutrition that preceded the presentation as marasmus or kwashiorkor rather than the effects of the severe episode. Learning and intellectual achievements are related to environmental stimulation and experience and to individual curiosity or 'drive'. Undernourished children are less active than adequately nourished children. They explore – and therefore learn from – their environment less than healthy children. Their misery and apathy may reduce parent–child interaction (Cravioto, DeLicardie and Birch, 1966; Grantham-McGregor, 1986).

It is clearly important from the above that recovery in PEM should not only supply extra nutrition for catch-up growth, but extra environmental stimulation for catch-up learning. Thus rehabilitation of the family and the environment as well as the child are important to complete recovery.

References

ANON (1970) Classification of infantile malnutrition. *Lancet*, **ii**, 302–303

ALLEYNE, G. A. O., HAY, R. W., PICOU, D. I., STANFIELD, J. P. and WHITEHEAD, R. G. (1977) *Protein–Energy Malnutrition*, pp. 122–132. London: Edward Arnold

ARNHOLD, R. (1969) The arm circumference as a public health index of protein-calorie malnutrition of early childhood. The Quac stick: a field measure used by the Quaker service team in Nigeria. *Journal of Tropical Pediatrics*, **15**, 243–247

BEISEL, W. R. (1982) Synergism and antagonism of parasitic diseases and malnutrition. *Reviews in Infectious Diseases*, **4**, 746–750

CAMERON, M. and HOFVANDER, Y. (1983) *Manual on Feeding Infants and Young Children*, pp. 19–32. Oxford: Oxford University Press

CRAVIOTO, J., DeLICARDIE, E. R. and BIRCH, H. G. (1966) Nutrition, growth and neurointegrative development: an experimental and ecologic study. *Pediatrics*, **38**, 319–372

DEAN, R. F. A. (1952) The treatment of kwashiorkor with milk and vegetable protein. *British Medical Journal*, **ii**, 792–796

DUGGAN, M. B., ALWAR, J. and MILNER, R. D. G. (1986) The nutritional cost of measles in Africa. *Archives of Disease in Childhood*, **61**, 61–66

FARTHING, M. J. G. and KEUSCH, G. I. (1986) Infection and Nutrition. In *Pediatric Nutrition*, edited by G. C. Arneil and J. Metcoff, pp. 194–218. London: Butterworths

FRANK, S. (1985) Protein-energy malnutrition. In *Pediatric Nutrition*, edited by G. C. Arneil and J. Metcoff, pp. 153–193. London: Butterworths

GOLDEN, M. H. M. (1985) The consequences of protein deficiency in man and its relationship to the features of kwashiorkor. In *Nutrition and Adaptation in Man*, edited by K. Blaxter and J. C. Waterlow, pp. 169–187. London: John Libbey

GOMEZ, F., GALVAN, R. R., FRENK, S., MUNOZ, J. C., CHAVEZ, R. and VASQUEZ, J. (1956) Mortality in second and third degree malnutrition. *Journal of Tropical Pediatrics*, **2**, 77–83

GRANTHAM-McGREGOR, S. (1986) The effect of malnutrition on mental development. In *Proceedings of XIII International Congress of Nutrition*, 1985, edited by T. G. Taylor and M. K. Jenkins, pp. 68–74. London: John Libbey

HABICHT, J. P., MARTORELL, R., YARBOROUGH, C., MALINA, R. M. and KLEIN, R. E. (1974) Height and weight standards for preschool children. *Lancet*, **i**, 611–615

HENDRICKSE, R. G., COULTER, J. B. S., LAMPLUGH, S. M. *et al.* (1982) Aflatoxins and kwashiorkor: a study of Sudanese children. *British Medical Journal*, **284**, 843–846

JACKSON, A. A. (1986) Severe undernutrition in Jamaica. *Acta Paediatrica Scandinavica*, Suppl. **323**, 43–51

MASAWE, A. E. J. and RWABWOGO-ATENYI, J. (1973) Serum protein and transferrin determinations to distinguish kwashiorkor from iron deficiency anaemia. *Archives of Disease in Childhood*, **48**, 927–931

MATA, L. J., URRUTIA, J. J. and GARCIA, B. (1967) Effect of infection and diet on child growth: experience in a Guatemalan village. In *Nutrition and Infection*, edited by G. E. W. Wolstenhome and M. O'Connor. Ciba Foundation Study Group, No. 31, pp. 112–134. London: Churchill

MURRAY, M. J., MURRAY, N. J., MURRAY, A. B. and MURRAY, M. B. (1975) Refeeding – malaria and hyperferraemia. *Lancet*, **i**, 653–654

PHILLIPS, I. and WHARTON, B. A. (1968) Acute bacterial infection in kwashiorkor and marasmus. *British Medical Journal*, **i**, 407–409

POSKITT, E. M. E. (1971) Measles in Ugandan village children. *Lancet*, **ii**, 68–70

POSKITT, E. M. E. (1972) Seasonal variation in infection and malnutrition in a rural clinic in Uganda. *Transactions of the Royal Society of Tropical Medicine and Hygiene*, **66**, 931–933

POSKITT, E. M. E. (1974) Clinical problems related to the use of drugs in malnutrition. *Proceedings of the Nutrition Society*, **33**, 203–207

PUFFER, R. R. and SERRANO, C. V. (1973) *Patterns of Mortality in Childhood*, Scientific Publication No. 262. Pan American Health Organisation. Washington: World Health Organisation

RAO, B. S. N. (1985) Metabolic adaptation to chronic malnutrition. In *Substrate and Energy Metabolism in Man*, edited by J. S. Garrow and D. Halliday, pp. 145–154. London: John Libbey

ROWLAND, M. G. M. (1986) The weanling's dilemma: are we making progress? *Acta Paediatrica Scandinavica,* Suppl. **323,** 33–42

ROWLAND, M. G. M., COLE, T. J. and WHITEHEAD, R. G. (1977) A quantitative study into the role of infection in determining nutritional status in Gambian village children. *British Journal of Nutrition,* **37,** 441–450

ROWLAND, M. G. M., GOH ROWLAND, S. G. J. and DUNN, D. T. (1986) The relationship between weaning practices and patterns of morbidity from diarrhoea: an urban Gambian case study. In *Diarrhoea and Malnutrition in Childhood,* edited by J. A. Walker-Smith and A. S. McNeish, pp. 7–13. London: Butterworths

STUART, H. and STEVENSON, S. S. (1964) Physical growth and development. In *Textbook of Pediatrics,* 7th edn., edited by W. E. Nelson, pp. 12–61. Philadelphia: W. B. Saunders

WATERLOW, J. C. (1972) Classification and definition of protein-calorie malnutrition. *British Medical Journal,* **iii,** 566–571

WATERLOW, J. C., GOLDEN, M. H. N. and PATRICK, J. (1978) Protein-energy malnutrition: treatment. In *Nutrition in the Management of Clinical Disease,* edited by J. W. T. Dickerson and H. A. Lee, pp. 49–71. London: Edward Arnold

WATERLOW, J. C. and RUTISHAUSER, I. H. E. (1974) Malnutrition in Man. In *Early Malnutrition and Mental Development,* edited by J. Cravioto, L. Hambraeus and B. Vahlquist, pp. 13–26. Stockholm: Almquist and Wiksell

WHARTON, B. A., HOWELLS, G. R. and McCANCE, R. A. (1967) Cardiac failure in kwashiorkor. *Lancet,* **ii,** 384–387

WHITEHEAD, R. G., FROOD, J. F. L. and POSKITT, E. M. E. (1971) Value of serum-albumin measurements in nutritional surveys: a reappraisal. *Lancet,* **ii,** 287–289

WILLIAMS, C. D. (1933) A nutritional disease of childhood associated with a maize diet. *Archives of Disease in Childhood,* **8,** 423–433

WORLD HEALTH ORGANISATION (1983) *Measuring Change in Nutritional Status.* Geneva: World Health Organisation

Chapter 9
Mineral deficiencies

With the exception of iron, clinical deficiencies of minerals and trace elements are rare in childhood. How frequently subclinical deficiencies occur is unknown (Söderhjelm, 1985) but certain situations predispose to deficiency of one or more minerals (*Table 9.1*). Causes of deficiency can be divided into those due to inadequate intake, inadequate absorption, increased requirements, failure to utilize, and increased losses, although there is considerable overlap of causes in any such classification.

Table 9.1 Conditions predisposing to mineral deficiencies

Domicile:	Local foods may be deficient in some minerals, particularly in mountainous areas (iodine, selenium)
Diet:	Prolonged breast feeding with no weaning. Monotonous diets, e.g. diet consisting of local staple only. Strict vegans. Prolonged total parenteral nutrition
Inborn errors of metabolism affecting absorption and metabolism:	Acrodermatitis enteropathica
Increased requirements:	Recovery from malnutrition, low birth weight, any cause of catch-up growth, recovery from trauma
Increased losses:	Chronic diarrhoea, exfoliative dermatitis, burns, increased urinary excretion

Iron

The prime need for iron is for haemoglobin synthesis, but iron is also required for synthesis of other proteins and enzymes. Deficiency causes many non-specific symptoms as well as those of anaemia.

Iron is widespread in foods, but the largest concentrations are in red meats, especially liver, and dark green leafy vegetables. Iron absorption from green vegetables is enhanced when vegetables are consumed with meat sources. By contrast, high phytate intakes, usually from consumption of unrefined flour, bind iron in the gut and high milk intakes may also inhibit absorption. Many young children eat meat and vegetables rarely, but have high milk and flour consumption. Their iron absorption may be poor even when their intake is quantitatively just adequate. The presence of reducing agents such as ascorbic acid in the diet facilitates absorption by converting available iron from ferric to ferrous forms.

Dietary iron intake in Western diets is usually about 89–107 mmol (5–6 mg)/ 4.2 MJ (1000 kcal) food energy per day. The margin between requirements and availability of iron is always small in childhood since iron requirements for growth are high. *Table 9.2* shows estimated stores and requirements for iron in childhood.

Table 9.2 Iron stores and requirements in childhood*

Age	Total body iron		Requirements		
	mg/kg body weight†	mg/total body	*For growth* (mg/day)	*Losses* (mg/day)	*RDA* (mg/kg)
28 weeks	74	80	0.3	0.2	2.0
Birth	75	250	0.3	0.2	1.5
6 months	37	290	0.5	0.4	0.9
1 year	38	390	0.3	0.5	0.8
2 years	39	490	0.2	0.6	0.8
8 years	39	990	0.2	0.6	0.8

* Smith and Rios, 1974; Widdowson, 1974; Wharton, 1987.
† Variation largely due to differences in fat:lean tissue.

The percentage of iron absorbed varies with the form of iron in the diet and with individual iron stores. Less than 10% of dietary iron may be absorbed but in iron deficiency and when iron is from haem or breast milk, absorption may be as high as 50%. Iron is absorbed chiefly as ferrous ions, but haem from meats may be absorbed intact. Absorption takes place in the duodenum and upper jejunum. Iron is lost from the body as gastrointestinal epithelial cells are shed. Only small quantities, amounting to 0.2–0.25 µmol (0.012–0.013 mg)/kg body weight/day are lost in urine or sweat (Smith and Rios, 1974; Lentner, 1981; Stekel, 1984).

Once in the body, iron is transported in the blood bound to transferrin. Transferrin levels vary, being low when there is infection or other chronic toxic condition but high in iron deficiency when percentage transferrin saturation is low. Transferrin levels are relatively low in neonates, particularly the preterm, but rise gradually over the first year of life to levels of 45–72 µmol/l (2.5–4.0 g/l). Transferrin saturation is relatively high (mean 65%) around 3 weeks of age owing to breakdown of red cells since birth but (at that age) low levels of haematopoiesis. Saturation falls again reaching about 36% at 6 weeks (Halliday, Lappin and McClure, 1984) and stays low in childhood.

Ferritin is present in blood in very small amounts but its presence directly parallels the extent to which iron is stored in the tissues, particularly in bone marrow. Levels are high in neonates but fall rapidly during early infancy and remain low throughout infancy and early childhood. Values below 10 µg/l at any age indicate depletion of iron stores.

Table 9.3 lists the clinical and haematological features of iron deficiency. The misery, apathy and pica of iron deficiency contribute to further inadequate iron intake and general malnutrition by inducing poor, often faddy, appetites. Pica may also lead to parasitic infestation, especially Ascariasis in areas where this is common, due to ingestion of infested earth. Gastrointestinal infestation may

Mineral deficiencies

Table 9.3 Clinical and haematological features of iron deficiency

Symptoms:	Misery, lethargy, apathy, bad temper, anorexia, pica, breathlessness, increased infections
Signs:	Pallor, especially nail beds, mucous membranes and palmar creases. Smooth tongue, flattened brittle nails, hyperdynamic circulation with bounding pulses and tachycardia, forceful apex beat, left ventricular failure
Haematological signs*:	Low haemoglobin: <10.5 g/dl Low mean corpuscular volume: <70 fl† Low mean corpuscular haemoglobin concentration <32% Blood film shows hypochromic, microcytic picture Serum iron <10 µmol/l (50 µg/dl) Transferrin saturation <10% Serum ferritin <10 µg/l

* Results should be compared with normal range for laboratory used.
† MCV varies through childhood and is high in early infancy, but direction of variations seems controversial (Stekel, 1984; Lentner, 1981).

Table 9.4 Clinical causes of iron deficiency and iron-deficiency anaemia in childhood

Inadequate intake:	Low dietary iron:
	   Faddy eater
	   Vegetarian diet
	   Cows' milk feeding in infancy
	   Anorexia
	   Persistent vomiting

Malabsorption:	Coeliac disease, high-phytate diet, hyperpyrexia, heavy infestation with Ascariasis
Failure to utilize (anaemias due to failure to incorporate iron into red cells rather than total body iron deficiency):	Chronic inflammation, infection, juvenile rheumatoid arthritis, pyridoxine deficiency, copper deficiency, other 'sideroblastic' anaemias
Increased requirements:	Prematurity, catch-up growth, pregnancy

Increased loss:	Blood loss:
	   Hookworm infestation
	   Oesophagitis
	   Meckel's diverticulum
	   Bleeding disorders
	   Exfoliative conditions

exacerbate dietary iron deficiency, through mucosal damage and reduced iron absorption. *Table 9.4* indicates some of the clinical causes of iron deficiency and iron deficiency anaemia.

Iron deficiency is common amongst children both in developed and in developing countries. In Britain iron deficiency is particularly common amongst toddlers from poor urban homes. Asian children are at great risk, possibly because of their poor environment but probably also because of the high-phytate, low-iron content of many of their traditional foods. In a recent survey of Asian children aged 22 months in Birmingham, UK (Grindulis *et al.*, 1986), over half (excluding children who had haemoglobinopathies and pathological cause for secondary iron deficiency) the group had haematological evidence of iron deficiency, and one-fifth had haemoglobin values less than 10 g/dl.

Diagnosis of iron deficiency is usually made by finding anaemia. The interpretation of haemoglobin levels in childhood is difficult since normal values vary with age and are different from those of adults. Haemoglobin levels at birth are high (18–20 g/dl) secondary to low intrauterine oxygen tension. Levels fall quite rapidly in the first months of life owing to relative bone marrow quiescence secondary to higher oxygen tensions of extrauterine life and to slightly shorter life span of neonatal red blood cells (70 days in term infants, 40 days in significantly premature infants). Thus in the term infant of about 1 month, reticulocyte counts are low (<1%) and haemoglobin has fallen to levels of 13–14 g/dl. By 2 months, in term infants, haemoglobin levels have often fallen to levels around 11 g/dl and are likely to remain in this region even if the infants are vigorously supplemented with iron. Rates of growth demand rapid red-cell production to maintain haemoglobin levels, and it is not usually until 6 or 7 years that haemoglobin levels begin to rise closer to adult values of 14 g/dl. Iron deficiency should be considered in those young children whose haemoglobin levels are below 10.5 g/dl or whose red-cell morphology strongly suggests iron deficiency (*Table 9.3*). A blood film usually shows a microcytic hypochromic anaemia with low serum ferritin, serum iron and transferrin saturation. Serum total iron binding capacity is normal or high.

Iron stores show a natural variation with age in childhood. As haemoglobin falls and the bone marrow shows little response in the first month of life, iron stores increase and iron deficiency is most unlikely (*Figure 9.1*). Once birth weight has

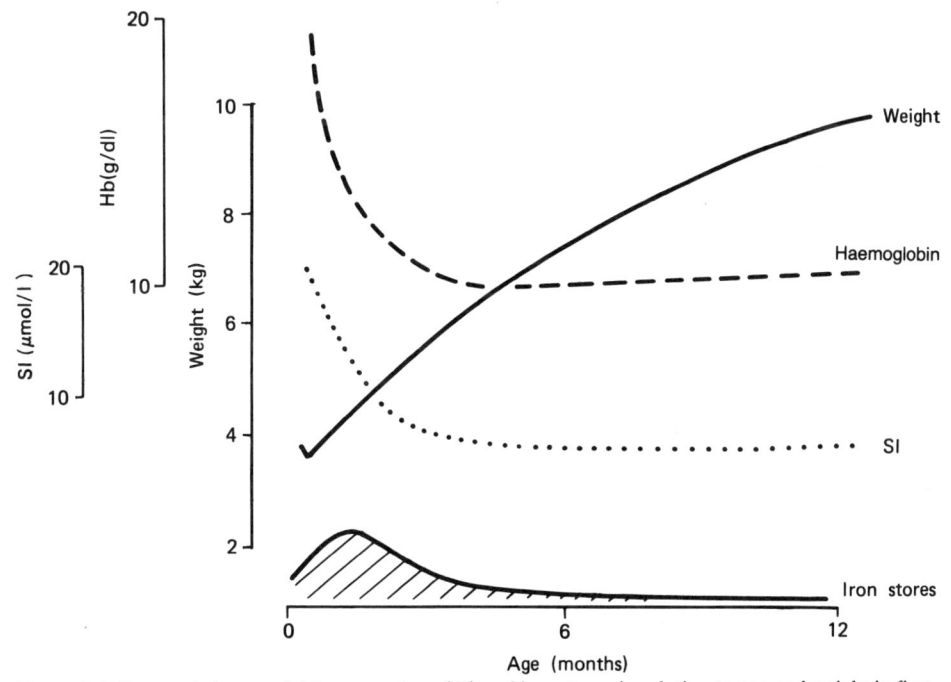

Figure 9.1 Changes in haemoglobin, serum iron (SI) and iron stores in relation to age and weight in first year of life. Haemoglobin drops and iron stores increase with bone marrow inactivity secondary to increased oxygen tension in tissues compared with fetus. Growth rapidly uses stores and haemoglobin synthesized by marrow does not keep pace with growth so haemoglobin levels stay low. Needs of growth keeps iron stores low throughout early childhood.

doubled and the blood compartment therefore also doubled, iron present at birth in the high neonatal haemoglobin and body stores will have been utilized in erythropoiesis, and the ability to maintain adequate iron nutrition thereafter is dependent on the ability to meet requirements through the diet. For practical purposes, iron stores can be regarded as minimal throughout early childhood. This can make it difficult to decide whether or not a child with low serum iron but acceptable haemoglobin level needs iron therapy.

Subtle evidence of iron deficiency is usually present before significant anaemia develops since iron is involved in enzymatic reactions in many cells. Iron-deficient children are often irritable or apathetic and anorexic. Many studies have tried to determine the relationship between iron nutritional status and intellectual activity, behaviour and learning. Some purport to show reduced attention span and learning abilities in iron-deficient children. However, the extent to which these findings can be attributed to iron deficiency are hampered by the association between socioeconomic status and iron deficiency. Primary behavoural disturbances may also directly affect the child's feeding behaviour and reduce the likelihood of the disturbed child consuming a diet adequate in iron. Most parents report considerable improvement in appetite, behaviour and well-being of their children after onset of iron therapy. These changes may be apparent before there has been significant change in haemoglobin level. Pollitt and Leibel (1976), in a review of the subject, stated that, 'it is unclear whether the poor performance, perceptual disturbance and conduct problems observed in anaemic subjects were consequences of anaemia, *per se*, of iron deficiency alone, or of a general nutritional inadequacy'. A more recent review suggests that if social-language tests are used (in older infants) greater differences between iron-deficient and non-iron-deficient children may be demonstrable. Iron repletion therapy tends to improve mental development scores in iron-deficient (both anaemic and non-anaemic) children. Children with iron deficiency appear less likely to pay attention to relevant cues in problem solving situations (Pollitt *et al.*, 1986).

In areas of overall poor nutrition, iron-deficient children are likely to be smaller and lighter than those without iron deficiency. However, these small, light iron-deficient children are less likely than better nourished iron-deficient children to show improvement with iron repletion. Selective deficits in attention and higher order cognitive functions are highly likely in this small and underweight iron-deficient group (Pollitt *et al.*, 1986). Clearly the relation of iron deficiency and behaviour is not one which can be separated easily or satisfactorily from the psychosocial and other nutritional aspects of nurture.

In a recent study from Britain, children aged 17–19 months in Birmingham, with haemoglobin in the ranges 8–11 g/dl, were assessed anthropometrically and developmentally using the Denver developmental scoring test (Aukett *et al.*, 1986). Children treated with iron showed slightly greater increase in weight over 2 months than those not treated with iron. However, they showed no significant differences in overall psychomotor development over the 2 months of study when compared with children who received no iron supplement. A significant number of children from the iron-deficient group who showed an increase in haemoglobin values of over 2 g/dl did, however, achieve average development over the period of study when compared with the groups who either had no iron or who did not show this rise in haemoglobin. Thus it would seem that treatment with iron can improve weight gain velocity in this age group but the evidence that iron repletion improves developmental progress in iron-deficient children is slight. This study only followed up children for a short period. Continued observation and a longer period of treatment might have shown more conclusive results.

The role of iron deficiency, *per se*, in causing or encouraging the delayed physical and intellectual development prevalent amongst children in deprived environments is questionable. There is nevertheless a suggestion from many of these studies that iron deficiency may at least have a role in the delayed growth and development of deprivation. Iron therapy is cheap and, provided dosages are not exceeded, safe. The advantages of minor iron deficiency, if any, are few. It would seem sensible, therefore, to recommend that iron deficiency is treated whenever it is suspected.

Treatment of iron deficiency is simple in theory, but quite difficult to achieve successfully in practice. Most iron preparations are not very palatable and they must be given for several months if iron stores are to be replenished satisfactorily. *Table 9.5* outlines some common preparations used to treat iron deficiency in children. Doses can be confusing since they may be quoted as the dose of a particular iron preparation or as the elemental iron equivalent. Therapeutic regimens suitable for children are usually total daily dose of 12 mg elemental iron for those under 6 months; 36 mg at 1 year; 72 mg for 1–5 years; 120 mg for 6–12 years; and 120–180 mg for adults. Parenteral iron is rarely necessary.

Table 9.5 Some iron preparations used frequently in childhood

		Contents of each tablet or 5 ml teaspoonful		Total daily dose (i.e. number of tablets or 5 ml teaspoonfuls)		
		Iron compound (mg)	Elemental iron (mg)	<1 yr	1–5 yr	6–12 yr
Ferrous sulphate	Tablets	200	60	½	1	2
Ferrous sulphate	Mixture	60	12	2–3	6	12
Ferrous glycine sulphate (Plesmet; Napp Laboratories)	Mixture	141	25	1	3	6
Sodium iron edetate (Sytron; Parke-Davis)	Mixture	190	27.5	1	3	6
Ferrous fumarate (Fersamal; Duncan, Flockhart)	Tablets	200	65	½	1	2
Ferrous fumarate (Fersamal; Duncan, Flockhart)	Syrup	140	45	½–1	2	3

It MUST be remembered that iron is a highly poisonous substance if taken in high doses. Tablets and medicines MUST be kept out of reach of children, preferably under lock and key.

Iron overload, apart from that occurring acutely when toddlers ingest large quantities of iron tablets or medicines, is rarely a problem in childhood except in conditions where frequent blood transfusion is necessary for survival – most notably as treatment for the thalassaemias. Each pint of blood delivers about 222 mg iron to the tissues and this cannot be excreted by physiological means. Iron accumulates and ultimately causes liver and cardiac damage. Affected children present with cardiomyopathy secondary to haemosiderosis and liver failure with portal hypertension. Infusion of desferrioxamine with each blood transfusion can certainly delay onset of transfusional siderosis in 'at risk' children and should be practised.

Zinc

Zinc is the metal perhaps secondary only to iron in importance for metabolism. It is involved in the action of many enzymes. Estimation of zinc status of the body is difficult. Levels in the blood do not reflect total body zinc well. Zinc hair levels have been – perhaps inappropriately – regarded as better indicators of the relative zinc concentration in tissues in the recent past (Dorea and Payne, 1985). Food sources of zinc are liver, shellfish, nuts, legumes, cocoa and even water supplies in high zinc environments.

Recognizable zinc deficiency is not common. There are two types of presentation. In acrodermatitis enteropathica, a congenital abnormality of zinc absorption leads to a severe and even lethal condition of infants where there is mucocutaneous ulceration, failure to thrive and susceptibility to infection (*Table 9.6*). This condition is discussed further in Chapter 15. In older children zinc deficiency is most likely in those on low-protein and strict vegetarian diets. Zinc absorption is inhibited by diets of high phytate and perhaps also high vegetable fibre content.

Table 9.6 Features of acrodermatitis enteropathica

Autosomal recessive condition
Reduced zinc uptake from gastrointestinal tract
Signs may not develop during breast feeding

Chronic diarrhoea
Characteristic severe skin rash around mouth and anus
Dermatitis of fingers and toes
Dystrophic nails and paronychiae
Alopecia
Reduced resistance to infection
Malnutrition and growth failure

Low plasma zinc
Low serum alkaline phosphatase
Low leucocyte zinc levels

Response to oral zinc therapy

Risk of fetal abnormality in affected mothers insufficiently supplemented with zinc during pregnancy

Clinical features of zinc deficiency are non-specific in most cases. There is growth retardation, anorexia and ageusia (loss of taste). Epithelial lesions with glossitis, alopecia and nail dystrophy indicate quite severe deficiency. Diarrhoea is common. Abnormalities of the immune system secondary to zinc deficiency lead to impaired resistance to infection. In older children there is delayed pubertal development and this has been described quite extensively in the Middle East. Whether the delay in growth relates to low levels of activity of serum hormones (insulin, growth hormone, cortisol) important in growth and maturation, or to more general effects on metabolism induced by widespread zinc deficiency, is not clear. Zinc-responsive growth retardation in weanlings from Mexican–American homes has also been described from Denver, USA. This problem may be more common and widespread than previously recognized (Hambidge, 1986).

Zinc requirements are in the region of 1 mg/kg/day in infancy; 10 mg/day between 1 and 10 years of age, and 15 mg/day in adults (Lentner, 1981). Absorption of zinc may be reduced in the presence of other metals in foods. However, this interference seems most likely with 'non-organic' minerals supplementing foods such as infant formulas. Absorption of naturally occurring zinc in food seems affected little by organically bound minerals such as iron in the haem form (Solomons and Jacob, 1981).

Copper

Copper is an important constituent of many enzyme systems, some of which (cytochrome oxidase and dismutase) occupy vitally important positions in metabolism. Yet clinical confirmation of copper deficiency is rare except in specific groups such as very low birthweight infants, protein-energy malnutrition and those on parenteral feeding. Evidence that copper deficiency is responsible for clinical signs and symptoms in other individuals is largely lacking, although there is concern in the United States that the national diet may be low in copper (Hambidge, 1985).

The term infant is born with substantial stores of copper in the liver. Neonatal hepatic copper concentration is about 10 times higher than that in the adult (200–400 µg/g dry weight in infants compared with 12–48 µg/g dry weight in adults) (Hambidge, 1985).

Copper accumulates in the liver over the last trimester of pregnancy bound to metallothionein and is released postnatally, thus protecting the full-term infants against copper deficiency. Serum copper levels increase with age. In breast-fed infants levels are independent of the copper concentration of the milk, maternal serum copper levels or whether or not mother is receiving copper supplementation (Salmenperä et al., 1986). Very low birthweight infants will be born with smaller liver stores of copper and may develop deficiency after about 2 months of age unless fed supplemented feeds. *Table 9.7* outlines copper requirements in childhood. For the preterm infant, there is no consensus on the minimal daily requirements for copper (Salim et al., 1986; Anon, 1987; Wharton, 1987).

Table 9.7 Recommended safe levels (mg daily) of copper intake in childhood*

28 weeks	0.20†
Term infant	0.25†
<6 months	0.5–0.7
6–12 months	0.7–1.0
1–3 years	1.0–1.5
4–6 years	1.5–2.0
>7 years	2.0–3.0

* Lentner, 1981; Hambidge, 1985; Wharton, 1987.
† There is no certainty that these levels of intake are necessary – *see* text.

Human milk contains about 0.6 μmol (39 μg)/100 ml of copper but levels fall in prolonged lactation. Cows' milk contains only about 0.13 μmol(9 μg)/100 ml. In the United States the Food and Nutrition Board has recommended that infant formulas should be supplemented with a minimum of 0.95 μmol (60 μg) copper/100 kcal (and higher concentrations in premature baby formulas). DHSS (1980) does not specifically recommend the addition of copper to cows' milk derived formulas, but states that the amount in feeds should not exceed 0.95 μmol (60 μg)/100 ml, nor be less than 0.16 μmol (10 μg)/100 ml – levels achieved by feeding cows' milk based formula. Nevertheless, many formulas are supplemented with copper. As with other minerals, absorption does not necessarily parallel intake. Absorption of copper from breast milk is high, possibly as a consequence of the high copper to zinc ratio and low iron content of human milk, but probably also because of the binding of minerals to protein ligands which facilitate absorption. In soya-based infant formulas, phytate binding inhibits absorption and mineral concentrations must be relatively higher than in cows' milk based formulas.

Although copper intake may seem low in young infants, serum copper levels rise after birth reaching adult levels around 4 months. In breast-fed infants levels are independent of the copper concentration of the milk, of maternal serum copper levels or of whether or not mother is receiving copper supplementation. The explanation for the dietary independence of serum copper in infants is due to mobilization of the liver stores of copper during early life. Premature infants, born with smaller livers and smaller total copper stores, are thus most likely to develop copper deficiency in the first months of life (see Chapter 5) particularly if fed breast milk or standard infant formula with low copper content.

Foods containing copper are oysters(!), nuts, liver, kidney, corn oil, margarine and dry legumes. Hard water and copper piping can make significant contributions to intake.

About 40% of ingested copper is absorbed, largely in the stomach and upper small intestine. Percentage absorption increases in deficiency states although, like iron, absorption is partly dependent on the form in which copper is presented to the gut. Other trace elements such as iron, zinc, cadmium, calcium, sulphur and molybdenum interfere with copper absorption. Copper is bound to albumin in the portal circulation; caeruloplasmin is formed in the liver and this is the form in which most copper circulates in the systemic circulation. The purpose of caeruloplasmin is not clear. Copper uptake by cells may occur more readily from copper bound to amino acids, but can also occur from copper bound to caeruloplasmin. Caeruloplasmin may be important in converting ferrous to ferric iron, an essential step for releasing iron from stores and binding it to transferrin for transport to bone marrow. A second copper-containing enzyme – ferroxidase II – may be important in Wilson's disease (an hereditary deficiency of caeruloplasmin) through preventing the anaemia usually seen with copper deficiency (Hambidge, 1985).

Copper deficiency leads to intracellular abnormalities of iron metabolism. Iron transport within cells is defective, thus leading to inefficient production of haem and a hypochromic, iron deficiency anaemia in association with copper deficiency.

Table 9.8 outlines some of the clinical features of copper deficiency. Copper deficiency is not easy to confirm since caeruloplasmin acts as an acute-phase reactant and tends to rise in circumstances of stress, particularly infection. Normally, however, serum copper (normal levels: 11–25 μmol/l, 0.7–1.6 mg/l); and caeruloplasmin (normal level 0.1–0.7 g/l) levels are depressed in copper deficiency. Normal levels are variable, but often low, in healthy term neonates (copper

Table 9.8 Clinical features associated with copper deficiency

Anaemia:	Hypochromic, unresponsive to iron therapy
Neutropenia:	Due to maturation arrest in bone marrow
Osteoporosis:	Especially of metaphyses and epiphyses, cupping of metaphyseal ends, fractures
Failure to thrive	
Decreased skin pigmentation	
Oedema	
Central nervous system involvement:	Hypotonia, apathy, psychomotor retardation
Hair changes and seborrhoeic dermatitis	

4.5 µmol/l, 0.3 mg/l; caeruloplasmin 0.05–0.265 g/l) and rise to adult levels in plasma over the first 6 months (Salmenperä et al., 1986). In premature infants, levels reach adult values at an equivalent gestational age irrespective of chronological age. Levels in children of 6 months to 10 years tend to be higher than in adults. The proof of copper deficiency as a cause of clinical signs is thus largely in the rapid remission of symptoms and signs with copper treatment.

Copper deficiency in premature infants may present as severe osteoporosis with cupping and flaring of the bone ends, periosteal reaction and sub-metaphyseal fractures (see Chapter 5). Older or full-term infants on bizarre diets may also present with severe bone disease and pathological fractures due to copper deficiency (Cordano, Baertl and Graham, 1964).

Subclinical copper deficiency has occasionally been raised as a possible explanation for the fractures in suspected non-accidental injury. In otherwise normal children this is not a tenable explanation. Dietary needs of copper in term infants are not great since copper is mobilized from liver stores. Well-documented cases of copper deficiency bone disorders in otherwise healthy, term infants are very rare and usually associated with grossly abnormal diet or malabsorption (Cordano, Baertl and Graham, 1964; Chapman, 1987). Thus to suggest copper deficiency developing without reason and causing bone fractures without other evidence (bony or systemic) of copper deficiency is unwise (Patterson, 1987). Non-accidental injury is a positive diagnosis based on suggestive clinical history (or lack of history) and clinical, radiological and social findings. It is not a diagnosis made because all other conceivable alternatives have been excluded. And it should not be a diagnosis that can be unsettled by suggestion of highly unlikely nutritional deficiencies which can also produce fractures but otherwise have many different features. If the diagnosis of non-accidental injury is a diagnosis made by exclusion because there is no other explanation for the findings, it should be a diagnosis made with extreme caution, if at all.

There may be occasional VLBW infants in whom copper deficiency presents in early infancy with fractures of ribs or metaphyseal fractures of the long bones. Because of the ease with which the bones fracture, the history of injury may, be obscure. However, radiological appearances are likely to show severe osteoporosis, metaphyseal cupping and metaphyseal sickle-shaped spurs. Other features of copper deficiency are also likely to be present (Table 9.8). Under these circumstances serum copper levels are likely to be extremely low, and a therapeutic trial of the effects of copper on the non-bony clinical features may be helpful. The bony changes are likely to improve so slowly that the effects of copper on the bones may be inconclusive. However, we regard *routine* serum copper estimation in cases of suspected non-accidental injury as a waste of resources and clinically both unjustified and unhelpful. Serum copper levels vary too much to be expected to give useful and consistent reassurance that copper deficiency is not present. Common sense should tell us whether that is likely or not.

Definite(!) copper deficiency can be treated with copper sulphate 2–3 mg daily as a 1% solution. The liver of premature infants may not tolerate copper very well, and these doses should not be exceeded.

Menkes' steely-hair or kinky-hair syndrome is a rare, sex-linked disorder due to severe abnormality of copper metabolism. There is gross osteoporosis and progressive neurological damage. Scalp hair is sparse and brittle and has a twisted appearance (pili torti) microscopically. Serum copper and caeruloplasmin levels are low. Sadly, administration of copper does not halt the downhill progression, and death usually occurs before the age of 1 year.

Selenium

Selenium levels in soil vary widely across the world and diseases secondary to either selenium excess (selenosis in Nebraska) or deficiency (muscular dystrophy in lambs and calves) have been recognized in animals for some time. By contrast, the role of dietary selenium deficiency in human disease, although widely studied, has only been related to one condition affecting otherwise normal individuals: Keshan disease.

The main physiological role for selenium is as a constituent of glutathione peroxidase. This enzyme is used in the conversion of hydrogen peroxide to water and catalyses the reduction of fatty acid hydroperoxides to hydroxy acids protecting the tissues from peroxidation. Selenium is thus important in maintaining cell membrane stability and controlling free radical damage.

Selenium is found in seafoods, kidney, liver, meats and whole grains but concentrations in food vary with geographic region and soil selenium content. Garlic is the only vegetable containing significant amounts of selenium. Human milk contains about 15–20 µg/l selenium. If comparison is made with other metals in human milk, selenium is probably very well absorbed; hence the levels in human milk may represent the minimum needs of human infants for selenium. The selenium content of cows' milk is lower than that of human milk. There are no recommendations for the minimum selenium content of cows' milk derived formulas. Recommended safe intakes for selenium at various ages are outlined in *Table 9.9*. Bioavailability of selenium in the diet is affected by the form in which it

Table 9.9 Suggested safe selenium intakes (mg daily) at various ages*

<6 months	0.01–0.04
6–12 months	0.02–0.06
1–3 years	0.02–0.08
4–6 years	0.03–0,12
>7 years	0.05–0.20

* Lentner, 1981.

is ingested and other dietary components – such as ascorbic acid. The factors controlling bioavailability are incompletely understood.

Keshan disease

Certain areas of the world, notably New Zealand and a belt of China running from the north-east to the south-west, have very low selenium concentrations in the soil. Population studies show low dietary intakes of selenium and low serum selenium levels. In New Zealand no clinical symptoms associated with these low levels of intake have been reported in man. In China an endemic cardiomyopathy – Keshan disease – affects women of child-bearing age and children in the selenium-deficient areas (Yang, 1986). In affected areas, dietary selenium supplementation reduces the prevalence of Keshan disease significantly. The established condition also shows some improvement with selenium supplementation. Why Keshan disease should be so prevalent in this one area is not clear. Neither is it clear why the condition tends to have a seasonal presentation. Because of its close association with vitamin E metabolism and because of selenium's role in control of free radicals, it may be that in the area where Keshan disease occurs, unrecognized lack, or even excess, of some other ions or vitamins predisposes to tissue damage caused by deficiency of selenium.

A very different condition – Kaschin–Beck disease – occurs in children aged 5–15 years in Keshan-endemic areas. Kaschin–Beck disease is an endemic osteoarthropathy with necrosis of cartilage and epiphyseal growth plates. It too is reported to improve with selenium supplementation (Diplock, 1986).

Suggestions that selenium protects against cancer in later life have not been substantiated. Heavy ingestion of selenium is toxic, and unnecessary prophylactic supplementation is not recommended.

Chromium

As with several other trace elements, chromium seems to have a clear-cut physiological effect in animals – so that symptoms and disease develop with deficiency – but a less well identified role and basic requirements in human nutrition. Chromium is essential for normal glucose metabolism in rats and appears to act as a co-factor for insulin. There have been suggestions, so far not well substantiated, that the widespread deterioration of glucose tolerance with age in Western society is tied up with falling total body chromium content. However, the levels of chromium observed in normal individuals in blood, urine and other tissues are close to the minimal sensitivity of the machines used to estimate them. It is extremely difficult to distinguish low normal values from deficiency. We do not know what the requirements for chromium are in man, nor the normal range of plasma values, except that plasma chromium levels appear to be in the region of 1 pg/ml. Suggested dietary intakes are indicated in *Table 9.10*.

Chromium may be involved in nucleic acid metabolism, but its main recognized role is as a co-factor for insulin. Here it may be facilitating attachment of insulin to receptors on the cell surface and within the cell at the peripheral sites for insulin action. Glucose tolerance factor, a chromium-amino-acid-nicotinic acid compound, may be the form in which chromium has this effect. It has been suggested that chromium can only pass to the fetus across the placenta as glucose tolerance factor.

Table 9.10 Suggested safe intakes of chromium (mg daily) at various ages*

<6 months	0.01–0.04
6–12 months	0.02–0.06
1–3 years	0.02–0.08
4–6 years	0.03–0.12
>7 years	0.05–0.2

* Lentner, 1981; Kelts, 1984.

Glucose tolerance factor is probably stored in the liver and released in parallel to insulin release. The mechanisms controlling this are not understood. Chromium is excreted through the kidney (Hambidge, 1984).

Chromium is poorly absorbed and may be absorbed predominantly as organic compounds found in brewer's yeast and other foods rather than as metallic chromium.

Although in elderly adults there is some evidence that glucose tolerance can be improved by chromium supplementation and that high-density lipoprotein concentration is increased by chromium supplementation, only two circumstances in childhood have produced symptoms suggestive of chromium deficiency: malnutrition and parenteral nutrition. Chromium deficiency seems to complicate PEM in some areas, notably Turkey (Gurson and Saner, 1973). Weight gain and glucose intolerance in children with PEM may improve following chromium supplementation. Long-term parenteral nutrition has also been associated with chromium-responsive weight loss, peripheral neuropathy and encephalopathy. These conditions were associated with abnormally low removal rates for glucose from plasma and low respiratory quotients suggesting difficulty in utilizing glucose for energy metabolism.

Iodine

Iodine deficiency presents as a syndrome of great antiquity unlike the other trace element deficiencies we have been describing. The effects of iodine deficiency in the mother on the fetus have been described in Chapter 2. Iodine deficiency can affect all age groups and has profound effects in infancy when normal thyroid hormone production is essential for normal brain development.

Endemic goitre has been recognized for centuries as a disease of certain regions of the world. Iodine supplementation of the diets of Ohio schoolchildren earlier this century confirmed the nature of the endemic goitre. Goitre arises when iodine is unavailable usually in areas far from the sea and in mountainous areas where rain has leached iodine out of the soil. The Andes, Himalayas, mountains of Central Africa and Papua New Guinea are particularly affected areas. Derbyshire in UK was badly affected with endemic goitre (Derbyshire neck) until relatively recently.

Table 9.11 lists recommended intakes of iodine. Minimal requirements are probably less than 50 µg/daily in adolescents and 20 µg/daily in infants and young children. Breast milk contains 40–90 µg/l. Iodine is well absorbed from all foods. In Western countries intakes may be seasonal with high winter levels when cattle are fed iodine-supplemented winter feed (Broadhead, Pearson and Wilson, 1965).

Table 9.11 Recommended intakes of iodine (μg daily) according to age*

<6 months	40
6–12 months	50
1–3 years	70
4–6 years	90
7–12 years	120
>10 years	150†

* Lentner, 1981; Kelts, 1984.
† Pregnancy and lactation demand extra intakes estimated at 25–50 μg daily.

Goitre occurs when iodine intake is less than 15 μg/daily. Serum thyroxine (T4) decreases but triiodothyronine (T3) may remain at normal levels. Thyroid stimulating hormone levels are high – causing the thyroid enlargement. When endemic cretinism occurs urinary iodine excretion is usually less than 20 μg/daily (Kavishe, 1986).

Access to iodized salt in the absence of natural sources of iodine is effective in preventing endemic goitre and cretinism. Quantities of iodine added to salt vary. In the USA iodized salt contains 75 μg/g iodine. In West Germany upper permissible levels are 5 μg/g. Intramuscular depot injections of 5 ml iodized oil containing 400 mg/ml iodine are effective goitre prophylaxis and the effects last about 4 years.

Infants fed iodine-deficient milk from iodine-deficient mothers may be unable to maintain adequate thyroid hormone production in early life, and thyroid deficiency may lead to cretinism. Later in childhood, brain damage is not a feature of inadequate thyroid hormone production but goitre, if associated with inadequate thyroid production, leads to poor growth and slowed metabolism. Goitres usually disappear in boys at puberty when the needs for iodine decrease as growth ceases, but remain in girls and even enlarge during pregnancy and lactation.

Certain substances – notably plants such as the brassicas – act as a goitrogens by inhibiting iodine uptake by the thyroid gland. The presence of these together with possible genetic differences in requirements may explain why some children develop goitre or inadequate thyroid hormone production on relatively low iodine diets and others do not.

Fluorine

Fluorine has assumed new importance over the last 20 years since its effect as a cariostatic substance has become generally accepted. In many areas of the world, the fluoride content of drinking water is sufficient to provide protective effects against dental caries (i.e. concentrations of 1 mg fluoride per litre drinking water). Breast-fed infants have low intakes of fluoride even though their mothers may be taking fluoride supplements. Intakes will be in the region of 4 μg in low-fluoride areas and 8 μg in high-fluoride areas, in comparison with calculated intakes of 320 μg in formula-fed infants.

Apart from its effect on the teeth (*see* Chapter 12) fluoride has no other known role in metabolism. In order to have maximum cariostatic effect, fluoride must come into contact with the teeth. Mothers giving their children fluoride drops or tablets should ensure that the substances are rolled around the cheeks and not just swallowed after being placed on the tongue. Supplements given before teeth appear are probably mainly useful in encouraging mothers and their infants in the practice of taking regular fluoride although fluorine is deposited in teeth and bones as fluorapatite. Drops containing 0.25 mg fluoride should be given to infants daily when at least one part per million of fluoride is not present in the drinking water. The quantities of fluoride given should increase gradually to 1 mg/day by 3 years of age.

Other trace elements

Molybdenum, manganese and cadmium are substances known to be necessary for health in animals. They probably affect human metabolism as well, but the nature of these effects has not yet been determined (Söderhjelm, 1985). VLBW infants and children on artificial diets or intravenous feeding are likely to be at risk of deficiency states for these minerals. Avoidance of deficiency of unspecified (trace) elements in parenterally fed individuals and those on elemental diets can be prevented by small weekly transfusions of fresh plasma.

References

ANON (1987) Copper and the infant. *Lancet*, **i**, 900–901
AUKETT, M. A., PARKS, Y. A., SCOTT, P. H. and WHARTON, B. A. (1986) Treatment with iron increases weight gain and psychomotor development. *Archives of Disease in Childhood*, **61**, 849–857
BROADHEAD, G. D., PEARSON, I. B. and WILSON, G. M. (1965) Seasonal changes in iodine metabolism. Iodine content of cows' milk. *British Medical Journal*, **i**, 343–348
CHAPMAN, S. (1987) Child abuse or copper deficiency? A radiological view. *British Medical Journal*, **294**, 1370
CORDANO, A., BAERTL, J. M. and GRAHAM, G. G. (1964) Copper deficiency in infancy. *Pediatrics*, **34**, 324–336
DEPARTMENT OF HEALTH AND SOCIAL SECURITY (1980) Artificial feeds for the young infant. *Report on Health and Social Subjects*, No. 18. London: Her Majesty's Stationery Office
DIPLOCK, A. T. (1986) Free radicals in medicine and the biological role of selenium. In *Proceedings of the XIII International Congress of Nutrition*, edited by T. G. Taylor and N. K. Jenkins, pp. 585–589. London: John Libbey
DOREA, J. G. and PAYNE, P. A. (1985) Hair zinc in children: its uses, limitations and relationship to plasma zinc and anthropometry. *Human Nutrition: Clinical Nutrition*, **39C**, 389–398
GRINDULIS, H., SCOTT, P. H., BELTON, N. R. and WHARTON, B. A. (1986) Combined deficiency of iron and vitamin D in Asian toddlers. *Archives of Disease in Childhood*, **61**, 843–848
GURSON, C. T. and SANER, G. (1973) Effects of chromium supplementation on growth in marasmic protein calorie malnutrition. *American Journal of Clinical Nutrition*, **26**, 988–991
HALLIDAY, H. L., LAPPIN, T. R. J. and McCLURE, G. (1984) Iron status and the preterm infant during the first year of life. *Biology of the Neonate*, **45**, 228–235
HAMBIDGE, K. M. (1985) Trace elements in human nutrition. In *Nutrition in Pediatrics: Basic Science and Clinical Applications*, edited by W. A. Walker and J. B. Wilkins, pp. 17–45. Boston: Little Brown
HAMBIDGE, K. M. (1986) Zinc deficiency in the weanling. *Acta Paediatrica Scandinavica*, Suppl. **323**, 52–58
KAVISHE, F. P. (1986) Endemic goitre and cretinism in Africa. In *Proceedings of the XIII International Congress of Nutrition*, edited by T. G. Taylor and N. K. Jenkins, pp. 487–491. London: John Libbey
KELTS, D. G. (1984) Normal diet and digestion. In *Manual of Pediatric Nutrition*, edited by D. G. Kelts and E. G. Jones, pp. 1–19. Boston: Little Brown

LENTNER, C. (ed.) (1981) Nutritional standards. In *Geigy Scientific Tables, Volume 1. Units of Measurement, Composition of the Body, Nutrition*, pp. 232–240. Basle: Ciba-Geigy

PATTERSON, C. R. (1987) Child abuse or copper deficiency? *British Medical Journal*, **295**, 213

POLLITT, E. and LEIBEL, R. L. (1976) Iron deficiency and behaviour. *Journal of Pediatrics*, **88**, 372–381

POLLITT, E., SACO-POLLITT, C., LEIBEL, R. L. and VITERI, F. E. (1986) Iron deficiency and behavioural development in infants and pre-school children. *American Journal of Clinical Nutrition*, **43**, 555–565

SALIM, S., FARQUHARSON, J., ARNEIL, G. C. *et al.* (1986) Dietary copper in artificially fed infants. *Archives of Disease in Childhood*, **61**, 1068–1075

SALMENPERÄ, L., PERHEENTUPA, J., PAKARINEN, P. and SIIMES, M. A. (1986) Copper nutrition in infants during prolonged exclusive breast feeding. *American Journal of Clinical Nutrition*, **43**, 251–257

SMITH, N. J. and RIOS, E. (1974) Iron metabolism, iron deficiency in infancy and childhood. In *Advances in Pediatrics*, Vol. 21, edited by I. Schulman, pp. 239–280. Chicago: Year Book Medical Publishers

SÖDERHJELM, L. (1985) Some reflections on trace elements in paediatrics. *Acta Paediatrica Scandinavica*, **74**, 17

SOLOMONS, N. W. and JACOB, R. A. (1981) Studies on the bioavailability of zinc in humans: effects of heme and non heme iron on the absorption of zinc. *American Journal of Clinical Nutrition*, **34**, 475–482

STECKEL, A. (1984) Iron requirements in infancy and childhood. In *Iron Nutrition in Infancy and Childhood*, edited by A. Stekel, pp. 1–10. New York: Raven Press

WHARTON, B. A. (1987) *Nutrition and Feeding of Preterm Infants*. Oxford: Blackwell Scientific

WIDDOWSON, E. M. (1974) Nutrition. In *Scientific Foundations of Paediatrics*, edited by J. A. Davis and J. Dobbing, pp. 44–55. London: William Heinemann

YANG, G. Q. (1986) Selenium – deficiency and endemic Keshan disease in China. *Proceedings of the XIII International Congress of Nutrition*, edited by T. G. Taylor and N. K. Jenkins, pp. 124–127. London: John Libbey

Chapter 10

Vitamin deficiencies

Minimal dietary requirements for many vitamins cannot be stated specifically since vitamin intakes from foods are readily affected by cooking processes and needs vary with state of health, rates of growth and intakes of other nutrients. Recommended dietary intakes vary widely and are probably greatly in excess of minimal needs. In general, vitamin requirements are highest during periods of rapid growth, during or following stress such as infection or surgery, and in children on unusual or restricted diets (*Table 10.1*). Extremes of cooking and processing tend to destroy vitamins although fermentation may increase the vitamin content of some foods.

Table 10.1 Conditions predisposing to vitamin deficiencies

Deficient intake:	Prolonged breast feeding without weaning: monotonous limited diets; unsupplemented elimination, elemental or specialized diets; destruction of vitamins in storage or cooking processes; strict vegan diets
Malabsorption:	Malabsorption syndromes; foods prepared so vitamins unattainable; binding of vitamins to food residues in gut; utilization of vitamins by organisms in the gut
Failed utilization:	Some inborn errors of metabolism; metabolic disorders, e.g. renal failure; defects of transport, e.g. low RBP in malnutrition
Increased losses:	Loss of vitamin D as inactive metabolites
Increased requirements:	Rapid growth, prematurity, stress, infection; some inborn errors of metabolism

Vitamin A deficiency

Vitamin A deficiency is rare in children on normal diets in Britain. In Asia, over ten million children are estimated to be affected by vitamin A deficiency, and many of these will become blind and – all too often – die secondary to infection (Sommer *et al.*, 1981). In the United States it is one of the three major nutrients most likely to be deficient in childhood (Schwarz, 1985). Sadly, sources of vitamin A are readily available within many of the environments that are associated with widespread clinical deficiency. Recommended safe intakes are outlined in *Table 10.2*.

The units used to quote intakes of vitamin A are confusing. It is probably most appropriate to quote Retinol Equivalents (RE) since these take into account the

Table 10.2 Recommended safe dietary intake of vitamin A as Retinol Equivalents (RE)/day*

Age	WHO/FAO†	FNB (RE/day)‡	DHSS§
Preterm infant	–	500	(800)
Term infant	300	420	450
1 year	300	400	300
1–3 years	250	400	300
4–6 years	300	500	300
7–10 years	400	700	400–575
11–14 years	575–750	1000	725–750

* *See* text for interpretation of retinol equivalents; 1 RE = 1 µg.
† WHO/FAO Ad Hoc Expert Committee (1973).
‡ Food and Nutrition Board (1975).
§ DHSS (1979).

low absorption and conversion of carotene to retinol: 1 RE = 1 µg retinol or 6 µg β carotene or 3.3 International Units. The main sources of animal (retinol) and plant (carotene) precursors of retinol in the body are indicated in *Table 10.3*. Since retinol is transported in the plasma bound to retinol binding protein (RBP), conditions that lead to low RBP (most notably protein-energy malnutrition) lead to low vitamin A activity and evidence of deficiency. Retinols are important for clearing free radicals and maintaining membrane stability; for normal epithelial structure; and for the formation of the eye pigments, rhodopsin and iodopsin.

Table 10.3 Main dietary sources of vitamin A

	Sources	*Metabolism*
Retinols and retinyl esters	Colostrum. Milk, cream, butter, cheese, margarine (fortified), egg yolk, liver, kidney, fish liver oils	Absorbed as retinol combined with palmitic acid in mucosal cells. Stored in liver. Transported bound to RBP in plasma
β carotenes	Dark green leafy vegetables, spinach, turnip tops, parsley, carrots, sweet potato, tomatoes, peppers, peas, red palm oil	Partially absorbed intact. Absorption increased in liver disorders, hypothyroidism, diabetes and high intakes
		Partially hydrolysed to two molecules of retinol and then absorbed. 50% efficiency in conversion. Absorption only about 33% (1 µg carotene = 0.167 µg retinol)

These protein-bound pigments are changed from cis- to trans-forms by light – a change that releases energy and stimulates retinal nerve endings. *Table 10.4* lists the varied problems associated with vitamin A deficiency.

In vitamin A deficiency states mucosal integrity is impaired and resistance to infection reduced. Infections, particularly persistent diarrhoea and measles, predispose to vitamin A deficiency (Tomkins, 1986). Diets low in fat and malabsorptive states also predispose to deficiency of vitamin A. Low levels of RBP

Table 10.4 Clinical manifestations of vitamin A deficiency

Visual and eye signs:	Reduced dark adaptation, night blindness. Drying of epithelial surfaces – xerosis conjunctivae, xerosis corneae. Wrinkling, clouding and softening of cornea – keratomalacia. Foamy silver grey epithelial plaques on lateral conjunctivae: Bitot's spots. Photophobia. Secondary infection. Trauma leading to scarring and blindness, extrusion of lens and loss of vitreous. Shrunken, useless eye – phthisis bulbae
Other epithelial surfaces:	Follicular hyperkeratosis especially of upper arms and thighs; overall dry, scaly skin
Growth:	Failure to thrive
Immunology:	Reduced resistance to infection due to damaged epithelial surfaces; reduced T-cell maturation
Blood levels:	Plasma vitamin A <100 µg/dl

in protein-energy malnutrition contribute to the prevalence of vitamin A deficiency in severe malnutrition. Unsupplemented premature infants are also at risk owing to poor fat absorption and rapid rates of growth (Stanton et al., 1986).

Management of vitamin A deficiency depends on whether therapy is preventive, treating mild signs or treating developing xerophthalmia. Water-miscible oral preparations are preferable since, if there is fat malabsorption, absorption of oily preparations may be poor.

Prevention
Deficiency can be prevented with the recommended daily intakes of 800 µg retinol palmitate in prematures, although much lower levels of intake (230 µg/kg) are probably safe (Wharton, 1987); 400 µg in term and older infants and 700–1000 µg daily in older children. The oral dose of 30 000–66 000 µg once, three to six monthly, is also effective prophylaxis and should be given to mothers postpartum in areas of prevalent deficiency to protect their breast-fed infants.

Mild deficiency without eye involvement
A 5–10 day course of 1000–2000 µg retinol daily followed by preventive therapy is usually adequate.

Eye involvement
Here treatment must be swift and effective. One dose of 35 000 µg of a water-miscible preparation of retinol palmitate intramuscularly followed by a 5–10 day oral course as above should be repeated if there is no improvement after a month.

It is important to keep to treatment guidelines since excessive intakes of vitamin A are almost as dangerous as the deficiency. Acute intoxication with vitamin A leads to vomiting, and signs of raised intracranial pressure (bulging fontanelle, diplopia and papilloedema). Chronic intoxication leads to anorexia, failure to thrive, alopecia, pruritis, seborrhoea, angular stomatitis, tender bony swellings with midshaft hyperostosis on X-ray, hepatomegaly and signs of raised intracranial pressure as in the acute form. Plasma retinol levels will be high (>80 µg/dl).

B vitamin deficiencies

The B vitamins are found widely in animal and vegetable foods. Deficiency of one B vitamin is commonly associated with deficiencies of others. Deficiencies resulting from inadequate dietary intakes of these vitamins are usually the consequence of famine, severely restricted diets, inappropriate preparation of food or excessive storage or cooking.

The main functions of B vitamins are as co-factors for metabolic processes or as precursors of essential metabolites.

Thiamine (vitamin B$_1$) deficiency: beri-beri

Table 10.5 outlines sources and metabolic effects of vitamin B$_1$. Deficiency is particularly common when the staple diet is polished rice unless the rice has previously been subjected to parboiling when B vitamins in the rice husks are absorbed into the grain and retained. (Parboiling comprises soaking, steaming and then drying the grains before removing the husks.)

Table 10.5 Sources and metabolic actions of vitamin B$_1$

Sources
   Widespread in foods: meat, fish, dairy produce, cereals, especially cereal husks
   Destroyed by heat and alkali
   Lost in polishing rice or refining flour

Metabolic action as thiamine pyrophosphate
   Decarboxylation of ketoacids
   Transketolase reactions in pentose phosphate shunt
   Oxidative decarboxylation acetyl CoA and α ketoglutarate to succinyl CoA
   Transketolase reaction in synthesis of ribose

Thiamine deficiency syndromes take two forms: 'wet' and 'dry' beri-beri. In 'wet' beri-beri there is high output cardiac failure and cardiac arrhythmias. In the 'dry' form – commoner after infancy – neurological symptoms and signs predominate.

Since requirements for B$_1$ are high in early infancy, and breast-fed infants derive the vitamin from the milk, beri-beri is common amongst breast-fed infants born to thiamine-deficient mothers. Symptoms usually develop at 2 or 3 months old.

Initially infants are restless, pale, vomiting and may have constipation. Their features are waxy and flabby. Pulses are bounding, and the infants are dyspnoeic. 'Wet' beri-beri with oedema and cardiac failure then develops secondary to the peripheral vasodilatation, high-output cardiomyopathy and salt and water retention by the kidneys. There is cardiomegaly and pulmonary oedema on chest X-ray. ECG shows prolonged QT interval, inverted T waves and overall low voltage. Pericardial, peritoneal and pleural effusions may develop. Tendon reflexes, especially at ankles and knees, are absent due to associated peripheral neuropathy.

'Wet' beri-beri can occur at any age but older children develop the 'dry' form initially more commonly. Here the clinical signs are neurological. There is peripheral neuritis with paraesthesiae, hyperaesthesia and burning sensations in the feet. Muscles are tender and weak, and the children may have difficulty rising from the floor. Tendon reflexes are absent and there is glove/stocking distribution of sensory loss and muscular weakness. Wernicke's encephalopathy may develop with confusion, meningism and signs of raised intracranial pressure.

Thiamine deficiency may be suspected when red blood cell transketolase levels are diminished. Lactate and pyruvate levels are raised after exercise or glucose load in thiamine deficiency, but care is needed in the collection and transport of blood specimens if accurate pyruvate and lactate levels are to be obtained. The most satisfactory demonstration of thiamine deficiency is to give a loading dose of thiamine (10 mg). Such a dose does not produce any measurable thiamine excretion in the urine in deficient infants. Normal levels of urinary thiamine are above 50 µg/day.

Treatment of B_1 deficiency is simple but urgent. Infants and young children should be given vitamin B_1 10 mg/daily and older children a somewhat higher level with 50 mg/daily for adults. Cardiac failure (wet beri-beri) should be treated with intravenous or intramuscular thiamine, 100 mg daily. This may produce considerable improvement very rapidly, although complete recovery may take many weeks.

Prophylaxis demands intakes of 0.5 mg/daily in infants; 0.7–1 mg/daily in older children. Pregnant and lactating women should take 1–1.5 mg/daily.

Riboflavin deficiency

Table 10.6 outlines the sources and metabolic action of riboflavin. Isolated riboflavin deficiency rarely occurs but it is common in association with deficiencies of other B group vitamins and with protein-energy malnutrition. Thus signs of deficiency are not very specific to this vitamin alone. Deficiency is usually secondary to inadequate intake, although malabsorption of riboflavin is common in association with biliary atresia and chronic hepatitis. Riboflavin tends to be lost in the urine in protein deficiency states. Transient depletion is common in low birthweight infants. Destruction of riboflavin in feeds on exposure to the bright lights of neonatal units may contribute to this (Lucas and Bates, 1984).

Clinical features of riboflavin deficiency are largely the non-specific signs seen in many B group vitamin deficiencies (*Table 10.7*). More specifically, riboflavin deficiency causes a seborrhoeic dermatitis with greasy, yellowish flaky scales on an erythematous base in the nasolabial folds and on the forehead, giving a 'hoar-frost' appearance. Equally characteristic is proliferation of the scleral blood vessels on to the cornea. This can result from trauma but is not a feature of other B vitamin deficiencies.

Table 10.6 Sources and metabolic action of riboflavin

Sources
  Widespread in animal products, especially liver, kidney, milk, cheese, eggs; plant sources (brewer's yeast, leafy vegetables)
  Light sensitive: easily destroyed
  Requirements increased with high carbohydrate intake

Action
  As riboflavin phosphate, is important in formation of co-enzymes flavin mononucleotide and flavin adenine dinucleotide; essential for oxidation pathways

  There may be increased urinary loss of riboflavin in conditions of protein deficiency owing to instability of flavoproteins

Table 10.7 Non-specific signs suggestive of B-group vitamin deficiency*

Cheilosis:	Pallor, thinning, maceration at angles of mouth, angular stomatitis
Glossitis:	Smooth tongue with loss of papillae, magenta colour; sore
Stomatitis:	Reddened, swollen oral mucosae
Conjunctivitis:	Sore eyes with photophobia and lacrimation
Anaemia:	Normochromic, normocytic anaemia, marrow hypoplasia
Dermatitis:	Dry, scaly hyperpigmented skin
Neurological involvement:	Peripheral neuritis, depression and confusion
Growth:	Failure to thrive

* B-group vitamin therapy in non-specific deficiency states should include thiamine, riboflavin, nicotinamide, biotin, pantothenic acid, inositol, folic acid, choline.

In deficiency states, urinary riboflavin excretion is less than 30 μg/day. Red blood cell glutathione reductase is low. Treatment should be with other B group vitamin supplements as well (Ketovite liquid and tablets; Paines & Byrne).

Niacin deficiency: pellagra

Table 10.8 presents the sources and metabolic action of niacin. Tryptophan can be converted to niacin in the body, and niacin deficiency is thus counterbalanced by high-tryptophan diets. Pellagra tends to occur when maize is the staple diet since maize is a poor source of tryptophan as well as niacin. Niacin is lost in milling or is unavailable as niacin unless the maize is prepared with alkali. Pellagra is also common when millet with high leucine content is consumed (sorghum vulgare or jowar). Jowar is not deficient in tryptophan or niacin, and it is not clear why it should predispose to pellagra.

Pellagra – the disease associated particularly with niacin deficiency – is classically described as diarrhoea, dermatitis and dementia. In children the diarrhoea may be replaced by constipation, and the dementia is less dramatic. There is a light-sensitive dermatitis which may develop rapidly on exposed areas with blistering or severe erythema which desquamates later. The skin is pigmented after healing. Oral lesions as described in *Table 10.7* are florid, and there may even be ulceration of the tongue. The children are apathetic or depressed.

Table 10.8 Sources and metabolic action of niacin (nicotinate, nicotinamide)

Sources
   Synthesized from tryptophan when sufficient in diet (60 mg tryptophan equivalent to 1 mg niacin); widespread in animal products, fish, crustacea; large amounts in many seeds, cereals, yeast.

   Lost in milling of grains; unavailable as niacytin in maize unless food prepared with alkali; antagonized by foods containing high leucine–low isoleucine ratios.

   Niacin content of foods may be increased by fermentation of grain or milk

Action
   Nicotinate converted to nicotinamide in body; precursor of co-factors nicotinamide adenine dinucleotide and nicotinamide adenine dinucleotide phosphate – co-factors for wide variety of essential metabolic processes

Diagnosis of niacin deficiency is by a therapeutic trial. N-methyl nicotinamide excretion in urine is low in niacin deficiency. A dose of niacin, 50–300 mg/daily by mouth or possibly smaller amounts intravenously, is not followed by increased N-methyl nicotinamide excretion in the urine if there is deficiency. Large doses of niacin produce flushing and burning sensations in the skin.

Requirements of the three B vitamins described above are possibly stated more appropriately in terms of energy intake since energy intakes affect the metabolic needs for these vitamins. Thus recommended intakes are: thiamine 0.4 mg/4.2 MJ (1000 kcal); riboflavin 0.55 mg/4.2 MJ; niacin or equivalent 6.6 mg/4.2 MJ.

Vitamin B_6 (pyridoxine) deficiency

Pyridoxine, combined with phosphate, functions as co-enzyme for many metabolic reactions, including:

1. Decarboxylation and transamination of amino acids.
2. Metabolism of glycogen and fatty acids.
3. Breakdown of kynurenine.
4. As co-enzyme for glutamic decarboxylase and gamma amino butyric acid (both used in normal brain metabolism).
5. In active transport of amino acids across cell membranes.
6. Chelation of metals.
7. Synthesis of arachidonic acid from linoleic acid.
8. Normal glycine metabolism (lack of pyridoxine phosphate results in oxaluria).

Vitamin B_6 deficiency is probably more common as a result of abnormalities in B_6 metabolism than as a direct result of dietary deficiency. Interference, either by drugs or genetic abnormalities, can affect the reaction of B_6 with apo-enzymes, or can alter enzyme–coenzyme interactions resulting in reduced availability of pyridoxine phosphate in the body. In certain inborn errors of metabolism where there are abnormalities of enzymes, high levels of pyridoxine may improve function in the abnormal enzymes or facilitate alternative pathways.

The clinical effects of pyridoxine deficiency or dependency include convulsions, peripheral neuritis, dermatosis and anaemia.

Infants fed diets deficient in B_6 from birth may develop convulsions 1–6 months after birth. Pyridoxine deficiency may also be associated with a dermatosis consisting of cheilosis, glossitis with seborrhoea around nose, eyes and mouth. A pyridoxine-responsive peripheral neuritis is common when isoniazid therapy is given without supplementary vitamin B_6. Pyridoxine deficiency is also associated with oxaluria, bladder stones, hyperglycinaemia, lymphopenia and decreased antibody production in response to infection. Microcytic anaemia with high serum iron and marrow haemosiderosis is a relatively common manifestation of pyridoxine dependency. *Table 10.9* lists deficiency and dependency syndromes associated with pyridoxine.

Pyridoxine-dependent convulsions usually occur between 3 hours and 2 weeks postnatally. When pyridoxine dependency is suspected, 100 mg pyridoxine, intramuscularly, followed by 2–10 mg intramuscularly or 10–100 mg by mouth daily should be given. If the convulsions do not cease or at least improve greatly within 24 hours, diagnosis is incorrect. There may be a history of high maternal intake of B_6 during pregnancy in which case the condition may resolve gradually.

Table 10.9 Conditions causing pyridoxine deficiency, dependency or both

Low intake:
    Due to deficienct diet, prolonged heat processing, unsupplemented milk formulas, unsupplemented elemental diets

    Inadequately absorbed due to malabsorption syndromes

Requirements increased:
    Owing to inborn errors of metabolism:
        Pyridoxine-dependent convulsions
        Pyridoxine-dependent anaemia
        Xanthurenic aciduria
        Cystathionuria
        Some forms of homocystinuria

    Dependency resulting from high maternal intake in pregnancy

    Owing to drug therapy:
        Isoniazid
        Penicillamine
        Oral contraceptives

Pyridoxine-dependent anaemia is a sideroblastic (microcytic, hypochromic anaemia with high iron stores) anaemia. Diagnosis is by trial of high doses of pyridoxine and elimination of other known causes of sideroblastic anaemias.

Type 1 homocystinuria (marfanoid features, malar flush, osteoporosis, ectopia lentis and thromboembolic episodes) may sometimes respond to pharmacological doses of pyridoxine, perhaps because the homocysteine is removed by other pathways than the defective cystathione synthetase pathway.

In another inborn error of metabolism, cystathioninaemia with cystathionuria, the enzyme that normally splits cystathionine to homoserine and cysteine is abnormal. Binding sites for the co-enzyme pyridoxine phosphate are altered, but increased enzymatic function occurs with the addition of vitamin B_6. Treatment with pharmacological doses of B_6 reduces blood and urinary levels of cystathione, although the ultimate effects on mental development are less clear.

Pyridoxine phosphate is involved in many aspects of tryptophan metabolism and several tryptophan metabolites are excreted in deficiency states. In pyridoxine-responsive xanthurenic aciduria there is no evidence of pyridoxine phosphate deficiency, but large doses of pyridoxine phosphate normalize the xanthurenic acid excretion. Liver biopsy shows that there is a defect in the binding of pyridoxine phosphate to the enzyme kynureninase.

Treatment of simple deficiency (i.e. not dependency) of pyridoxine phosphate is by 10 mg by mouth daily. Dependency requires doses ranging from 10 to 100 mg daily.

Folic acid deficiency

Dietary deficiency of folic acid is relatively common and the variety of ways in which metabolism can be affected or requirements increased means that folic acid deficiency is one of the commonest vitamin deficiencies. Although widely present in animal and plant products, particularly green vegetables, folic acid is readily destroyed by cooling and storage processes.

Conditions presenting with folic acid deficiency are varied:

Dietary inadequacy – This occurs when excessive cooking or storage destroys folate. Shortage of fresh foods and dairy products and especially fresh vegetables may lead to deficiency.

Malabsorption – Folate is absorbed in the jejunum and readily becomes deficient in malabsorptive states. In coeliac disease loss of epithelial cells in the jejunum and rapid cell turnover leads to increased folate requirements as well as malabsorption. In situations where the small intestine is colonized by bacteria, folate is diverted into bacterial metabolism.

Abnormal metabolism – In protein-energy malnutrition there is a block in the conversion of dihydrofolate to the active form tetrahydrofolate. Clinical deficiency of folate is common.

Drug therapy – Anticonvulsants cause increased metabolism of folate in the liver and thus increased requirements. (Contraceptive treatment also leads to increased folate requirements.) Folic acid antagonist drugs are an important part of the armamentarium for treating malignancies.

Increased requirements due to rapid growth or increased cell turnover – Folate is essential for nucleoprotein synthesis and thus for normal cell division. Deficiency is likely to develop in any state where there is rapid growth (prematurity; catch-up growth; pregnancy) or where there is increased cell loss (eczema; exfoliative dermatitis; haemolytic anaemia).

Failure of utilization – In vitamin B_{12} and vitamin C deficiencies, folate metabolism is affected and megaloblastic macrocytic anaemia occurs.

Evidence for folate deficiency occurs within a month of onset of inadequate intake. Megaloblastic anaemia and pancytopenia are classical features, but the importance of folate in the synthesis of the purines and pyramidines essential for nucleoprotein formation results in reduced growth as well as reduced haematopoiesis. Folic acid deficiency presents as a megaloblastic, macrocytic, anaemia with neutropenia and thrombocytopenia. Neutrophils are large with hypersegmented nuclei and this may

Table 10.10 Biochemical tests of folate status (Oski, 1985)

Test	Normal values (ng/ml)	Comments
Serum folate	>3	Falls before anaemia develops. Low levels indicate recent low intake but not necessarily deficiency state
Red-cell folate	>75	Better indication of deficiency since indicates deficient state of >60 days duration

be the earliest clinical finding. Bone marrow is hypercellular because of erythroid hyperplasia. Reticulocyte count is low and nucleated red cells appear in the peripheral blood about 20 weeks after onset of inadequacy. The significance of circulating folate levels depends on the measurement used (*Table 10.10*). Treatment is with folic acid orally or parenterally, 2–5 mg daily. Response to treatment is usually rapid.

B_{12} deficiency

Vitamin B_{12} is present in many animal foods. Dietary deficiency of B_{12} is thus unlikely except in strict vegans who consume no milk, eggs or animal products. Deficiency most commonly results from failure to absorb or transport the vitamin (*Table 10.11*).

Table 10.11 Causes of vitamin B_{12} deficiency

Type of defect	Causative conditions
Inadequate intake	Strict vegans, breast milk from vegan mother

Malabsorption	Lack of intrinsic factor
	  Congenital
	  Acquired (often associated with autoimmune endocrinopathies)
	Familial malabsorption of B_{12} – intrinsic factor complex (Imerslund–Gräsbeck syndrome)
	Disease or resection of terminal ileum

Increased requirements	Bacterial or parasitic colonization of small bowel in blind loops, diverticula, or anastomoses Fish tapeworm: *Diphyllobothrium latum*
Defective transport	Transcobalamin II deficiency

Vitamin B_{12} combines with a glycoprotein (intrinsic factor) secreted by the parietal cells of the gastric fundus prior to absorption at specific sites in the terminal ileum. Transport of the vitamin in the blood is by two binding proteins – transcobalamins I and II. Deficiency of transcobalamin II is recorded. Lack of intrinsic factor, consumption of B_{12} in the gut or splitting of the vitamin-intrinsic factor combination by intestinal organisms, can all produce B_{12} deficiency (Oski, 1985).

Since Crohn's disease frequently involves the terminal ileum, vitamin B_{12} deficiency is a common association of this condition. Children (and adults) with terminal ileitis or resections of the terminal ileum for Crohn's disease must receive replacement B_{12}.

In the inborn error of metabolism methylmalonic acidaemia (inability to metabolize the amino acids valine, isoleucine and methionine), accumulation of proprionate and methylmalonate causes metabolic acidosis, protein intolerance, mental retardation, failure to thrive and occasionally hyperammonaemia, pancytopenia and hypoglycaemia. Fifty per cent of the children with methylmalonic acidaemia respond to vitamin B_{12} 1–2 mg/daily. In several of the varieties of methylmalonic acidaemia, cobalamin cannot be converted into either the adenosyl nor the methyl form. Large doses of B_{12} presumably facilitate conversion of some of the vitamin to more active forms.

Vitamin B_{12} deficiency leads both to haematological and to neurological abnormalities. The haematological abnormalities may respond to folate therapy but the neurological problems do not. There is a megaloblastic, macrocytic, anaemia with nucleated red cells but reticulocytopenia. Neutropenia, thrombocytopenia and hypersegmentation of the white-cell nuclei occurs. Bone marrow shows a megaloblastic, erythroid picture with giant metamyelocytes.

The neurological signs are those of subacute combined degeneration of the cord, namely peripheral neuritis, degeneration of the dorsal columns and cortico-spinal tract involvement. Occasionally blindness secondary to retrobulbar neuropathy develops.

Treatment of B_{12} deficiency depends on the cause. Where straightforward dietary deficiency is the cause, oral supplementation is satisfactory (1–3 μg daily). In other situations, inadequate absorption usually requires treatment with intramuscular injections. Initially 1000 μg daily is given and followed by 100–1000 μg 1–3 monthly when there is clinical improvement. Treatment will probably have to continue for life. Complete resolution of anaemia and total or near-total resolution of the neurological abnormalities are usual.

Vitamin C deficiency (scurvy)

Scurvy was common in Europe until this century. Children were particularly likely to be affected. The deficiency was largely seasonal since fresh fruits and vegetables were often in short supply in winter, and the need for vitamin C to cope with the stress of infection was greater during the winter. Children are now rarely seen with scurvy in developed countries unless they are on artifical diets from which vitamin C has been omitted. Scurvy is still liable to occur when diets are limited in food variety, where cooking is excessive, or where children are exceptionally faddy. It is not always recognized that only a few varieties of 'squash' and 'pop' fruit juices contain vitamin C so drinking 'orange squash' does not necessarily maintain the ascorbic acid content of a diet.

The clinical features of scurvy involve many systems:

Skin – Typically the skin is dry with hyperkeratosis of hair follicles and perifollicular petechiae so the follicles are surrounded by a red halo. More extensive bruising and ecchymoses may occur. There is loss of hair.

Mucous membranes – The mouth and conjunctivae are dry, the gums swollen and bleeding, and the teeth become loose. These changes are less dramatic than in adults and may be minimal in infants with no teeth or children with good dental hygiene.

Skeletal system – The typical lesions are separation of epiphyses and subperiosteal haemorrhages (*Figure 10.1*). Scorbutic rosary results from costal epiphyseal separation. Callus formation is florid, and the bones are painful. The child adopts a recumbent frog-like posture to reduce pain in bones and joints.

General – Malaise, weakness, arthralgia and joint effusions contribute to an intensely miserable child who may fear being handled because of pain.

Immunology – Mucosal integrity and several immunological processes are affected. Infection is common and often overwhelming. T-cell maturation is reduced. Abnormalities of collagen formation probably contribute to reduced resistance to infection at cutaneous portals of entry.

Both oxidized and reduced forms of ascorbic acid are found in tissues, suggesting that ascorbic acid has a role in reactions involving electron transfer. Along with vitamin E, riboflavin, selenium and glutathione, ascorbic acid controls the generation of free radicals.

In the absence of vitamin C normal collagen is replaced by a non-fibrous precursor. The hydroxylation of proline to form hydroxyproline, an important

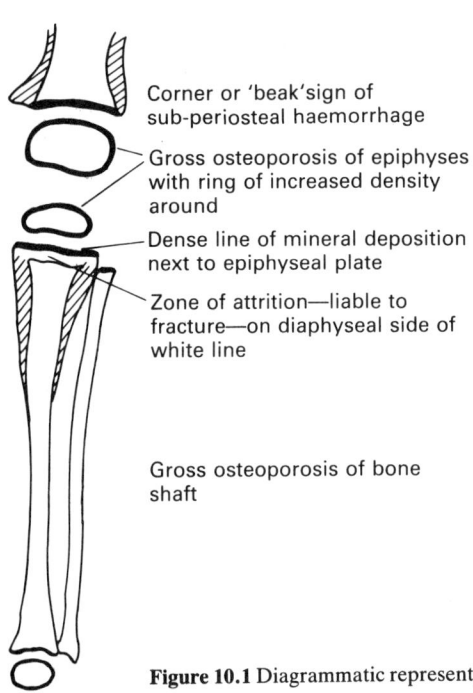

Figure 10.1 Diagrammatic representation of skeletal changes of scurvy.

Labels on figure:
- Corner or 'beak' sign of sub-periosteal haemorrhage
- Gross osteoporosis of epiphyses with ring of increased density around
- Dense line of mineral deposition next to epiphyseal plate
- Zone of attrition—liable to fracture—on diaphyseal side of white line
- Gross osteoporosis of bone shaft

constituent of collagen, requires transfer of a free hydroxy radical from ascorbic acid.

In premature infants transient neonatal tyrosinaemia may develop with high protein intakes and relative vitamin C deficiency. Reducing protein intake to 2–3/kg/day and ascorbic acid supplementation to 50–100 mg/kg/day usually cures the tyrosinaemia. The condition appears to be due to inhibition of p-hydroxyphenylpyruvic acid oxidase in the presence of either a build-up of substrate or a deficiency of vitamin C (Wharton, 1987).

Deficiency of vitamin C takes several months to develop since body stores are extensive. Thus it is usually infants in the second half of the first year of life who develop signs unless the mother is herself vitamin C deficient. Stores are depleted

Table 10.12 Diagnostic tests for ascorbic acid deficiency

Test	Normal result	Comments
Plasma ascorbic acid	>0.6 mg/dl	Indicates inadequate recent intake *not* necessarily deficiency state when low
Buffy coat (white cell and platelet) ascorbic acid	>0.1 mg/dl	Better indicator of true deficiency than plasma level. More difficult to measure
Effect of loading dose of ascorbic acid	>80% test dose excreted within 3–5 hours after parenterally administered dose	Delayed excretion demonstrates true tissue deficiency

more rapidly in trauma, burns, infection or other conditions leading to rapid cell turnover and increased tissue growth. Diagnosis is made by demonstrating absence of vitamin C in the buffy coat (white cell and platelet layer) of centrifuged blood (*Table 10.12*).

Treatment of scurvy is with oral ascorbic acid 200 mg daily for a week followed by 25–50 mg daily by mouth. Response is dramatic but radiological changes may take a year to resolve.

Vitamin D deficiency: nutritional rickets

Rickets should be considered as a clinical syndrome for which there are a variety of causes, not all of which relate to nutrition or to vitamin D metabolism. *Tables 10.13* and *10.14* list the various disease processes leading to the rickets syndrome. Nutritional- or sunlight-deficiency rickets was exceedingly common in temperate Europe until the 1950s but has rapidly become a condition seen only in those with malabsorption, those on abnormal diets or in immigrants with inappropriate customs and diets for the European climate. Outside Europe, however, 'nutritional' rickets is still a common disease of early childhood. Its adult counterpart, osteomalacia, is important for paediatric nutrition since infants born to affected women are likely to show congenital rickets (*see* Chapter 2).

Vitamin D has two main sources. It can come from the diet or from synthesis in the skin. Dietary sources are relatively few. Vitamin D is found in mammalian and fish liver, the flesh of oily fish (herring, mackerel, sardine, salmon), egg yolk, foods which are fortified with vitamin D such as margarine, tinned milks and infant foods, and – to a lesser extent – dairy produce, particularly where there has been fat concentration as in cheese and cream. Butter and milk contain relatively small amounts of vitamin D. Animal products contain the cholecalciferol form of vitamin

Table 10.13 'Nutritional' rickets

Clinical condition	Aetiology

Vitamin D deficiency rickets	Insufficient vitamin D from diet or skin synthesis to meet needs for metabolism and growth
	May be exacerbating conditions:
	  Malabsorption: cystic fibrosis; coeliac disease; cholestasis.
	  Gut binding of 25 (OH)D or calcium by phytates.[*][†]
	  Increased metabolism: anticonvulsants[‡] – phenytoin, phenobarbitone, carbamazepine; steroids.
	  Increased requirements with catch-up growth

Substrate deficiency rickets: 'rickets of prematurity', 'bone disease of VLBW'	May be due to inadequate vitamin if infant not supplemented; commonly results from deficiency of phosphate; calcium; protein; copper[§]; calcium loss may be exacerbated by diuretics
Alkali-induced rickets	More common in adults; phosphate binding in gut due to excessive aluminium hydroxide ingestion

[*] Robertson *et al.*, 1981.
[†] Wills *et al.*, 1972.
[‡] Hunter *et al.*, 1971.
[§] Brooke and Lucas, 1985.

Table 10.14 Non-nutritional rickets syndromes

Clinical condition	Aetiology
Congenital	
Familial vitamin D dependency	Presents as severe infantile rickets. Inborn error in one hydroxylation of 25 (OH)D. Responds to high dose vitamin D or to 1 α (OH)D. Autosomal recessive condition
Familial hypophosphataemic vitamin D resistance	Tubular disorder of phosphate retention. Loss of phosphate in urine. Sex-linked dominant so boys more affected than girls. Presents as rickets in second year of life with bone changes but no hypotonia. Very low serum phosphate. Normocalcaemia
Other tubular disorders	Tubular loss of phosphate and other metabolites such as water, sodium, potassium, amino acids, glucose
Acquired:	
Tubular disorders secondary to renal damage	Presentation similar to congenital tubular disorders.
Renal rickets	See Chapter 17.
Tumour rickets	Aetiology uncertain. Tends to improve with resolution of tumour

D – vitamin D_3. Fortified foods may be fortified with cholecalciferol or, more commonly, with an irradiated derivative of plant ergosterols – ergocalciferol (vitamin D_2). Although New World monkeys cannot utilize ergocalciferol, there is no evidence for this limitation in man.

The other, and in most cases much more important, source of vitamin D is by synthesis in the skin following sunlight irradiation. The vitamin D precursor in the skin, 7-dehydrocholesterol, is converted to cholecalciferol when subjected to ultraviolet light of wavelength around 300 nm. Sunlight of this wavelength is only present in the higher latitudes of Europe in the summer months. Thus not only the extent of exposure to sunshine but the timing of exposure is significant for the formation of vitamin D in the skin.

Both ergo- and cholecalciferol are transported to the liver where they are hydroxylated to 25 hydroxy vitamin D (25(OH)D). From the liver 25(OH)D is transported bound in plasma to 25(OH)D binding protein. In the kidney further hydroxylation results in the formation of the chief active metabolite, 1–25 dihydroxy vitamin D (1–25(OH)$_2$D), as required (*Figure 10.2*).

1–25(OH)$_2$D is probably formed in the mitochondria of cells lining the proximal renal tubule. It may also be formed in the placenta and in some sarcoid granulomata (Weisman *et al.*, 1979). One-hydroxylation is stimulated by low levels of 1–25(OH)$_2$D, parathormone, low serum calcium and low serum phosphate. The effects of the active hormone are to increase calcium absorption in the small intestine both directly and through stimulating synthesis of calcium binding protein. 1–25(OH)$_2$D, together with parathormone, also stimulates osteoclast activity in bone. Reorganization of bone and mineralization of osteoid take place thus enabling bone growth.

Stimulation of osteoclastic activity may seem curious since this resorbs bone. But the combination of increased calcium from the gut and calcium and phosphate from bone, raises the calcium phosphate product in active areas of bone and cartilage and results in deposition of new mineral.

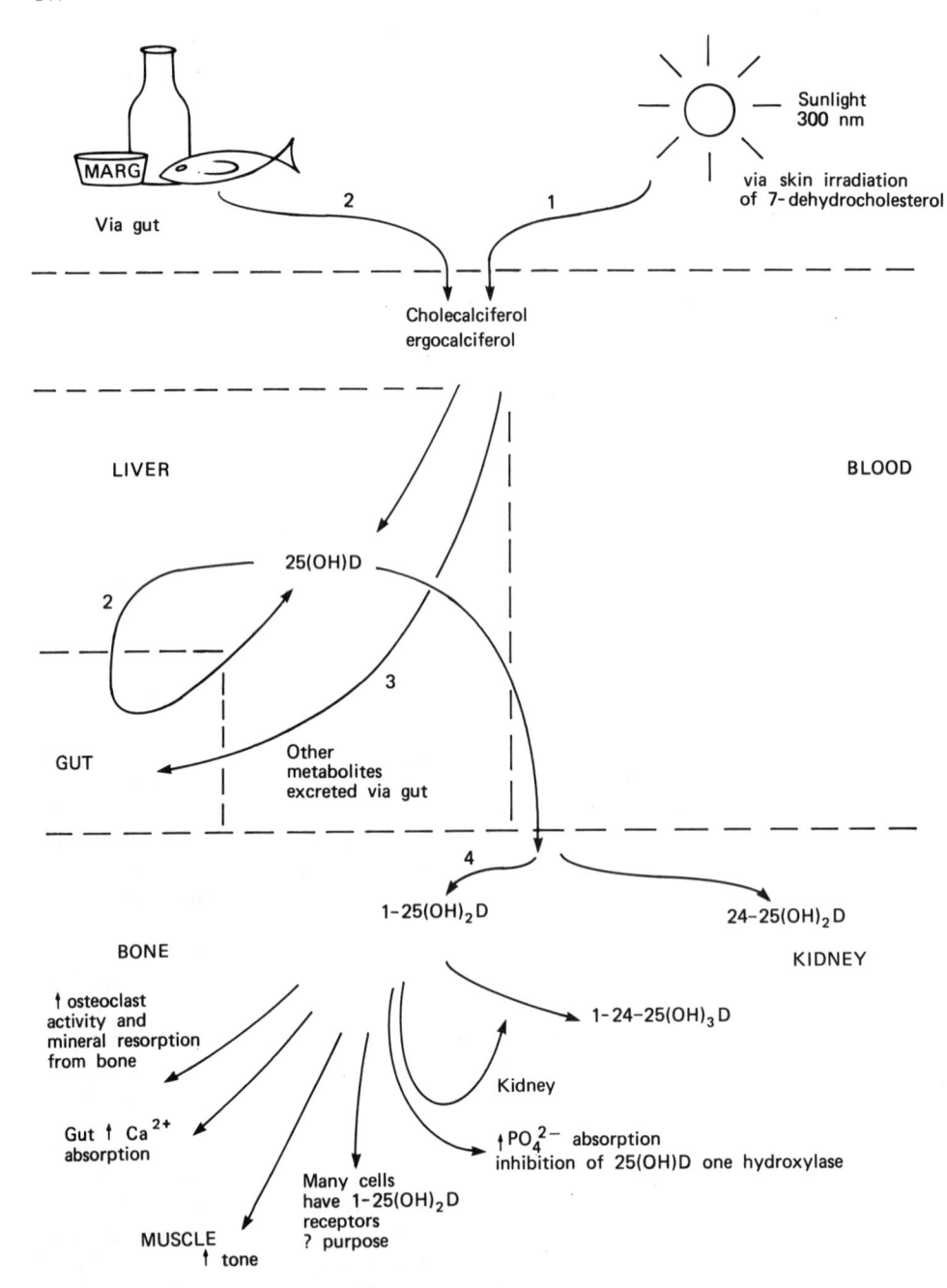

Figure 10.2 Vitamin D metabolism (simplified!). 1 = Skin pigmentation may influence conversion of 7 dehydrocholesterol under conditions of minimum sunlight exposure. 2 = High phytate content of diet or poor fat absorption binds vitamin D and metabolites in gut thus increasing requirements. 3 = Excretion of inactive polar metabolites increased by anticonvulsants. 4 = Reduced 1-hydroxylation in chronic renal failure; 1-hydroxylase stimulated by parathormore therefore low in hypoparathyroidism. Net effect of 1–25 (OH)$_2$D: increased Ca and phosphate in blood and at bone surface leading to bone mineral deposition.

The presence of 1–25(OH)$_2$D, high calcium levels and diminished parathormone, reduce synthesis of 1–25(OH)$_2$D from 25(OH)D and encourage formation of 24–25(OH)$_2$D and other metabolites in the kidney. Some of these metabolites, including 25(OH)D, can exert similar effects to 1–25(OH)$_2$D when administered in pharmacological doses (*Figure 10.2*). Whether they have physiological effects on metabolism is not certain.

The effects of 1–25(OH)$_2$D are chiefly on calcium and phosphorus regulation and the mineralization of bones, but the presence of receptors in many cells suggests that the vitamin-pro-hormone (i.e. 1–25(OH)$_2$D) has more widespread effects than have been previously considered.

Since the work of Chick in 1919 (Chick, 1976) in Vienna after the First World War, when it was shown that both dietary vitamin D and summer sunlight could cure rickets, there has been debate about whether sources from the diet or from the skin are more important for maintenance for normal D metabolism. It seems clear that where there is deficiency of either sunlight or diet, rickets can be prevented by a sufficiency of the other vitamin source. However, plasma 25(OH)D levels show a marked seasonal variation in temperate latitudes with peak values in Britain in late August and lowest values in late February. There seems little evidence that dietary intakes vary sufficiently to account for this pattern and thus skin synthesis of the vitamin appears most relevant to maintenance of adequate circulating 25(OH)D levels (Poskitt, Cole and Lawson, 1979).

Features of rickets: clinical findings

Rickets in the premature has been described in Chapter 5 but it seems likely that many of the cases of 'rickets' in that age group are due to deficiency of substrate rather than of vitamin D provided basic supplementation with vitamin D is provided. The condition may be more appropriately termed 'bone disease of prematurity'.

Rickets due to vitamin D deficiency occurs in newborn infants when mothers have osteomalacia. The condition is manifest in swellings at the end of the metaphyses of the limbs, 'rickety rosary' due to swelling of costochondral junctions, soft skull with large fontanelles and generalized hypotonia. Hypotonia and soft ribcage may lead to respiratory distress syndrome. These infants often present with jitteriness and convulsions secondary to hypocalcaemia. In the newborn period and in early infancy, infants either do not mount significant parathyroid response to falling calcium or they are unable to respond to parathormone secretion by increased calcium mobilization. Consequently, calcium levels fall and convulsions occur. The situation may be exacerbated in the neonatal period by maternal secondary hyperparathyroidism induced by maternal vitamin D deficiency. Increased parathormone crosses the placenta so that at birth infants have relatively suppressed parathyroids and consequently severe rebound hypocalcaemia in the neonatal period.

Classically, the child with rickets is around 1 year of age and weaned. The history of exposure to summer sunlight is poor. Children who have not been weaned and who are totally breast fed, particularly by D-deficient mothers, or who are being fed unsupplemented cows' milk, are also likely to develop rickets in the absence of adequate sunlight exposure, since vitamin D concentrations both in breast milk and in cows' milk are low. Vitamin D in breast milk seems adequate to maintain normal mineral absorption from human milk in early infancy. Thus vitamin D deficiency rickets is usually a complication of infants breast fed for *prolonged* periods only, provided mothers have adequate vitamin D nutrition.

The symptoms of rickets are generalized, with apathy and misery secondary to bone pain. There may be recurrent chest infections due to hypotonia and the soft bony ribcage prevents adequate clearing of secretions from the chest by coughing. Classical signs are illustrated in *Figure 10.3*. The soft bony skeleton tends to be

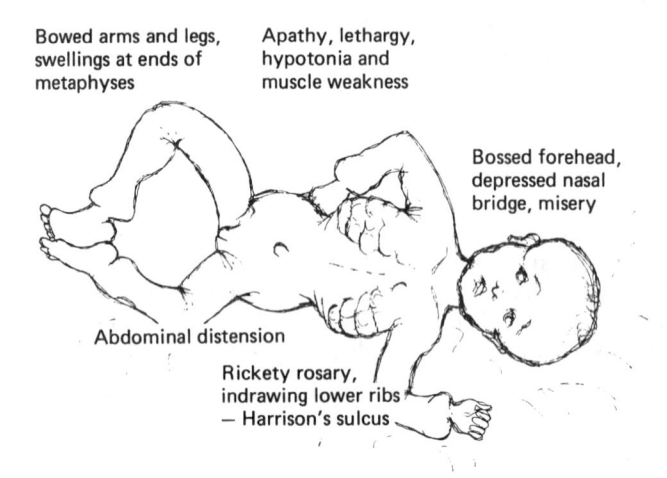

Figure 10.3 Clinical features of rickets.

pulled in around the attachment of the diaphragm, creating Harrison's sulcus. The children are reluctant to walk and weight bear, although they may have been walking prior to the development of rickets. Weight-bearing bones tend to be bowed so that in infants around 6 months the arms are typically bowed; whereas in children over a year, bowing of the legs may be more obvious. There is swelling at the end of the metaphyses showing as lumps just proximal to the joints at the wrists, knees and ankles particularly. Flaring at the end of the bony ribs creates the knobbly appearance of the costochondral junctions – the rickety rosary. Softening and poor development of the skull bones leads to bulging of the skull anteriorly and posteriorly – craniotabes. There is overall poor muscle tone, and abdominal distension may be marked. Linear growth is retarded, and short stature may be marked. Other nutrient deficiencies may be present.

In older children the symptoms and signs are less dramatic, although poor linear growth is usual and there is considerable bone pain. The tendency for the legs to bow may be counteracted by internal rotation of the limbs and a knock-knee posture.

Biochemical findings

The usual findings in nutritional rickets are serum calcium levels which are low or in the low normal range; low serum phosphate and greatly raised alkaline phosphatase. In young infants hypocalcaemia may be more marked and hypophosphataemia less marked. As already explained, young infants may be relatively resistant to the secondary hyperparathyroidism that accompanies most vitamin D deficiency rickets and which tends to restore calcium to more or less normal levels whilst increasing phosphaturia. Generalized aminoaciduria occurs in nutritional rickets as well as being a feature of some of the vitamin D resistant rickets syndromes (*see Table 10.14*).

Radiological appearances

Figure 10.4 delineates the features of classical 'nutritional' rickets seen on X-ray. Whereas the changes in gross cases are obvious and indisputable, controversy often reigns over whether changes are present in borderline cases. The changes are due to failure of calcification of osteoid tissue and build-up of osteoid at the metaphyses. Healing produces zones of provisional calcification at the ends of the metaphyses.

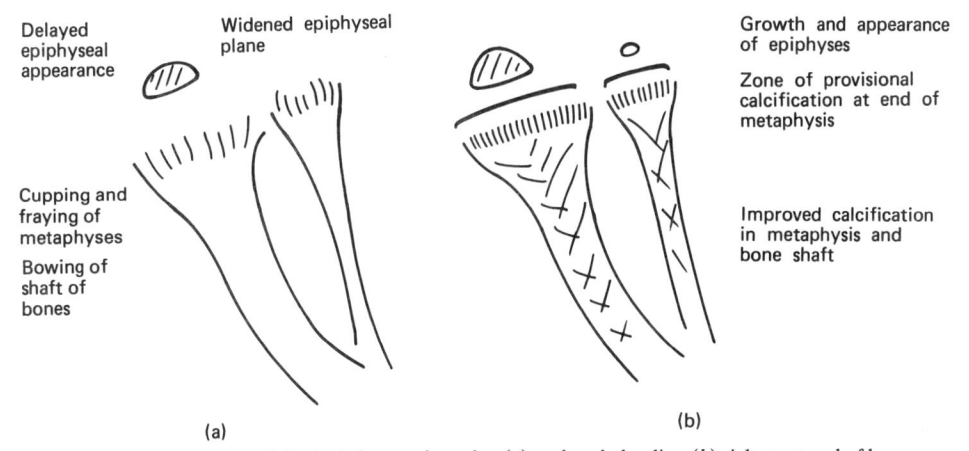

Figure 10.4 Diagram of radiological changes in active (*a*) and early healing (*b*) rickets at end of long bones.

Rickets in British immigrants

Whereas 'nutritional' rickets is seen rarely in otherwise healthy Caucasian infants in Britain, it has until recently been exceedingly common in immigrants from the Indian sub-continent resident in Britain. Probably as the result of a widespread public health campaign, rickets in this particular group seems to be declining in prevalence, and many of the cases now seen are in other immigrants from the Horn of Africa and the Arabian peninsula. Why should these groups be so susceptible to rickets? This issue has never been completely resolved, partly because it seems likely that the cause of the prevalence of rickets in these groups is multifactorial. A genetic predisposition may be particularly common in these racial groups, but there has been no substantial evidence to support this view. Rickets is seen quite commonly in India. Almost certainly the predisposition to rickets depends on environmental factors, most notably diet and those customs that influence the amount of summer sunlight exposure.

Dietary factors
The diets of many British children are low in vitamin D. Whilst children from the Indian subcontinent and the Middle East may have even lower intakes of vitamin D, it seems unlikely that the level of intake is the most relevant factor in their predisposition to rickets. It is sometimes stated that West Indians in Britain tend to eat more margarine (which is supplemented with vitamin D) and this is why, despite their dark skins, they do not seem to be particularly at risk of rickets. This may be true, but in many ways West Indians have integrated more into the British way of life than families from the Indian sub-continent and cultural rather than dietary factors may still be very relevant to the differences in the prevalence of rickets.

With the exception of rickets of prematurity, the rickets syndrome, when its causes are dietary, is usually considered to be due to deficiency of vitamin D. Yet it is almost impossible to make young rats develop rickets unless they are not only vitamin D but phosphate deficient as well. The importance of calcium and phosphate in the development or prevention of rickets in the presence of inadequate vitamin D in man is not determined. In Ireland in the Second World War, increased extraction of the flour (resulting in greater phytate or fibre content) was associated with an increased prevalence of rickets in children over a year of age (Robertson *et al.*, 1981). Infants still predominantly breast-milk fed and not eating cereal or bread did not show the same increase in prevalence. The prevalence of rickets declined again with calcium supplementation of the flour. It has been suggested that the high phytate content of unrefined flour such as that used in wartime or used for making the typical Indian breads (chappatis, parathas, popadums, etc.) causes binding of calcium in the gut and relative calcium malabsorption, thus contributing to the development of rickets. Under such circumstances an increased vitamin D intake may be necessary to mobilize calcium from the gut.

It has also been suggested that phytate in the small intestine binds 25(OH)D secreted into the bile within the gut lumen and prevents its reabsorption from the jejunal and ileal mucosa. Thus requirements for vitamin D are increased again. Whilst phytate may bind calcium in the gut, there is little evidence that it has a significant effect in interfering with the enterohepatic circulation of 25(OH)D.

Environmental factors
Asian and Arab immigrants to this country live in relatively poor circumstances and occupy the older areas of British cities. Old city-centre houses rarely have gardens and are close together. Opportunities for children to be exposed to significant amounts of British summer sunlight may be restricted. Traditional customs and religious attitudes encourage girls to remain covered up and small children to stay at home with their mothers who remain predominantly indoors and well covered against sun or public gaze when they are outside.

Whilst the European child with pale skin may synthesize sufficient cholecalciferol in a poor summer, the pigmented skin of Asian and African peoples may act as a limiting factor to the rate at which cholecalciferol is synthesized when ultraviolet light of the appropriate wavelength is present in small quantities. These families may be unable to afford, or unwilling to enjoy, seaside holidays (where children and adults are most likely to expose themselves to sunshine), choosing either to return to their homeland and, coincidentally, build up their reserves of vitamin D; or to visit friends in other industrial towns in Britain. In our experience, summer holidays are important for maintaining reasonable circulating levels of 25(OH)D throughout the year (Poskitt, Cole and Lawson, 1979). The tendency of the British to brave the weather at the seaside, exposing their bodies in bathing costumes despite the cold, could be an important contributing factor to maintenance of sufficent cholecalciferol synthesis even in cool, wet summers!

These explanations can be used to account for rickets in Britain, but do not explain the presence of rickets amongst children in Nigeria, India and other sunny tropical countries. In southern Nigeria, the skies are frequently overcast and families may live in large, shady compounds so that exposure of small children to sunlight may be inadequate. Deficiency of minerals as well as dietary vitamin D could contribute to the development of rickets.

Treatment of nutritional rickets

Table 10.15 indicates relative needs for prevention and treatment of rickets. Where rickets has been produced by the metabolic effects of drugs or secondary to malabsorption, requirements are increased. In all these conditions treatment is with cholecalciferol, vitamin D. Synthetic 1-hydroxy vitamin D – alfacalcidol – (One Alpha; Leo) is very effective in controlling vitamin D resistant rickets, but is unnecessary and, due to its expense, unjustified, as treatment for *nutritional* rickets.

Table 10.15 Prevention and treatment of vitamin D deficiency rickets

	Dose of vitamin D (cholecalciferol or ergocalciferol)*†
Prevention	
Premature infants	10–20 µg/day
Infants <1 year	10 µg/day
Children/adolescents	2.5 µg/day
Treatment	
Daily regimen	100 µg daily for 4 weeks then daily preventive therapy
Single dose (stoss therapy)	10 mg once orally. May be repeated after 1 month if no healing

* These preventive recommendations probably greatly in excess of needs if child exposed to sunlight of appropriate wavelength for skin synthesis of vitamin D.
† 1 µg = 40 International Units.

Bone pain and hypotonia in children with nutritional rickets improve after about a week of treatment with vitamin D. Biochemistry takes a long time to return to normal as bone remodelling may take place over years. Initially, plasma calcium level may fall and alkaline phosphatase activity increase as bone mineralization occurs. Calcium and phosphate levels then gradually return to normal but alkaline phosphatase levels may remain elevated for a year or more as growth, healing and remodelling occur.

Treatment of non-nutritional rickets

Management of these conditions varies. Alfacalcidol (One Alpha; Leo), a 1-hydroxylated synthetic vitamin D, should be used for treatment instead of vitamin D since huge pharmacological doses of vitamin D derivatives are usually required and the shorter half life of alfacalcidol means that overdoses can be rapidly corrected. In familial vitamin D dependency rickets relatively low levels of alfacalcidol may be effective since the condition appears to be due to abnormalities in synthesis or response to 1–25(OH)$_2$D. Management of renal tubular defects and hypophosphataemic vitamin D resistant rickets is through phosphate replacement with alfacalcidol to encourage bone mineralization. Alfacalcidol is essential therapy for renal rickets (where shortage of 1–25(OH)$_2$D is part of the explanation for the bony disease) since poor renal function is usually the cause of deficiency of 1-hydroxylated vitamin D (*see* Chapter 17).

In large doses vitamin D has major side effects. The effects of large doses on calcium levels must be monitored. In Britain in the 1950s supplementation of infant foods with vitamin D was excessively enthusiastic, and infants and young children occasionally received very high daily intakes. Some infants appeared hypersensitive to vitamin D and developed hypercalcaemia on relatively small vitamin D supplements. All individuals if grossly overtreated with vitamin D can show symptoms of vitamin D intoxication: anorexia, constipation, polydipsia, polyuria, failure to thrive, ectopic calcification and renal failure. Infants who were over-treated with vitamin D in the 1950s tended to present with failure to thrive, vomiting, constipation and hypercalcaemia. Some of these children improved when their vitamin D intakes were reduced, but others, who classically showed characteristic facies and cardiac defects, had more resistant symptomatology. This latter group of children has now been described as the Williams–van Beuren–hypercalcaemia–abnormal facies syndrome complex (Williams' syndrome for short!).

Williams' syndrome

These are children with characteristic facies of high forehead, epicanthic folds, depressed nasal bridge with anteverted nostrils, long upper lip with pronounced bow, mental retardation, short stature, supravalvular aortic stenosis and hypercalcaemia in early life. Hypertension may also be present. Some children show these phenotypic features but do not show hypercalcaemia. In the classic Williams' syndrome, treatment of the hypercalcaemia with a low-calcium diet improves vomiting, constipation and polyuria, but does not affect mental development nor the cardiac problem significantly. Hypercalcaemia when present should be treated with a low-calcium, low-vitamin D diet (Locasol New Formula; Cow & Gate). Normal vitamin preparations must be excluded. Vitamin A supplementation is advisable for older children on weaning diets since the vitamin A from the milk may be inadequate. Ro-A-Vit (Roche) as 400–800 RE/day is suitable. Dietary management (Francis, 1987) should be maintained until at least 6 months after the return of serum calcium to normal values. Vitamin D supplementation must *not* be given.

Recent studies have variously suggested that abnormalities in 25(OH)D, calcitonin or parathormone metabolism may be responsible for the hypercalcaemia of Williams' syndrome (Taylor, Stern and Bell, 1982; Culler, Jones and Deftos, 1985).

Immobilization

Children with vitamin D resistant rickets syndromes or other conditions requiring high doses of vitamin D or alfacalcidol are likely to develop hypercalcaemia on their *usual* daily dose of vitamin during periods of immobilization. This is particularly important in the case of children with vitamin D resistant rickets where they may be on very high doses of alfacalcidol and where immobilization following surgery for correction of bony deformity is likely. Vitamin D preparations should stop a few weeks before immobilization is anticipated. Alfacalcidol has a shorter duration of action and can be stopped 1 week before immobilization. Serum calcium levels during immobilization and orthopaedic manoeuvres must be closely monitored. Calcium levels above 2.5 mmol/l suggest that the vitamin D preparation dosage should be reduced.

Vitamin E deficiency

Neonatal vitamin E deficiency has been discussed in Chapters 4 and 5. In older children vitamin E deficiency has only been shown recently to have clinical manifestations (Harding *et al.*, 1982). In abetalipoproteinaemia (*see* Chapter 15) correction of low circulating levels of vitamin E modifies or prevents the development of neurological signs of the later stages of the condition (Muller, Lloyd and Bird, 1977). Children with abetalipoproteinaemia have steatorrhoea. Since vitamin E is a fat-soluble vitamin, malabsorption is likely.

More recently, some older children and adults with cystic fibrosis have developed neurological signs similar to those that develop in abetalipoproteinaemia (Bye *et al.*, 1985). It is now felt advisable for children with cystic fibrosis and other fat malabsorption syndromes to receive supplementary vitamin E from the time of diagnosis (*see* Chapter 15).

Vitamin K deficiency

Haemorrhagic disease of the newborn has been described in earlier chapters. Vitamin K deficiency in older children is rare except in those on unsupplemented parenteral feeding: on artificial diets; with heavy antibiotic therapy; or with severe steatorrhoea, liver disease or both. Treatment is with supplementary vitamin K 2–5 mg daily either orally or by intramuscular injections, depending on the principal cause. Intramuscular injections are best avoided when there is overt bleeding. Intravenous injections (phytomenadione) should be given very slowly.

References

BROOKE, O. G. and LUCAS, A. (1985) Metabolic bone disease in preterm infants. *Archives of Disease in Childhood*, **60**, 682–685

BYE, A. M. E., MULLER, D. P. R., WILSON, J., WRIGHT, V. H. and MEARNS, M. B. (1985) Symptomatic vitamin E deficiency in cystic fibrosis. *Archives of Disease in Childhood*, **60**, 162–164

CHICK, H. (1976) Study of rickets in Vienna, 1919–1922. *Medical History*, **20**, 41–51

CULLER, F. L., JONES, K. L. and DEFTOS, L. J. (1985) Impaired calcitonin secretion in patients with William's syndrome. *Journal of Pediatrics*, **107**, 720–723

DEPARTMENT OF HEALTH AND SOCIAL SECURITY (1979) *Recommended Amounts of Food Energy and Nutrients for Groups of People in the United Kingdom*. London: Her Majesty's Stationery Office

FOOD AND NUTRITION BOARD (1975) *Recommended Dietary Allowances*, 8th edn. Washington: National Academy Press

FRANCIS, D. E. M. (1987) *Diets for Sick Children*, 4th edn., p. 330. Oxford: Blackwell Scientific

HARDING, A. E., MULLER, D. P. R., THOMAS, P. K. and WILLISON, H. J. (1982) Spinocerebellar degeneration secondary to chronic intestinal malabsorption: a vitamin E deficiency syndrome. *Annals of Neurology,* **12,** 419–424

HUNTER, J., MAXWELL, J. D., STEWARD, D. A., PARSONS, V. and WILLIAMS, R. (1971) Altered calcium metabolism in epileptic children on anticonvulsants. *British Medical Journal,* **ii,** 202–204

LUCAS, A. and BATES, C. (1984) Transient riboflavin depletion in preterm infants. *Archives of Disease in Childhood,* **59,** 837–841

MULLER, D. P. R., LLOYD, J. K. and BIRD, A. C. (1977) Long term management of abetalipoproteinaemia: possible role for vitamin E. *Archives of Disease in Childhood,* **52,** 209–214

OSKI, F. A. (1985) Nutritional anaemias. *Nutrition in Pediatrics: Basic Science and Clinical Applications,* edited by W. A. Walker and J. B. Watkins, pp. 707–726. Boston: Little Brown

POSKITT, E. M. E., COLE, T. J. and LAWSON, D. E. M. (1979) Diet, sunlight and 25-hydroxyvitamin D in healthy children and adults. *British Medical Journal,* **i,** 221–223

ROBERTSON, I., FORD, J. A., McINTOSH, W. B. and DUNNIGAN, M. G. (1981) The role of cereals in the aetiology of nutritional rickets: the lesson of the Irish National Nutrition Survey, 1943–8. *British Journal of Nutrition,* **41,** 17–22

SCHWARTZ, K. B. (1985) Vitamins. *Nutrition in Pediatrics: Basic Science and Clinical Application,* edited by W. A Walker and J. B. Watkins, pp. 47–75. Boston: Little Brown

SOMMER, A., TARWOTJO, I., HUSSAINI, G., SUSANTO, D. and SOEGIHARTO, T. (1981) Incidence, prevalence and scale of blinding malnutrition. *Lancet,* **i,** 1407–1408

STANTON, B. F., CLEMENS, J. D., WOJTYNIAK, B. and KHEIR, T. (1986) Risk factors for developing mild nutritional blindness in urban Bangladesh. *American Journal of Disease in Children,* **140,** 584–588

TAYLOR, A. B., STERN, P. H. and BELL, N. H. (1982) Abnormal regulation of circulating 25-hydroxyvitamin D in the Williams' syndrome. *New England Journal of Medicine,* **306,** 972–974

TOMKINS, A. (1986) Intestinal parasites: nutritional importance. *Diarrhoea and Malnutrition in Childhood,* edited by J. A. Walker-Smith and A. S. McNeish, pp. 60–67. London: Butterworths

WEISMAN, T., HARELL, A., EDELSTEIN, S., DAVID, M., SPIRER, Z. and GOLANDER, A. (1979) 1–25 dihydroxyvitamin D3 and 24–25 dihydroxyvitamin D3 *in vitro* synthesis by human decidua and placenta. *Nature,* **281,** 317–319

WHARTON, B. A. (1987) *Nutrition and Feeding of Preterm Infants.* Oxford: Blackwell Scientific

WHO/FAO AD HOC EXPERT COMMITTEE (1973) *Energy and Protein Requirements.* WHO Technical Reports, Series No. 522. Geneva: World Health Organisation.

WILLS, M. R., DAY, R. C., PHILLIPS, J. B. and BATEMAN, E. C. (1972) Phytic acid and nutritional rickets in immigrants. *Lancet,* **i,** 771–773

Chapter 11
Problems of vegetarian and unusual diets

The mixing of races and religions that has taken place in this and other countries, particularly over the past 40 years, has led to great changes in national diets (Carlson, Kipps and Thomson, 1984). Curry, yoghurt, pizza, boiled rice and similar foods are now 'everyday' British food when they used to be exotic menu items. The increased variety these foods bring to the national diet are likely to benefit children since eating a variety of foods is the best way to avoid deficiencies of trace nutrients. Appreciation of variety in food taste and consistency might also reduce the faddy and finicky appetites shown by many children. The interest and inspiration from other races and religions which have come with some of the searches for new and exotic foods have also brought an increase in the numbers of people who see dietary regimens as providing purpose and meaning to life through self-discipline. At times this leads to the adoption of very restrictive, bizarre diets. It is these unusual and rigid diets that may present risks for children, rather than the inclusion of foreign foods or adoption of well-established but foreign dietary practices within the traditional diet.

Vegetarian diets

Vegetarian implies avoidance of meat but the term encompasses a number of dietary practices, the main examples of which are outlined:

Semi-vegetarian — Often eat meats other than red meat, e.g. fish, chicken; usually individual preferences.
Lacto-ovo-vegetarian — Eat no meat but eat dairy products and eggs.
Lactovegetarian — Eat dairy products but no eggs.
Total vegetarian (vegan: non lacto-ovo-vegetarian) — Eat neither dairy products nor eggs; no animal products.
Yogic vegetarian — Lacto-ovo-vegetarians but stress natural and unprocessed foods.
Hare Krishnas — Lactovegetarians but stress natural and unprocessed foods.
Rastafarian — Orthodox avoid all animal products, alcohol, salt, canned foods and concentrate on chemical-free, organic, foods; some drink milk.
Macrobiotics (Zen) — Ten dietary regimens (-3 to +7), all naturally grown foods; gradual exclusion of many foods as dietary regimens increased; liquids used sparingly.

Additive avoidance, non-allergenic diets — Concentrate on naturally grown 'additive free', foods; should only be adopted after medical advice.

Groups and individuals who for emotional, religious or personal reasons avoid eating meat have probably existed since man first became a hunter as well as gatherer. Vegetarian diets which include milk products and eggs carry little risk of nutrient deficiency for children. Since such diets are usually rich in fibre, relatively low in saturated fat, and not energy dense, they may even carry advantages for health (*see* Chapter 21). Many toddlers on normal diets are reluctant to eat meat so lacto-ovo-vegetarian diets may differ little from those of children not on specifically meat-free diets. Well-planned lacto-ovo-vegetarian diets with pulses, cereals, cheese, milk and eggs, may even result in diets that approach nutrient requirements for a wider variety of nutrients than many typical toddler diets. It may be helpful to design diets using the food grouping method outlined in *Table 8.9*.

General problems in relation to vegetarian diets

Energy
The relatively low energy density of many vegetarian foods can cause problems for young children who are only able to consume the necessary bulk to meet requirements if fed frequently (Shull *et al.*, 1977; McLean and Graham, 1980). Weanlings and toddlers reared on these diets should be fed at least four times a day with meals containing a substantial source of energy.

Protein
Vegetarian diets require more planning than omnivorous diets. Many plant proteins do not contain all the essential amino acids and their protein is of relatively low biological value. The biological value of vegetable proteins can be increased by combining poor sources of particular essential amino acids with good sources of these amino acids so that the protein value of the meal is enhanced. This is easier if milk, other dairy products and eggs are consumed since the essential amino acid content of these products is high and thus the need for other essential amino acid sources less.

Milk and dairy products should be eaten in combination with plant protein sources. With vegans, the need to mix or complement proteins to increase the net protein utilization of the diet becomes critical to the nutritional adequacy of the dietary regimen (*Table 11.1*). Considerable nutritional knowledge or adherence to

Table 11.1 Complementary protein combinations for vegetarian diets

Dairy products:	High in lysine and isoleucine; use with cereals or nuts and seeds*
Legumes	Low in tryptophan and sulphur-containing amino acids; use with grains, seeds and potatoes
Grains:	Low in isoleucine and lysine; use with milk and yeast or with legumes, potatoes, vegetables
Dark green, leafy vegetables	Overall protein content fairly low (5%) but relatively high concentration of sulphur-containing amino acids; use with legumes. Good source of vitamin A

* Nuts and seeds (unless well ground into forms such as peanut butter) should only be fed to older children because of the risks of choking and aspiration in small children.

dietary traditions which have allowed successful nutrition on these diets is necessary to avoid the risk of inadequate protein intake in vegan children, particularly amongst those in the weaning period. This diet has other problems also (*see below*).

Minerals
Iron deficiency is a greater risk for vegetarian than non-vegetarian children since meats are a good source of available iron. Haem iron is readily absorbed intact and facilitates the absorption of non-haem iron from many vegetable foods. This is in contrast to the iron in eggs which appears to inhibit iron absorption from non-haem-containing foods. Curry powder contains a very high level of iron (75 mg/100 g) but it is not certain how well it is absorbed. Vegetarian children should be encouraged to ensure a good intake of iron-containing foods (dark green vegetables and legumes, particularly lentils, chick peas and peas). When iron-containing foods are mixed with ascorbic-acid-containing fruits, absorption of iron is facilitated. Milk and cheese products should also be encouraged where acceptable. Children should be encouraged to continue to drink 500 ml of milk a day to maintain calcium intake. In infants this should be formula rather than cows' milk because of the added iron. Vegan children should be encouraged to take a soya-based *infant* formula as this helps meet needs for calcium and iron as well as protein. Very large intakes of milk reduce intakes of other foods and encourage iron deficiency due to dietary imbalance and even insidious blood loss due to cows' milk protein allergy, so should be discouraged. The phytate and fibre of vegetable products decreases the availability of calcium, zinc and other minerals for absorption so higher intakes of minerals are necessary than for children on mixed diets.

Vitamins
Two vitamins are obtained more or less entirely from animal products: B_{12} and D. Vitamin D is present in dairy products, although only in small amounts unless the products contain concentrated milk fat (cheese, cream). However, vitamin D is also added to margarines and to infant cereals. Moreover, the main source is probably skin synthesis in children beyond early infancy (who may have little sunshine exposure). Rickets is thus not very common in vegetarian children. Vitamin B_{12} is present in milk and eggs but without these the diet is likely to be deficient in B_{12}. Seaweed B_{12} content is very variable and extracts are unreliable sources.

Lactovegetarianism

Lactovegetarians eat dairy products but no eggs. Their diet is therefore slightly more restricted than the lacto-ovo-vegetarian diet. Ensuring adequate protein intake requires careful mixing of pulses, grains and dairy products in the diet. Adequate exposure to summer sunlight is important for maintaining vitamin D nutrition since its only source in the diet will be dairy products and fortified margarine and cereals.

Vitamin B_{12} is not found in plant foods except in fermented soy products and seaweed, when amounts may be variable. In pregnancy vitamin B_{12} is not readily mobilized from maternal stores and needs for both mother and fetus must be met from the maternal diet. The vitamin B_{12} content of milk and dairy products is not high. Mothers and children eating diets containing no animal products other than dairy produce should be given supplementary vitamin B_{12}, 1–3 µg daily, which (assuming intrinsic factor production is normal) can be given orally.

Vegans

Here the potential problems are great. Vegans consume no animal products and thus egg and dairy products are excluded from the diet. Children may have difficulty consuming adequate protein, energy, calcium, minerals (especially iron and zinc), vitamins B_{12} D and even riboflavin to meet requirements. Vitamin (including B_{12}) and iron supplements are advisable for all vegan children.

Vegetable protein sources must be varied and should include grains and legumes as frequent meals together with mixed coloured vegetables and fruits. Soya flour is high in energy, protein and minerals but relatively low in methionine. Rice is, however, quite rich in methionine. They complement one another. Mixing different grains, as well as mixing grains with legumes and pulses, is also important (Lappe, 1974). Many legumes and pulses require prolonged soaking and cooking before they are digestible.

Growth of vegan children should be monitored regularly and parents advised on ways of increasing energy intakes by adding vegetable fats and oils to the diet and feeding frequent energy-dense snacks to small children.

Studies from the United States suggest that vegan children do have some restriction of growth – presumably nutritional in origin – in the post-weaning period (Hardinge and Stare, 1954; Shull *et al.*, 1977). There are few comparable studies of vegan children in UK since these children are commonly of different racial origins than other British children and may consequently have different growth patterns.

Rastafarians are one of the groups in Britain who may follow a vegan diet. Not all Rastafarians pursue strict meat-, salt- and alcohol-free diets, but those who do follow any dietary practice normally make a point of eating 'whole', organic or chemical-free foods (Springer and Thomas, 1983). This may lead them to avoid giving infants readily available tinned and packaged weaning foods. Foods that are acceptable may be more expensive since they are bought in small, often 'health food' stores rather than big supermarkets. The nutritional quality of infant foods from these stores is variable. Lack of variety in infant foods on sale may mean the diet is nutritionally very limited. If these alternative foods are nutritionally deficient, it is the weanlings who are at particular nutritional risk. Since many Rastafarians in Britain come from poor inner-city environments, these infants may become caught in a vicious circle of deficient diet, infection and deteriorating nutrition (*see* Chapter 6).

Zen macrobiotic diets

The Zen way of life does not have a large following in Britain so far, but followers are not uncommon in the United States. Major nutritional problems – kwashiorkor and marasmus – are seen in children whose parents adhere to strict Zen regimens. The way of life demands ever-increasing levels of dietary restriction with gradual elimination of foods until the highest level of brown rice and limited water intake is reached. Children should remain at the lower levels of the dietary regimens in order to prevent dietary deficiencies and restricted growth. The traditional infant formula for children of Zen adherents is a gruel of cereal, beans and water and is of very low energy density. It is thoroughly dangerous for infants and puts them at risk of major malnutrition (Roberts et al., 1979; Zmora, Gorodischer and Bar-Ziv, 1979) or death from overwhelming infection secondary to poor nutrition. The addition of honey to this formula in order to increase its energy content has been associated with cases of botulism in infants in the USA and is also undesirable (Arnon et al., 1979). Where parents insist their children adhere to these regimens, growth must be very closely monitored and vitamin and mineral supplements provided. Breast milk from mothers on strict regimens may be relatively low in protein and vitamins. If they will accept them, these mothers should be given supplementary vitamins, including B_{12}, during breast feeding. When breast feeding ceases, parents should be encouraged to allow their children to accept soya infant formulas since these are reasonable sources of protein and are supplemented with iron and vitamins. Formula S (Cow & Gate) and Prosobee (Mead Johnson) are totally animal-product-free infant formulas. Soya 'milks' available in health food shops are not adequate alternatives since they are deficient in methionine, vitamins and iron.

Parents who wish their children to adhere to totally inappropriate dietary regimens are usually individuals who have 'opted out' of traditional society to a considerable degree and many neither seek advice about feeding their children, nor accept such advice when given. They have often rejected formal medical services and may practise herbal or spiritual healing. Education of sect leaders, healers and herbalists with whom the parents have contact and reasonable support may be the only practical line of approach for preventing malnutrition in the children. The alternative, if children's growth and health are suffering significantly from parental persistence with inappropriate diets, is to consider removing children from their families by legal intervention. This is not a happy conclusion nor an action to be undertaken lightly and is likely to increase the alienation of relevant groups.

Immigrant groups at risk of nutritional deficiency in Britain

The racial groups most at risk of childhood nutritional deficiencies in Britain today remain those whose origins, or parental origins, were the Indian subcontinent (Jivani, 1978). As these families become more integrated into British society and establish themselves in business, the risks diminish to some extent. Family traditions are maintained more readily than in some immigrant groups and change is often slow, particularly for girls and mothers who have less contact with other groups and may have their traditional ways reinforced by arranged marriages with men brought up in their home country (not easy given present immigration laws!). Family traditions probably help maintain traditional dietary practices where the use of mixed vegetable proteins and appropriate preparation of foods are likely to provide an adequate diet. However, traditional foods may be expensive in this country and poverty can be a relevant contributing factor to poor nutrition.

Many Asian groups are lacto-vegetarians or even vegans and thus subject to the problems discussed earlier. Their dark skin and usually urban habitat predispose to sunlight deficiency. Their diets are low in vitamin D – fats used tend to be ghee (clarified butter) rather than supplemented margarine – and have a high phytate content (from unrefined flour) which binds calcium, phosphate and vitamin D in the gut. Nutritional rickets has been, and still is, common in young Asian children in Britain. Nutritional education programmes within Asian communities have had only limited effect on circulating levels of 25(OH)D in Asians. The full explanation for the prevalence of rickets/osteomalacia in children and adults from the Indian subcontinent remains uncertain (Stephens et al., 1982).

Less well educated Asian women often continue to feed their children large volumes of milk rather than provide weaning diet late into the first year or even into the second and third years of life (Jivani, 1978). If children appear to refuse new foods, little effort is made to encourage acceptance. This has two effects. If the children eat very little except milk – usually by this stage cows' milk – marasmus and iron deficiency are common. If, on the other hand, the children consume large quantities of milk and also take substantial solids, they may present with obesity. The problem may arise from traditions of late weaning for children in the country of origin together with a belief that milk is good for children and therefore to be encouraged. Apathy towards making efforts to wean small children who are addicted to feeding from bottles may contribute to the problem. Sadly, the prevalence of breast feeding amongst Asian families in Britain is particularly low (Evans et al., 1976; McNeill, 1985).

West Indian children do not show the same risk of rickets as Asian children. The reasons for this are not obvious since their darker skin would seem to increase the risk of vitamin D deficiency. However, many West Indians follow British dietary habits such as consumption of margarine and white bread – which has less binding effect on vitamin D and calcium than the unrefined flour of Indian breads – as well as following more outdoor activities for the children, more Western clothes and occasionally greater prosperity. The cultural habit of a summer holiday by the sea seems relevant to the maintenance of adequate vitamin D nutrition throughout the year (Poskitt, Cole and Lawson, 1979). Perhaps the practice of seaside holidays has yet to spread to the Asian groups in this country.

Another nutritional risk for immigrant groups is the potentially greater risk of contamination of meat products obtained from traditional 'halal' butchers than from formal meat selling businesses. Episodes of gastroenteritis secondary to food-acquired infection may threaten nutritional status. Poor hygiene may also be relevant to diarrhoea and failure to thrive in toddlers who have prolonged bottle feeding. Bottles containing milk, formula or 'juice' and carried around by 2–3-year-old children have plenty of opportunity for contamination of teats or contents when put down, thrown down, offered to pets or carried around in mothers' shopping bags – happenings common with *any* mobile children still being fed from bottles.

Megavitamins and other eccentric diets

An alternative to the restrictive diets described above is the potentially more dangerous enthusiasm for vitamin supplements in 'mega' doses to prevent various perceived problems (Hanning and Zlotkin, 1985; Evans and Lacey, 1986). The tendency for vitamins to inspire this devotion to excessive intake probably dates from the time of their discovery. Vitamin C is perhaps the vitamin most widely abused in this way, although others, particularly E, D, B_6 and A are also used excessively. *Table 11.2* lists the complications of excessive vitamin intakes. There is no evidence that any of these vitamins have significantly useful effects in normal individuals in these large doses, except that the ingestion of large doses of vitamin C may have some slight effect in lessening, but *not* preventing, the symptoms of the common cold. Even this finding is highly suspect.

Table 11.2 Complications of excessive vitamin intakes

Vitamin	Clinical features
A Carotenaemia:	Yellow skin; high plasma carotene
Excess retinol	*Acute*: nausea, vomiting, bulging fontanelle, pseudotumour cerebri. *Chronic*: anorexia, failure to thrive, alopecia, tender bony swellings, hyperostosis, raised intracranial pressure, hypercalcaemia, increased plasma retinol, fetal abnormality
B Niacin:	Paraesthesiae, itching, skin flushing, hepatotoxicity
Pyridoxine dependency	Withdrawal convulsions, especially in neonates
C	Haematuria due to cysteine and oxalate stones; diarrhoea; interference with vitamin B_{12} absorption
D Hypercalcaemia (of infancy)	Anorexia, constipation, failure to thrive, polyuria, hypercalcaemia, hyperostosis, renal deposition of calcium, hypertension and renal failure
E	Increased necrotizing enterocolitis; increased susceptibility to infection; interference with vitamin K metabolism – bleeding tendencies

Successful books have been written advocating particular regimens of therapy using vitamins, minerals, seaweeds and herbal mixtures rather than conventional medical practices. Such books are mostly rich in anecdote but have little analytical scientific support for the therapies they advance. Little can be done to suppress publications by devotees or by the unscrupulous if they are not liable to disciplinary action from professional organizations. Attempts to assign books and pamphlets on eccentric diets to their appropriate level may be met by litigation. And to devotees, such attempts only enhance the popular image of professional nutritional scientists deliberately obstructing promulgation of whatever diet is under discussion. Apart from the risks already described for high-dose vitamin therapy, these diets and treatments often include self-dosing with minerals and have risks of intoxication, due to high intakes of potassium particularly.

Home-prepared mixtures of vitamins and minerals, even if the doses recommended are safe, are potentially very dangerous since it is easy for quantities (sometimes described in terms of fractions of a teaspoon) to be wrongly measured. The Hippocratic aphorism 'First, do no harm' should apply to unconventional, as well as conventional, preventive and therapeutic measures. Nevertheless, this search for home remedies, diets to prevent illness, herbalism and other 'fringe' medical activities reflects public dissatisfaction with the cost of treatment, and the gulf between what the general public wants from the health services and what the health services provide. The formal medical system would be wise to consider the implications of this and temper health education programmes and methods of management of illness appropriately.

References

ARNON, S. S., MIDURA, T. F., DAMUS, K., THOMPSON, B., WOOD, R. M. and CHIN, J. (1979) Honey and other environmental risk factors for infant botulism. *Journal of Pediatrics*, **94**, 331–336

CARLSON, E., KIPPS, M. and THOMSON, J. (1984) Influences on the food habits of some ethnic minorities in the United Kingdom. *Human Nutrition: Applied Nutrition,* **38A,** 85–98

EVANS, C. D. H. and LACEY, J. H. (1986) Toxicity of vitamins: complications of a health movement. *British Medical Journal,* **292,** 509–510

EVANS, N., WALPOLE, I. R., QURESHI, M. U., MEMON, H. M. and EVERLEY JONES, H. W. (1976) Lack of breast feeding and early weaning of infants of Asian immigrants to Wolverhampton. *Archives of Disease in Childhood,* **51,** 608–612

HANNING, R. M. and ZLOTKIN, S. H. (1985) Unconventional eating practices and their health implications. *Pediatric Clinics of North America,* **32,** 429–445

HARDINGE, M. G. and STARE, F. J. (1954) Nutritional studies of vegetarians: 1. Nutritional, physical and laboratory studies. *American Journal of Clinical Nutrition,* **2,** 73

JIVANI, S. K. M. (1978) The practice of infant feeding among Asian immigrants. *Archives of Disease in Childhood,* **53,** 69–73

LAPPE, J. M. (1974) *Diet for a Small Planet.* New York: Ballantine Books

McLEAN, W. C. and GRAHAM, G. G. (1980) Vegetarianism in children. *American Journal of Diseases of Children,* **134,** 513–519

McNEILL, G. (1985) Birth weight, feeding practices and weight-for-age of Punjabi children in the U.K. and in the rural Punjab. *Human Nutrition: Clinical Nutrition,* **39C,** 69–72

POSKITT, E. M. E., COLE, T. J. and LAWSON, D. E. M. (1979) Sunlight, diet and 25 hydroxyvitamin D in healthy children and adults. *British Medical Journal,* **i,** 221–223

ROBERTS, I. F., WEST, R. J., OGILVIE, D. and DILLON, M. J. (1979) Malnutrition in infants receiving cult diets: a form of child abuse. *British Medical Journal,* **i,** 296–298

SHULL, M. W., REED, R. B., VALADIAN, I., PALOMBO, R., THORNES, H. and DWYER, J. T. (1977) Velocities of growth in vegetarian preschool children. *Pediatrics,* **60,** 410–417

SPRINGER, L. and THOMAS, J. (1983) Rastafarians in Britain. *Human Nutrition: Applied Nutrition,* **37A,** 120–127

STEPHENS, W. P., KLIMIUK, P. S., WARRINGTON, S. and TAYLOR, J. L. (1982) Observations on the dietary practices of Asians in the United Kingdom. *Human Nutrition: Applied Nutrition,* **36A,** 438–444

ZMORA, E., GORODISCHER, R. and BAR-ZIV, J. (1979) Multiple nutritional deficiencies in infants from a strict vegetarian community. *American Journal of Diseases of Children,* **133,** 141–144

Chapter 12
Nutrition and the teeth

Teeth are important for nutrition once children change from a totally liquid diet to one requiring biting and chewing. Nutrition is also important for teeth. Development, growth and maintenance of normal healthy teeth require good nutrition both during fetal life when the primary dentition is being formed and postnatally when the secondary dentition is being calcified. Nutrition is also relevant in protecting or predisposing teeth to caries.

The first teeth to erupt are the deciduous (milk or primary) teeth. These erupt from 6 months onwards and are shed from the age of 5 years. Secondary teeth are erupting from the loss of the deciduous teeth until 14 years, except for eruption of the third molars which may not occur until the third decade. Since the deciduous teeth are shed, their health may seem less important than that of the secondary or permanent teeth. However, the deciduous dentition is important for consumption of a healthy diet, for development of the jaws, for acting as a framework for alignment of the permanent teeth and for effective speech. Moreover, severe disease of the deciduous teeth can spread to affect the permanent teeth developing behind them.

Maternal nutrition and the teeth

Table 12.1 outlines conditions present at birth that affect the teeth. Anatomical positioning of the teeth will be affected by abnormalities of the jaws and palate and later health of the dentition affected since malocclusion encourages dental caries. Anatomical malpositioning of the teeth may be sufficiently bad to affect the ability of the teeth to perform biting tasks effectively (consider, for example, biting into an apple when upper and lower incisors cannot oppose).

The most common dental complication of problems *in utero* is enamel hypoplasia. Mineral is deposited in the matrix formed by ameloblastic activity from the fourth month of intrauterine life to form the enamel of the deciduous teeth. Any severe illness in the mother is likely to be reflected in diminished ameloblastic activity. When the period of illness or insult is short, ameloblasts return to normal activity quickly, and any defects in the enamel become covered with normal healthy enamel. If the period of restricted ameloblastic activity is prolonged, more profound defects may occur which lead to obvious abnormalities on the teeth when they erupt (Lecine, Turner and Dobbing, 1979).

The main effects on enamel production are in late pregnancy, perhaps because mineral deposition is important for enamel formation and in the last trimester

Table 12.1 Congenital dental problems affecting nutrition

Condition	Aetiology	Nutritional effects
Cleft lip and/or cleft palate	Associated with many genetically determined and multifactorial syndromes. May be a manifestation of maternal alcoholism or anticonvulsant therapy	Major feeding difficulty in young infants: require tube feeding, artificial palate or cup and spoon feeding. Will require surgical correction. Malalignment of the teeth later leads to difficulties biting and chewing and increased caries; require orthodontic treatment
Absent or partially absent teeth	Various genetically determined ectodermal dysplasias	Difficulty chewing. Capping available teeth and dentures necessary at young age
Enamel hypoplasia	Amelogenesis imperfecta: manifestation of genetically determined osteogenesis imperfecta.	Discoloured poorly formed teeth. Severe caries
	Maternal illness and maternal vitamin D deficiency in pregnancy. Any cause of intrauterine growth retardation	Patchily discoloured teeth susceptible to caries
Severe discoloration of teeth	Maternal tetracycline ingestion during pregnancy	Greenish brown staining to deciduous teeth. Poorly grown, caries-susceptible teeth

mineral demands of the fetus for growth of all tissues are high. The effects may be subtle and result from trivial but specific upsets to maternal nutrition. There is evidence that changes in maternal circulating vitamin D levels such as occur in Northern Europe in winter are sufficient to cause increased enamel hypoplasia in low birthweight infants born in winter (Purvis et al., 1973; Cockburn et al., 1980). One study suggests that early infant nutrition may be even more important than intrauterine events for these small infants (Mellander et al., 1982). Optimal calcium and phosphate nutrition seem important for normal enamel formation both in fetus and in neonate. By 6 weeks of postnatal age enamel formation of the deciduous teeth has almost ceased although the teeth continue to grow for a couple of years.

Postnatal problems affecting the teeth

Ameloblastic activity can be affected by any systemic illness. During illness, ameloblasts function poorly. If the situation persists for any length of time there will be areas of developing teeth where the enamel is thin and the teeth ridged or pitted. Enamel hypoplasia leads to discoloration, pits, grooves and rough surfaces on the teeth. When severe the dark brown of the underlying dentine shows through the enamel. The severity of enamel hypoplasia is a consequence of the duration of illness rather than the severity of illness, since, once the general health improves, enamel deposition returns to normal and new enamel may cover the hypoplastic areas. The importance of enamel hypoplasia is largely in the way it predisposes teeth to carious damage.

Caries

Caries is infection involving the substance of the teeth which destroys the dentine and the structure of the tooth if uncontrolled. It arises after destruction of the calcium salt enamel on the surface of the tooth by acid of pH <5.5. Areas of low pH develop under plaque – a gel-like mat that adheres to the tooth surface especially at the gum margins. Plaque is formed from salivary secretions colonized by *Streptococcus mutans*. As plaque increases, food debris and other micro-organisms accumulate. Sucrose and fermentable carbohydrates are digested to form dextrans by oral flora and these contribute to plaque formation. *Lactobacilli*, spirochaetal organisms and *Candida* accumulate under the plaque together with *Streptococci*. Enamel is eroded, and bacteria gain access to the tooth substance. The situation is exacerbated by the acidity of sweetened carbonated drinks –'pop'.

Caries requires a combination of circumstances: suitable oral flora; suitable substrate for micro-organism activity; susceptible teeth and an environment that encourages multiplication of micro-organisms. *Figure 12.1* outlines predisposing and protecting factors.

Food and the individual's nutritional status have a profound effect on the development of caries. Sucrose not only provides a substrate for bacteria, but

BACTERIA

Streptococcus mutans
Neisseria
Lactobacilli
Spirochaetes

SUBSTRATE FOR PLAQUE AND CARIES FORMING ORGANISMS

Sucrose, especially separate from main meals, encourages cariogenic organisms

Acids in diet (carbonated drinks) encourage cariogenic organisms

Fats and proteins discourage plaque formation

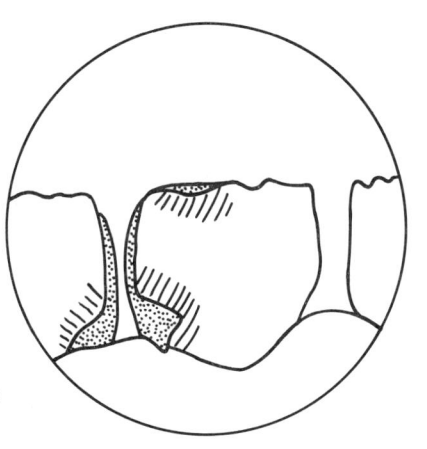

SUSCEPTIBILITY OF TEETH

Genetic factors
Enamel hypoplasia, ridges, pits predispose

Fluorapatite in teeth reduces susceptibility to decay

ENVIRONMENT

Physical

Plaque discouraged by brushing and flossing teeth

Nutritional

Sucrose induces small volumes of viscid saliva which encourage plaque formation

Poor nutrition encourages oral infection

Figure 12.1 Factors protecting against, or predisposing to, dental caries.

induces flow of only small amounts of viscid saliva which adhere to teeth and begin plaque formation. Chewing and fats and proteins in the diet lead to increased salivary flow and help cleanse the teeth. Fats also lubricate the mouth and deposit a protective film over the teeth which prevents plaque adhesion. Malnutrition, with parotid hypertrophy but poor salivary secretion and reduced resistance to infection, encourages caries development although in severely malnourished young children tooth eruption is delayed, thus preserving the teeth to some extent. Inflamed gums due to vitamin C deficiency or dry abnormal mucosa due to B vitamin deficiencies encourage the development of caries. Tooth brushing can cleanse the teeth of plaque but many small children have difficulty manoeuvring the toothbrush to clean the teeth adequately. The practice of finishing meals for small children with cheese, crisps, apples or carrots may be helpful in reducing the caries-favouring environment even without tooth cleansing as well (Lewis, 1978; Edell, 1984).

'Nursing bottle' syndrome

Young children are occasionally seen with complete carious destruction of their upper deciduous incisors. Whilst the condition may be the result of any poor oral hygiene coupled with enamel hypoplasia, many of these children have a history of prolonged contact with bottles of sweetened juices. These may have been the juice-containing dummies fashionable some years ago ('dinky' feeders). Sometimes the child has been put to bed with a bottle of juice as 'comforter' propped up so the child can suck at the bottle throughout the night. Reduced salivary flow and lip and tongue movements at night encourage prolonged contact of the acid juice with the teeth. Enamel destruction begins. Prolonged bottle feeding is inadvisable for many reasons, and 'nursing bottle' syndrome is one of them.

Fluoride

The most significant factor to affect the prevalence of caries is the use of fluoride in the drinking water. Areas that have a naturally high concentration of fluoride in the water (about 1 ppm) have been recognized for some time as having a low prevalence of dental caries. Many regions of the affluent world now add fluoride to the level of 1 ppm to the drinking water if the level is not naturally in this range. Where this is not done, it is often recommended that children receive regular fluoride supplementation: 0.25 mg/day for those aged 0–1 years; 0.5 mg/day when aged 1–3 years and 1.0 mg/day when aged over 3 years (Committee on Nutrition, 1972, 1979).

Fluoride is deposited in the enamel of developing teeth to form fluorapatite. Fluorapatite forms larger, more stable enamel crystals which are less soluble. The teeth also have fewer cusps and shallower grooves and pits and are thus less likely to allow plaque to adhere. The main protective effects of fluoride are thus during tooth development. However, fluoride also acts on the surface of teeth by ionic exchange so strengthening surface enamel. It disrupts plaque formation and discourages growth of plaque bacteria. Its local and continuing effect is also important. Fluoride toothpastes and fluoride supplementation of the water have effects for older children and adults as well as for those with developing teeth. Fluoride supplementation appears to have little effect on the fetus since transmission across the placenta is only slight.

Absorption of fluoride is reduced when there is food in the stomach. It is difficult to know how this affects absorption of fluoride from the water supply or the use of fluoride toothpaste to clean teeth after meals when some fluoride is likely to be swallowed. In areas where water is not supplemented and children are given fluoride supplements it seems appropriate to offer the supplements separate from mealtimes.

Does fluoride supplementation have any risks? This is a politically emotive subject. Supplementing drinking water seems – to some – an infringement of personal liberty. Views differ on this and we would not wish to argue the issue here (Margolis and Cohen, 1985). The level of 1 ppm fluoride in drinking water is equivalent to one drop in 17 gallons of water or the amount of water used in one cycle of a washing machine. Mottling of the teeth is most unlikely at this level and harmful side effects impossible. If, however, children are also being supplemented with fluoride tablets or drops and swallowing considerable amounts of fluoride from their toothpaste there is a theoretical risk of children receiving unnecessarily large doses of fluoride although intakes are still unlikely to amount to more than 5 mg per day, the level at which marked tooth mottling and weakening of tooth structure may occur. Fluorosis of the bones usually occurs with levels of over 10 mg/day. Small children cleaning their teeth twice a day could consume as much as 0.66 mg/day (Heifetz and Horowitz, 1986). It may be advisable for parents to put paste on toothbrushes so the basic quantity is small and to assist their small children to brush their teeth without swallowing a lot of paste.

Vitamin deficiencies and the teeth

Several vitamin deficiency diseases produce dramatic oral changes, most notably vitamin C deficiency and the reddened smooth tongue and angular stomatitis of combined riboflavin and niacin deficiencies. Conditions affecting the mouth are likely to affect production of saliva, local resistance to infection and thus encourage the development of caries even if not directly involving the dentition.

Classically, the vitamin deficiency state most commonly associated with dental effects is scurvy. Here the basic condition is gingival hyperplasia and bleeding. Interdental gingival papillae form tumour-like masses and there is commonly bleeding at the gingival margins. The condition is exaggerated by pre-existing caries, damaged teeth or periodontal disease. It is often stated that there are no oral manifestations of scurvy in very young edentulate infants. Such infants have relatively low density of micro-organisms in the mouth.

The increased susceptibility to infection which is a manifestation of scurvy contributes to increased oral infection both with organisms causing caries and those causing stomatitis. The combination of invasive organisms and reduced resistance may, in situations of poor hygiene and poor salivation due to protein-energy malnutrition, lead to the devastating condition of cancrum oris. Here infestation with fusiform bacilli and spirochaetal organisms leads to necrotizing gingivitis, osteomyelitis of the jaw and destruction of the cheek and face.

Vitamin D deficiency might be expected to have profound effects on the teeth since it is concerned with mineralization of bone. However, rickets developing in young children after the stage when the main deposition of tooth mineral has occurred has little effect on the primary dentition. The permanent teeth erupting after rickets has been treated are likely to show enamel hypoplasia and abnormalities of the dentine. Delayed tooth eruption is another manifestation of rickets.

It is a general impression in Britain that children's teeth are showing less caries than 20 years ago. It is difficult to know how much this can be attributed to fluoridation of the water, greater use of fluoride supplements and the almost universalization of fluoride toothpaste. Improved nutrition by reduced refined sugar in the diet and increased intake of chewable whole foods might be responsible if there were significant evidence that children's diets have changed in this way. Many parents are concerned to preserve their children's teeth but there is little evidence that the national diet has improved significantly in these respects. Changes will, no doubt, be attributed to each commentator's own particular hobby-horse for good dental health.

References

COCKBURN, F., BELTON, N. R., PURVIS, R. J., et al. (1980) Maternal vitamin D intake and mineral metabolism in mothers and their newborn infants. *British Medical Journal*, **281**, 11–14

COMMITTEE ON NUTRITION (1972) Fluoride as a nutrient. *Pediatrics*, **49**, 456–460

COMMITTEE ON NUTRITION (1979) Fluoride supplementation. Revised dosage schedule. *Pediatrics*, **63**, 150–152

EDELL, M. K. (1984) Dental nutrition. *Manual of Pediatric Nutrition*, edited by D. G. Kelts and E. G. Jones, pp. 85–98. Boston: Little Brown

HEIFETZ, S. B. and HOROWITZ, H. S. (1986) Amounts of fluoride in self administered dental products: safety considerations for children. *Pediatrics*, **77**, 876–882

LEVINE, R. S., TURNER, E. P. and DOBBING, J. (1979) Deciduous teeth contain histories of developmental disturbances. *Early Human Development*, **3**, 211–220

LEWIS, D. H. (1978) The prevention of dental disease in childhood. *Journal of Maternal and Child Health*, **3**, 184–186

MARGOLIS, F. J. and COHEN, S. M. (1985) Successful and unsuccessful experiences in combatting the antifluoridationists. *Pediatrics*, **76**, 113–118

MELLANDER, M., NOREN, J. G., FREDEN, H. and KJELLMER, I. (1982) Mineralisation defects in deciduous teeth of low birth weight infants. *Acta Paediatrica Scandinavica*, **71**, 727–733

PURVIS, R. J., BARRIE, W. J., MacKAY, G. S., et al. (1973) Enamel hypoplasia of the teeth associated with neonatal tetany: a manifestation of maternal vitamin D deficiency. *Lancet*, **ii**, 811–814

Chapter 13
Inborn errors of metabolism

Inborn errors of metabolism are genetically determined disorders usually resulting from single enzyme defects determined by single, abnormal, autosomal recessive genes. Some inborn errors are responsive to nutritional management. Management of the more important of these will be outlined here. Those caring for children with inborn errors of metabolism must consult experienced clinicians and dieticians and more authoritative manuals before undertaking management. It cannot be overstressed how important it is that management is co-ordinated by specialist teams of doctors, biochemists and dieticians experienced in this field.

Newborn infants in Britain are screened for hypothyroidism (not usually considered an inborn error of metabolism), for phenylketonuria and possibly for other inborn errors. Methods of screening and conditions screened vary according to the Regional Centre performing the screening tests (*Table 13.1*). Blood is

Table 13.1 Inborn errors of metabolism screened in the newborn period in Britain

All children:
 Phenylketonuria
 Congenital hypothyroidism

Other conditions that may also be diagnosed*:
 Maple syrup urine disease
 Tyrosinaemia
 Hyperprolinaemia
 Histidinaemia
 Galactosaemia

Conditions screened according to local interest:
 Cystic fibrosis
 Adreno-genital syndrome
 Thalassaemias
 Sickle cell disease

* The method of detecting phenylketonuria will influence the ease with which other inborn errors are detected.

collected between 6 and 10 days of age from heelprick onto circumscribed areas on cards which are then sent to the screening laboratory. Infants should be established on milk feeds for several days before screening. Infants on intravenous drip or not receiving significant amounts of dietary protein are likely to show false-negative results. Infants who were sick in the early neonatal period and premature infants who may have taken over a week to reach full feeds should have tests repeated after they have been fully enterally fed for at least a week. Infants, particularly preterm, who are parenterally fed occasionally have plasma phenylalanine levels that are sufficiently high to give false-positive results. Thus results must be interpreted cautiously until opportunity for repeat testing during full enteral feeding arises. Ideally, the screening, follow-up and management of inborn errors of metabolism should be regionally based. This allows the development of units with clinical expertise and technical support to manage complicated dietary therapy optimally.

Table 13.2 Examples of inborn errors of metabolism benefiting from nutritional management

Conditions manageable by total elimination of a non-essential nutrient: galactosaemia, hereditary fructose intolerance

Conditions controlled by restricted intake of an essential nutrient(s): classical phenylketonuria, maple syrup urine disease

Conditions involving abnormal metabolic processes sensitive to enzymatic co-factor or other nutrient supplementation: homocystinuria, phenylketonuria secondary to abnormalities of biopterin metabolism

Conditions where management depends on indirect control through major nutrients: defects of urea cycle, glycogen storage disease type I, familial type IIa hyperlipidaemia

Conditions where malabsorption or defective transport of a nutrient can be resolved by nutritional supplementation or parenteral administration: acrodermatitis enteropathica (*see* Chapter 15), transcobalamin II deficiency (*see* Chapter 10)

Table 13.2 outlines the types of inborn erros of metabolism which may benefit from nutritional management. With the exception of those conditions where pharmacological doses of nutrients overcome enzymatic deficiencies, these conditions are managed by diets that either eliminate non-essential nutrients or reduce intakes of one or more essential nutrients. Elimination is not always effective management since endogenous synthesis of causative nutrients may defeat the effects of dietary manipulation. The potential limitations of strict dietary regimens are covered by supplementary essential fatty acids, special vitamin preparations and/or special mineral preparations. The response to dietary treatment is monitored by regular assessment of general health, mental development and blood biochemistry. Many of the dietary regimens, if applied too rigidly, endanger normal growth. Thus regular monitoring of growth is also vital to ensure that the appropriate balance between limiting and excluding essential nutrients is maintained.

Conditions that can be managed by elimination of a non-essential nutrient

Galactosaemia

This condition affects approximately 1 in 70 000 children. The classical condition is severe but milder cases do occur. Details of the disease variants will not be discussed further.

Classical type
In classical galactosaemia, deficiency of galactose-1-phosphate uridyl transferase prevents conversion of galactose-1-phosphate to glucose. Galactose, galactitol and

galactose-1-phosphate accumulate in the blood. Newborns with classical galactosaemia fed breast or formula milk rapidly become ill with vomiting, failure to thrive, lethargy and hepatomegaly and may die from overwhelming infection. If the condition is either mild or partially treated, late effects include cataracts, mental retardation, ovarian dysgenesis and cirrhosis of the liver. Diagnosis is made initially by finding galactose (a reducing sugar) in the urine. Abnormal renal tubular function usually leads to glycosuria as well. Urine is thus positive both with Clinitest tablets (Ames: test for reducing sugars) and Clinistix (Ames: test specifically for glucose).

Confirmation of the diagnosis is demonstration of deficient or absent galactose-1-phosphate uridyl transferase activity in the red cells. Management is by avoiding lactose- and galactose-containing foods (Francis, 1987). Lactose-free milks are listed in *Table 13.3*.

Table 13.3 Some lactose-free formulas suitable for treatment of galactosaemia in infancy

Formula	Manufacturer	Relevant points
Galactomin 17*	Cow & Gate	Requires additional minerals and vitamins. Cows' milk protein. Sucrose free. Traces of lactose (0.1%)
Nutramigen	Bristol-Myers	Contains sucrose. Hydrolysed cows' milk protein
Pregestimil	Bristol-Myers	Sucrose free. Hydrolysed cows' milk protein
Prosobee	Bristol-Myers	Soya protein base with added methionine. Sucrose free
Formula S	Cow & Gate	Soya protein base with added methionine. Sucrose free
Wysoy	Wyeth	Soya protein base with added methionine. Contains sucrose

* Advertised for management of galactosaemia but not ideal due to traces of lactose and need for supplementary vitamins and minerals. Is being reformulated.

Milk products should still be avoided at weaning. Dietary advice is necessary to distinguish lactose- and galactose-free foods. Lactose is used as a filler in many products, including tablets. Whey containing some lactose is widely used as a sweetener and may occur in unexpected foods such as soft margarine. Management of galactosaemia must be strict in the first year of life but it is not clear how much postnatal dietary management affects intellectual development (*see below*). Any foods containing even small amounts of lactose should be avoided fastidiously. In the past, the diet was often relaxed after the age of 10. Neurological function may deteriorate if the diet is relaxed substantially, and dietary relaxation may also predispose to cataract formation. Minor indiscretions from small quantities of lactose received unexpectedly in foods (e.g. from butter and margarines) or in tablets will probably cause no harm to older children or adults but milk and milk products should be avoided for life.

It has been suggested that galactosaemic infants should be given small quantities of galactose in order to meet requirements for synthesis of galactose-containing cerebrosides but sufficient galactose can be synthesized from glucose within the body to meet requirements in classical galactosaemia (although not in epimerase deficiency). Exclusion of plant products containing galactosides was also recommended in the past, but vegetable galactosides are not broken down to galactose in the human intestine and remain unabsorbed so they present little risk and need not be excluded (Clothier and Davidson, 1983).

Long-term studies of the intellectual development of children with galactosaemia treated strictly from shortly after birth indicates that, despite adequate dietary management, mean IQ is below that expected from a normal population. The reasons for this are not totally clear, but brain damage may occur *in utero*. Raised erythrocyte galactose-1-phosphate levels can be demonstrated in the fetus during the second and third trimesters of pregnancy. For this reason it may be reasonable to recommend that where antenatal diagnosis has been made, the heterozygote (and therefore clinically normal) mother should avoid milk and milk products in order to minimize intrauterine brain damage to her fetus. There is, however, no substantial evidence that this improves the outlook for the fetus.

Intrauterine high levels of galactose-1-phosphate in the fetus may also be responsible for the other abnormalities found in effectively treated girls. As many as 60% of female patients with galactosaemia show evidence of primary ovarian failure, delayed puberty and primary amenorrhoea. These girls have abnormally high gonadotrophin levels indicating end organ failure. The reason for ovarian failure is not known but may result from the toxic effects of galactose and metabolities on ovarian parenchyma *in utero* so that normal ovarian growth and development in response to increased gonadotrophin secretion with puberty do not occur. There is no evidence for gonadal damage in boys with galactosaemia.

Galactosaemic women of childbearing age should continue a strict diet. High maternal galactose levels cross the placenta and may affect the fetus even though the fetus is likely to be heterozygous rather than homozygous for the galactosaemic gene. The risks to the fetus are probably less than expected from maternal galactose levels since fetal metabolism of the increased galactose load is efficient.

Siblings of confirmed cases of galactosaemia have a one in four chance of being affected with the condition. They should be treated with a lactose- and galactose-free diet until red cell galactose-1-phosphate uridyl transferase levels have been measured and galactosaemia either diagnosed or excluded. Diagnosis can be made rapidly with the Beutler test on a heelprick blood sample and does not require the child to be on a galactose-containing diet.

Galactokinase deficiency
In galactokinase deficiency galactitol and galactose accumulate in tissues. Cataract occurs in early life but development is otherwise normal. This condition should also be treated with a galactose-free diet since the cataracts may become less dense if treatment begins early. Mothers of affected children should probably avoid lactose and milk in subsequent pregnancies.

In galactokinase deficiency, unlike classical galactosaemia, galactose-1-phosphate does not accumulate. This suggests that galactose-1-phosphate is the toxic metabolite in galactosaemia, and these toxic effects may be due to the inhibitory effect of galactose-1-phosphate on other enzymes such as phosphoglucomutase. Alternatively, liver damage may be due to depletion of uridyltriphosphate. The presence of galactose-1-phosphate traps high-energy phosphate without converting galactose to glucose and thus restricts the availability of ATP for further UTP synthesis.

Hereditary fructose intolerance

In this condition, fructose-1-phosphate cannot be metabolized due to a deficiency of fructoaldolase activity. Glucose cannot be synthesized from fructose; and the ingestion of fructose is likely to be followed by vomiting, lethargy, hypoglycaemia and coma. Continued exposure to fructose results in failure to thrive, hepatomegaly and liver failure with ascites, oedema, jaundice and a bleeding diathesis.

Diagnosis is by studying the metabolic effects of a fructose load or by measuring liver fructose-1-phosphate activity.

Management of hereditary fructose intolerance is by removal of fructose and fructose-containing sugars (i.e. sucrose) from the diet. Paediatric dietetic advice must be sought since providing a fructose-free diet with adequate nutrition for growth and development is difficult. Sorbitol is metabolized through fructose and is dangerous. Breast-fed infants and those on sucrose-free formulas may remain undiagnosed until the introduction of weaning foods and drinks. Where the diagnosis has been made infants should be fed sucrose-free formulas if they are not breast fed (*Table 13.4*). At weaning, the diet becomes extremely difficult since a wide variety of foods contain sucrose, fructose or sorbitol. Confusion may arise because sucrose is described under a number of different terms when food ingredients are listed. Invert sugar, laevulose, honey, syrup, beet sugar and fruit sugar all indicate sucrose.

Table 13.4 Some sucrose- and fructose-free infant formulas

Formula	Manufacturer
Cows' milk protein base: Galactomins 17, 18	Cow & Gate
Hydrolysed milk protein base: Pregestimil	Bristol-Myers
Soya protein base:	
Formula S	Cow & Gate
Prosobee	Bristol-Meyers

Tremendous care is needed to advise on these children's diets. Home-prepared foods are advisable since then mothers know exactly what the children are receiving. Many foods normally used in home cooking, such as many fruits and vegetables, contain fructose or sucrose and must be avoided. Foods that unexpectedly contain sucrose or substances metabolized through fructose include tinned meats and fish pastes, peas and beans (not french or mung beans), baked beans, nuts, many diabetic products (because they contain sorbitol), tinned soups, drinking chocolate, breakfast cereals and tomatoes.

Children on sucrose-fructose free diets must be given supplementary vitamin C. Vitamin A is also necessary unless fortified margarine is used.

Conditions where partial elimination of an essential nutrient is necessary for management

Phenylketonuria

Phenylketonuria (PKU) is often cited as the classic example of an inborn error of metabolism. It was one of the earliest inborn errors to be treated nutritionally, and it is commoner than many inborn errors (about 1 in 10000 British children). Management illustrates many of the points that make dietary control of children with inborn errors a difficult process for the inexperienced. As with so many inborn errors of metabolism, time has demonstrated that PKU is not a single entity but encompasses a number of inborn errors, more or less sensitive to dietary management.

Table 13.5 outlines the causes of hyperphenylalaninaemia and atypical PKU. Atypical forms of PKU probably result from gene alleles which lead to less complete deficiency of phenylalanine hydroxylase than the classical PKU. Between 1% and 2% of PKU children have abnormalities of biopterin metabolism and do not respond to classical dietary measures. Screening urine for abnormal pteridine metabolites is advisable before defining dietary management. Abnormalities in biopterin metabolism can also be detected on white cell enzyme estimations.

Table 13.5 Conditions giving rise to hyperphenylalaninaemia*

Congenital:
  Phenylhydroxylase deficiency in liver:
    Severe deficiency – classical PKU.
    Less severe deficiency – atypical variant PKU, mild or transient hyperphenylalaninaemia.
  Phenylalanine metabolism dependent on co-factors (not responsive to diet):
    Deficiency of dihydropterin reductase.
    Defective biopterin synthesis.
Acquired:
  Transient hyperphenylalaninaemia of newborn (combination of high protein intake and immature metabolism)
  Liver disease
Drugs: co-trimoxazole, methotrexate

* After Smith (1985).

In classical PKU there is deficiency of the liver enzyme phenylalanine hydroxylase, which converts phenylalanine to tyrosine. Phenylalanine accumulates in the blood and is excreted in the urine along with abnormal metabolites such as phenylpyruvic acid and phenylacetic acid. Blood tyrosine levels are low. Without treatment these children develop severe mental retardation. They also have failure to thrive, fair hair, blue eyes and eczema. Lack of tyrosine may contribute to the deficiency of pigmentation. Fits, particularly infantile spasms, are frequent. Body and urine have a musty smell due to the presence of large quantities of abnormal metabolites. If treated early, the mental retardation, growth retardation and other signs of the condition can be totally prevented.

Phenylalanine is an essential amino acid and cannot be excluded from the diet altogether. Sufficient must be provided in the diet for normal growth and metabolism, yet insufficient to allow metabolites to accumulate and cause damage. Adequacy of the diet is monitored using plasma phenylalanine levels which should be kept between 180 and 360 μmol/1 (3 and 6 mg/dl) in the first 2–3 years of life, during the period of maximum brain growth. Thereafter levels may be allowed to rise to 500 μmol/1.

The principles of management of phenylketonuria can be listed as follows:

1. The majority of the protein in the diet is provided by special phenylalanine-low foods.

2. Phenylalanine requirements are provided by regulated amounts of natural protein-containing foods in 'portions' containing 50 mg phenylalanine, equivalent to approximately 1 g of protein in most cases (Francis, 1987).
3. The total protein requirements should be higher than usually expected for children of the same age because of the artificiality of the amino acid content of the protein supplied and its consequent low biological availability.
4. The energy of the diet is supplied from fat and carbohydrate sources which may have to be provided from supplements if sufficient cannot be taken from natural protein free sources.
5. Phenylalanine intakes should be reduced during periods of illness. Energy intakes should be maintained in order to minimize tissue protein catabolism.
6. Supplementary essential fatty acids, vitamins and minerals are required with some phenylalanine-low preparations.
7. Regular monitoring of phenylalanine levels in the blood, growth, general health, and intellectual development are essential.
8. Plasma phenylalanine levels should be kept between 180 and 360 μmol/l (3–6 mg/100 ml) in the first years of life.
9. Some relaxation of diet is usually allowed for teenage children but these children must be watched carefully for deterioration in growth and particularly in intellectual ability (Smith et al., 1978). Some children may be more affected by slightly raised phenylalanine levels than others.
10. Women anticipating childbearing should go back onto strict PKU diet prior to conception (see below).
11. Maternal requirements for phenylalanine increase in late pregnancy and supplements with tyrosine are also necessary. Careful dietary control is essential and should be supervised by those experienced in managing pregnancy in women with PKU.

Table 13.6 lists some phenylalanine-free and phenylalanine-low preparations currently available. Most of these cannot be regarded as complete formulas and must be provided with energy, vitamin, essential fatty acid and mineral supplements (*Tables 13.7* and *13.8*).

At diagnosis the first aim for treatment of the child with phenylketonuria is to restore phenylalanine levels in the blood to values under 360 μmol/l (6 mg/dl). This

Table 13.6 Some phenylalanine-low food preparations currently available in Britain*

Preparation	Manufacturers	Phenylalanine content (mg/100 g)
Albumaid XP	Scientific Hospital Supplies	10
Albumaid XP Concentrate	Scientific Hospital Supplies	25
Aminex biscuits†	Cow & Gate	21
Aminogram	Allen and Hanbury's	–
Lofenalac	Bristol-Myers	80
Maxamaid XP	Scientific Hospital Supplies	–
Minafen	Cow & Gate	20
P.K. Aid 1	Scientific Hospital Supplies	–

* These are NOT complete foods in themselves and MUST only be used as part of a prescribed diet.
† Other low-protein foods in the Aproten (Ultrapharm) and Rite-Diet (Welfare Foods) *Low Protein* range are suitable components of a prescribed diet.

174   Inborn errors of metabolism

Table 13.7 Energy supplements to protein controlled diet in PKU and similar conditions

Supplement	Manufacturers	Composition	Energy/100 g (100 ml) kJ	kcal
Fat:				
Calogen	Scientific Hospital Supplies	Both 50% arachis oil in water	1700	400
Prosparol	Duncan Flockhart			
Carbohydrate:				
Caloreen	Roussel	Glucose polymers	1674	398
Maxijul powder	Scientific Hospital Supplies	Water soluble maltodextrins	1570	375
Maxijul liquid	Scientific Hospital Supplies	Liquid = 50% solution of powder	800	187
Polycal	Cow & Gate	Glucose, maltose and polysaccharides	1610	380
Polycose powder	Abbott	Glucose polymer powder	1600	380
Polycose liquid	Abbott	Liquid = 50% solution of powder	840	200

Table 13.8 Non-energy supplements for PKU and other restricted diets

Supplement	Manufacturer	Composition
Vitamins:		
Ketovite Liquid	Paines & Byrne	Liquid and tablets must be taken together as complementary to one another
Ketovite tablets	Paines & Byrne	Mixture of vitamins A, B_1, B_2, B_6, B_{12}, nicotinamide, pantothenic acid, inositol, biotin, folic acid, choline, C, D, E and K
Minerals:		
Metabolic Mineral Mix	Scientific Hospital Supplies	Mixture of minerals and trace elements suitable for use with artificial and elemental diets
Aminogram	Allen & Hanbury	As above

involves feeding a phenylalanine-free preparation as a liquid formula, for example Albumaid (the child is normally a young infant), together with energy, vitamin and mineral supplements. Once plasma phenylalanine level has been brought within the normal range, supplementation with portions of normal infant formula or food containing phenylalanine should begin. Phenylalanine-low preparations tend to be salty, and these infants require above average fluid intakes. Total fluid intake should be 150–180 ml/kg/day in early infancy.

Portions vary in size depending on the food but each contains 50 mg phenylalanine. Human milk contains 75–100 mg phenylalanine/100 ml. Most formula milks also contain 70–100 mg phenylalanine/100 ml. Phenylalanine forms approximately 5% of most other proteins. Examples of phenylalanine 'portions' are indicated in *Table 13.9*. The table is not complete, but gives illustrative examples only. More details of diets can be found elsewhere (Francis, 1987).

Table 13.9 Examples of equivalent phenylalanine portions (50 mg)

Food	Approximate weight	Household measure
Cornflakes	15 g	3 rounded tablespoonfuls
Milk	30 ml	2 tablespoonfuls
Potatoes	70 g (boiled or roast)	1 hen's egg size
Rice (raw)	15 g	1 level dessertspoonful

Portions should be distributed over the course of a day since the phenylalanine-free protein cannot be utilized properly unless given with small amounts of phenylalanine as well. In infants the portions come from normal infant formula or from breast milk.

Breast feeding infants with PKU is difficult to maintain without good maternal motivation. Unless mothers are willing to express breast milk and then feed regulated amounts to their infants from bottles (which defeats much of the convenience and satisfaction of breast feeding), the infants should be fed the phenylalanine-free mixture prior to breast feeding so that hunger is largely sated. With careful monitoring of plasma phenylalanine levels it should be possible to estimate how frequently an infant should feed from the breast in order to get sufficient, but no more than sufficient, breast milk to maintain normal phenylalanine levels. This is clearly difficult to supervise, and mothers' milk production is likely to be low or to dry up if infants are not allowed to suckle freely.

Individual tolerance of phenylalanine varies and introduction of phenylalanine-containing 'portions' must be by careful biochemical supervision. Most infants require around 80 mg phenylalanine/kg/day during health. Slowing growth rates in infancy reduce phenylalanine tolerance and phenylalanine requirements per kg drop dramatically as infants grow although total phenylalanine requirements per day will probably increase as weight increases. Requirements may be only 20 mg/kg/day by the age of 2 years. The fluid bulk of the mixtures used to feed infants is such that toddlers may not tolerate the required volumes of infant phenylalanine-free preparations. Albumaid XP can be made up with smaller volumes of water or children may be changed to other phenylalanine-free preparations which are less bulky (e.g. P.K. Aid 1). Some of these preparations have added vitamins and minerals but specific needs with each dietary change must be checked with feed manufacturers, experienced nutritionists, dietitians and/or biochemists. Extra fluids should be offered freely after meals to prevent hyperosmolality which might result from the high nitrogen and mineral content of the diet.

Once weaning starts, foods such as meat, fish, cheese and eggs which are rich in protein and phenylalanine must be avoided. Vegetable products such as peas, beans, spinach and dried fruit also contain quite high levels of phenylalanine but can be used in the phenylalanine-containing protein allowances. The National Society for Phenylketonuria and Allied Disorders (*see* Appendix) can be very helpful with guidance on phenylalanine content of foods, recipes and general advice.

The effect of the diet in PKU and similar inborn errors of metabolism is assessed from several clinical aspects. General health and appearance of child and healthy family dynamics usually provide superficial indication of reasonable management. Assessment of weight gain, linear growth and growth of skull circumference provide further indications of progress since with appropriate dietary control these should be within the normal range. Poor growth may reflect inadequate control of phenylalanine levels, insufficient energy intake or too rigid a limitation of phenylalanine since small amounts are required for normal growth rates even in PKU children. Too great a restriction on phenylalanine will also lead to eczema, other skin rashes and later mental retardation. Blood phenylalanine levels will be a guide to whether diet is too lenient or too strict and must be measured frequently in early life. Finally, developmental and intellectual progress should be assessed regularly as further indication of the success – or otherwise – of treatment.

Children will require frequent review in infancy. Once growth rates are less rapid and toddler diet established review may not need to be so frequent, although this is dependent on the individual's progress. Monitoring may then be possible at home with mothers collecting blood samples on filter paper which are sent in to the laboratory and families advised on dietary adjustments according to results.

Some relaxation of the PKU diet is common in older children, especially teenagers. Occasional children show intellectual deterioration with time and may even develop a Parkinsonian-like condition with tremor and rigidity (Smith *et al.*, 1978; Holtzman *et al.*, 1986). Others show no ill effects. Girls and women wishing to become pregnant should return to strict control of phenylalanine intake with regular measurement of blood phenylalanine levels. There is considerable evidence that non-phenylketonuric infants born to phenylketonuric mothers who were not controlled in pregnancy have an increased incidence of intrauterine growth retardation, microcephaly, mental handicap and congenital heart disease. High maternal phenylalanine levels cross to the fetus and cause intrauterine damage. Although dietary control should be resumed before conception, introduction of strict diet early in pregnancy is not necessarily followed by fetal abnormality.

Pregnancy in PKU requires close supervision since phenylalanine requirements rise, particularly in the second and third trimesters, as the fetus grows. Moreover, tyrosine requirements also increase, since tyrosine is an essential amino acid in PKU. Tyrosine supplements are necessary and tyrosine levels in the blood should be monitored together with phenylalanine levels.

We have not dealt here with the forms of PKU not responsive to diet but modified by additional co-factors: 'malignant' PKU (Smith, 1985). These are the minority of PKU and present difficult management problems. Their existence means that diagnosis of the specific enzyme defect in new cases of PKU is important so that appropriate management can be instituted from the time of diagnosis.

Tyrosinaemia

There are different forms of tyrosinaemia which are variably sensitive to dietary management. In tyrosinaemia type I there is both hypertyrosinaemia and hypermethioninaemia with metabolic breakdown products of tyrosine in the urine. In the acute form children present with hepatocellular liver damage, aminoaciduria, glycosuria and hyperphosphaturia, vomiting, oedema and ultimately death from liver failure. More chronic forms of the disease develop vitamin D resistant rickets, nodular liver cirrhosis and again death from either liver failure or liver carcinoma. Management is similar to the management of PKU, although both tyrosine and phenylalanine intakes must be restricted and, since phenylalanine can be converted to tyrosine, it is the overall intake of both amino acids rather than the intake of either individually that matters. There is also associated hypermethioninaemia, and it is advisable to limit methionine intake as well. Dietary management does not seem to slow the progression of the liver disease and the overall outlook for these children is gloomy. Management – both general and dietary – is similar to that of PKU, using tyrosine, phenylalanine-free and methionine-low or methionine-free preparations (Albumaid XPXT, Scientific Hospital Supplies; Maxamaid XPXTXM, Scientific Hospital Supplies) and restricting these amino acids in the protein portions.

In tyrosinaemia type II there are very high levels of tyrosine in the blood and tyrosine metabolites in the urine, but no hypermethioninaemia. Children present with painful hyperkeratoses on palms and soles, keratitis with photophobia and lacrimation and mental retardation. The condition may not present until the second decade and treatment then has little effect on the mental retardation, although diet may be effective if started early.

Transient neonatal tyrosinaemia
Newborn infants, particularly the premature, sometimes show raised tyrosine levels in the blood and tyrosine metabolites in the urine. The administration of vitamin C (50–150 mg/day) causes these abnormalities to disappear. Presumably there is delayed maturation of an enzyme.

Maple syrup urine disease (MSUD)

This rare condition follows a rapid downhill course with failure to thrive, acidosis, hypoglycaemia and progressive neurological damage unless treatment is instituted. Oxidative decarboxylation of the branch chain amino acids – leucine, isoleucine and valine – is defective. Levels of branch-chain amino acids are elevated both in blood and in urine. Urine contains abnormal quantities of keto acids derived from these amino acids (hence the smell of maple syrup). MSUD can be controlled by diets low in branch-chain amino acids. However, these infants are usually acutely ill when first seen, and emergency management is needed to reduce branch-chain amino acid values in the blood and to lower branch-chain keto acid levels. Dietary management avoiding all branch-chain amino acids with high carbohydrate and fat intakes may be insufficient. Peritoneal dialysis, intravenous feeding, or both, but avoiding branch chain amino acids in the infusion until the neurological condition is brought under control, are often necessary. After restoration of branch-chain amino acids to normal levels, management of MSUD resembles that of phenylketonuria with low branch chain amino acid milks (MSUD Aid; Scientific Hospital Supplies) and small quantities of branch-chain containing foods to provide essential requirements. Total protein intakes need to be greater than expected for normal children because of the poor protein utilization from elimination diets. In older children solid intake is determined by leucine exchanges as with phenylalanine in PKU, or from lists containing the leucine, isoleucine and valine contents of foods. Either way, branch-chain amino acid levels in blood must be monitored carefully and growth and intellectual development assessed regularly. Dietary control requires monitoring blood leucine levels and keeping them between 2 and 5 mg/dl. When leucine levels rise above 10 mg/dl, acidosis, ataxia and branch-chain ketoacidosis develop. Leucine tolerance varies, usually between the range of 200 and 600 mg/day with isoleucine and valine tolerance at about 60–70% of this. Tolerance tends to fall with age but so do branch-chain amino acid requirements per kg, although total intake may increase slightly due to growth.

Conditions where enzymatic defects are sensitive to co-factor or other nutrient supplementation

Several inborn errors of metabolism are responsive to abnormal intakes of vitamins or other trace nutrient co-factors. *Table 13.10* lists some of the commoner or more readily treated conditions. It will be seen that in some of these conditions there are resemblances to inborn errors responsive to restriction diets. It is obviously essential in the management of children with inborn errors that the precise diagnosis and the exact enzyme defect is elucidated since management may vary widely depending on the nature of the enzyme defect.

Table 13.10 Some inborn errors of metabolism which may be responsive to nutritional co-factors

Vitamin dependency:	
B_1 – thiamine	Maple syrup urine variant
Niacin	Hartnup disease
B_6 – pyridoxine	Pyridoxine dependency convulsions
	Pyridoxine responsive anaemia
	Cystathionuria variant
	Hyperxanthurenic aciduria
	Homocystinuria variant
Biotin	Multiple carboxylase deficiency
	Proprionic acidaemias
Biopterin	Phenylketonuria variants
Folic acid	Homocystinuria and cystothioninuria
B_{12} – cobalamin	Methylmalonicaciduria
	Transcobalamin II deficiency
	Homocystinuria and hypomethioninaemia
D – calciferol	Familial vitamin D dependency rickets
Trace elements:	
Zinc	Acrodermatitis enteropathica

In some of these conditions the defect may relate to absorption or rate of metabolism of a nutrient and increased intake of the particular nutrient may overcome the problem. Examples of these latter conditions are acrodermatitis enteropathica and vitamin D dependency rickets (*see* Chapters 9 and 10).

Conditions where management depends on restricting major nutrients

Protein – defects of the urea cycle

Children with defects of the urea cycle usually present soon after birth with intractable vomiting, lethargy and neurological damage or death unless treatment is instituted. In arginase deficiency onset may be later and brought on by stress, surgery or infection. Hyperammonaemia is the most obvious toxic feature of these conditions and is at least partly responsible for the neurological damage. Vigorous treatment with peritoneal dialysis and meticulous dietary supervision has enabled these children to survive beyond the neonatal period.

Initial management of these infants is an emergency procedure. Plasma ammonia must be brought down to normal levels rapidly. Peritoneal dialysis or haemodialysis may be necessary in this acute phase. Adequate energy intakes in the form of high-carbohydrate and fat diets reduce protein breakdown. The management of these children is greatly helped by intravenous dietary supplementation with products that either drive the urea cycle beyond the deficient enzyme or which utilize waste nitrogen in synthesis or excrete it by pathways other than ureagenesis. Examples of these are:

1. In argininosuccinase deficiency supplementary arginine provides substrate for the urea cycle, and waste nitrogen is excreted through argininosuccinate which has an even greater renal clearance than urea.
2. In enzyme deficiencies occurring beyond the synthesis of ornithine from arginine, benzoate supplementation provides the substrate benzoyl CoA which transacylates glycine to yield hippurate. This has excellent renal clearance and diverts nitrogen away from the ureagenic pathway. Glycine is a non-essential amino acid and can be resynthesized using further nitrogen.
3. Phenylacetate is also useful in conditions where benzoate is useful. It reacts with glutamine to form phenylacetyl glutamine which is excreted via the kidney.

Immediate management remains vigorous dialysis to bring ammonia levels down to normal. The benefits of arginine, benzoate and phenylacetate in the treatment of the acutely sick neonate have not been fully evaluated but their use is justified. Meanwhile, precise diagnosis is established by measuring the relevant enzyme levels. Following diagnosis, children are fed a high-calorie (at least 502 kJ/kg/day, 120 kcal/kg/day), low-protein, diet supplying 0.5–1 g protein/kg/day of which a high proportion will be as essential amino acid containing formula, and supplemented with arginine and citrulline, benzoate or phenylacetate as appropriate. Supplementary vitamins will be required.

Where there is a family history of a normal full-term infant dying shortly after birth with progressive hypotonia and drowsiness despite normal delivery, inborn errors such as defects of the urea cycle or organic acidaemias should be suspected and newborn siblings monitored closely. Argininosuccinase and argininosuccinic acid synthetase deficiencies can be diagnosed in the fetus by amniocentesis. Arginase deficiency can be detected on enzyme analysis of fetal erythrocytes. Chorionic villous biopsy is helpful in diagnosing some of these disorders, most notably ornithine transcarbamylase deficiency, in early pregnancy. Neonates thought to be at risk of disorders of the urea cycle should be treated from birth with low-protein, high essential amino acid, high-calorie diets. Deficiency or accumulation of urea cycle intermediates will be apparent after about 48 hours but, on this sort of diet, plasma ammonia levels will not have risen to dangerous levels by that age (Brusilow, 1985).

Arginase deficiency
The presentation of this condition is rather different from that of the other disorders involving deficiency of enzymes in the urea cycle. Hyperammonaemia is mild or absent, and these children do not show the same acute neonatal presentation as children with other abnormalities of the urea cycle, but present as mental retardation and cerebral palsy in early life. Levels of arginine in the blood are greatly increased. Lysine, ornithine, cystine and orotic acid are excreted in the urine. Management is with a diet providing no more than 300 mg/kg/day of arginine.

Carbohydrates – Lacticacidaemias

There are a wide variety of disorders involving enzyme defects which lead to accumulation of lactic acid and severe illness with either death or neurological damage in early life. Most of these conditions are not immediately responsive to dietary management although in multiple carboxylase deficiency shortage of biotin due to re-utilized biotinidase may be overcome by giving supplementary biotin (Robinson, 1985).

Glycogen storage disorders

There are a number of inborn errors of metabolism involving glycogen. Not all these are affected by nutritional management, but glucose 6 phosphatase deficiency (von Gierke's: type I), debrancher enzyme deficiency (type III) and phosphorylase deficiency (Hers' disease: type VI) are to some extent amenable to nutritional management, particularly since hypoglycaemia, hyperuricaemia and hyperlipidaemia are major features.

In type I disease there is failure of gluconeogenesis and glycogenolysis. Children develop enormous livers owing to storage of unmovable glycogen and suffer profound hypoglycaemia. Nutritional management is aimed at controlling the hypoglycaemia and at the same time providing carbohydrate sufficient only to meet immediate requirements so that glycogen storage is diminished. Hyperuricaemia is another complication which may be improved by dietary manipulation but also responds to treatment with allopurinol.

The principles of management are to provide a regular source of carbyhydrate so that the body has no need either to store spare carbohydrate nor to obtain carbohydrate from liver glycogen (Williams, 1986). Carbohydrate should be provided in the form of glucose or starch. Sucrose and lactose should be avoided in type I glycogen storage disease since fructose and galactose are converted to glycogen and lactate in the liver and may contribute to the lactic acidosis these children show. Children are fed frequently, and excessive energy intakes are avoided since these only lead to further glycogen storage in the liver or to hyperlipaemia. Carbohydrate energy should form about 50%, protein 15% and fat no more than 35% of the diet and preferably less, since hypertriglyceridaemia and hypercholesterolaemia are associated problems. Low-cholesterol polyunsaturated fats may be helpful in controlling hypercholesterolaemia.

Nocturnal intragastric feeding in type I glycogen storage disease
Until recently this was the most effective form of management. For some time it has been recognized that a regular supply of glucose by intravenous drip to children with glycogen storage disease reduces the hypoglycaemia, hyperlipidaemia and acidosis of type I disease. Optimal rates of glucose or glucose polymer infusion are approximately 8–9 mg carbohydrate/kg/minute (Schwenk and Haymond, 1986). Blood lactate levels are inversely proportional to plasma glucose levels. By maintaining satisfactory glucose levels, intravenous infusion reduces lactate levels and acidosis, although the lactate levels always remain slightly raised, perhaps because the deficient enzyme, glucose-6-phosphatase, is necessary for recycling lactate formed by glycolysis. Trials of nocturnal nasogastric feeding showed a considerable improvement in affected children with less hypoglycaemia, reduced lactate levels, better growth, reduced liver size, falls in uric acid levels, less osteoporosis (perhaps because of reduced acidosis) and reduced hypertriglycer-

idaemia. The lowered triglyceride level may result from a reduced rate of free fatty acid release to the liver as a response to hypoglycaemia.

Nocturnal feeding of type I disease is not without problems. Type I disease children are usually fairly resistant to symptomatic hypoglycaemia, perhaps because their brains utilize lactate readily in the absence of glucose. With reduction in lactate levels the children adapt to some extent and become less resistant to hypoglycaemia. Sudden cessation of continuous nocturnal feeding due, for example, to disconnection of the drip, failure of the infusion pump or similar occurrences, may result in severe, profound and symptomatic hypoglycaemia. Thus continuous nocturnal infusion is a procedure that should not be introduced lightly. It is very demanding for parents and children, and the psychosocial stress may be excessive. Moreover, if the family are incapable of maintaining a satisfactory feeding programme during the day, there is probably little point in imposing a troublesome regimen at night which they may only follow intermittently and which could therefore by very dangerous.

Uncooked corn starch therapy
Recent developments in the management of glycogen storage disease type I suggest that feeding uncooked corn starch as a source of carbohydrate sustains more normal metabolic indices of adequate therapy such as glucose and lactate levels, than with other sources of carbohydrate (Chen, Cornblath and Sidbury, 1984). Corn starch is usually fed at a rate of 1.75–2.5 g/kg every 6 hours, although the optimal dose for maintaining normoglycaemia needs to be assessed in each patient prior to starting regular therapy. Curiously perhaps, corn starch has to be fed uncooked and should not be made up in warm water or with lemonade since these procedures disrupt starch granules and make them more accessible to hydrolysis by amylase. It is probably the slow breakdown of corn starch by pancreatic amylase and intestinal glucoamylase that is responsible for a gradual release of carbohydrate and maintenance of reasonably normal glucose levels.

Pancreatic amylase activity is low in the newborn, and the effect of this regimen on young infants is not known. If diagnosis of glycogen storage disease is made early in infancy and the infants have never been fed starch, pancreatic amylase activity may be relatively low but induction of the enzyme should occur with feeding starch. There is, however, little experience using this diet in very young infants and it is doubtful whether it is appropriate.

This regimen is difficult to follow but seems to present considerable hope for the management of these children (Williams, 1986). However, as with other conditions described in this chapter, help must be sought from those experienced in management before therapeutic diets are initiated.

Type III glycogen storage disease presents clinically as a milder form of type I and may respond satisfactorily to nocturnal feeding if this is considered necessary. Similarly, type VI may be improved by nocturnal feeding as far as hypoglycaemia is concerned but here hypertriglyceridaemia is the main problem, and fat intake must be carefully controlled.

Fat – hyperlipidaemia

The hyperlipidaemias are another group of inborn errors of metabolism where dietary therapy is helpful in control of some of the conditions. Diagnosis of hyperlipidaemia is made from a suspicious history with a personal or family history of early-onset atherosclerosis and coronary thrombosis or from clinical signs such as xanthelasmata (deposits of cholesterol on knees, elbows and below eyes) and/or corneal arcus (white ring at periphery of cornea). Diagnosis is made on fasting lipid profile which indicates different patterns of abnormal and normal lipids according to the type of hyperlipidaemia. 'Fasting' should mean that the child has been without food for at least 6 hours before blood is taken (Lloyd, 1984).

Serum lipid levels (cholesterol, triglyceride, chylomicrons and lipoproteins) are usually compared against normal ranges for the laboratory where they are measured. Often normal ranges for children have to be taken from work published by others. The mean and range for normal lipid levels is influenced by diet, age, race and nutritional status. Abnormal levels are above the 95th centile for age but, since 5% of normal children will be above this centile, it may be difficult to decide whether or not the child has pathological hyperlipidaemia if there is no supportive family history or clinical findings.

Classification of the hyperlipidaemias is confused since changes in diet, body weight or drug therapy may change the lipid profile abnormalities – and give the individual an apparently different disease (Thompson, 1985). Most familial hyperlipidaemias, with the exception of familial hypercholesterolaemia (familial type IIa hyperlipoproteinaemia) are rare. Management centres on adapting the fat intake (in quantity and quality) to suit the metabolic abnormality.

Familial hypercholesterolaemia

Homozygous type II hyperlipidaemia is rare and has a very poor prognosis. Premature ageing and very early atherosclerosis lead to death in the first or second decade of life. Dietary management is a more rigid adherence to the diet advised for the heterozygous child.

Heterozygous type II hyperlipidaemia (familial hypercholesterolaemia: FH) affects about one in 500 children although relatively few of these children will be recognized as having the condition. Lipid profile shows high plasma cholesterol and high betalipoproteins even in the non-fasting state. The hypercholesterolaemia is largely secondary to accumulation of endogenously produced cholesterol. Cholesterol cannot be metabolized at the cell surface. Dietary fat, particularly cholesterol, restriction and cholesterol elimination by binding agents in the gut (e.g. cholestyramine) can help reduce circulating cholesterol levels.

FH is usually recognized when a relative, often father, develops ischaemic heart disease in the third or fourth decade of life. High cholesterol levels in the relative may prompt a search for other affected family members. The heterozygous condition – FH – is inherited as an autosomal dominant condition.

Vigorous efforts to control hypercholesterolaemia do seem to have some effect in reducing the severity of atherosclerotic change and delaying the age at which ischaemic heart disease develops. These efforts should include other coronary prevention procedures (weight control, no smoking) as well as dietary management. The former may have as much influence on the prognosis as the latter since even rigorous dietary management and use of hypocholesterolaemic agents rarely lowers plasma cholesterol by more than 15%. *Table 13.11* outlines treatment suitable for affected children. High cholesterol foods are indicated in *Table 13.12*.

Cholestyramine (Questran; Bristol-Myers) is a resin which binds bile salts and thus cholesterol in the gut. It can induce nausea, diarrhoea or constipation, and through its binding effects lead to folic acid and fat-soluble vitamin deficiencies. It

Table 13.11 Management of heterozygous familial hypercholesterolaemia

General aspects:
  Avoid overweight
  Maintain reasonable levels of activity
  No smoking – ever!

Dietary aspects:
  Energy intake: modest; keep fat intake <35% total energy
  Polyunsaturated to saturated fat: >1:1
  Moderately high fibre intake to increase cholesterol binding in gut
  Cholestyramine: 4–24 g/day given in two doses
  Supplements: folic acid 5 mg weekly
  ? No added salt to diet

Table 13.12 Foods with particularly high cholesterol content (to be avoided in familial hypercholesterolaemia)

Cholesterol is found in animal products

Meats:
  Beef, lamb, pork, offal
  Prepared meats: liver sausage, tongue
  Fish: fish roe

Dairy products: cheese, butter, cream, lard

Eggs – yolk only

is unpleasant to take as it consists of quite large packets of granules which are mixed with water and swallowed several times a day. Doses for children are usually 1–3 sachets (4–12 g daily). Cholestyramine potentiates the effects of some drugs and reduces the absorption of others so it must be used carefully in association with other drug treatment. It has an effect on blood cholesterol levels but few children tolerate cholestyramine for periods longer than 2 years so the effect is almost invariably of short duration. Despite an often appalling family history of cardiovascular disease, these families are not impressive for the effort and enthusiasm with which they follow management regimens. Perhaps they recognize the limited effect of dietary manipulation when the primary problem is in endogenous cholesterol utilization.

References

BRUSILOW, S. W. (1985) Inborn errors of urea synthesis. In *Genetic and Metabolic Disease in Pediatrics*, edited by J. K. Lloyd and C. Scriver, pp. 140–165. London: Butterworths

CHEN, Y-T., CORNBLATH, M. and SIDBURY, J. B. (1984) Cornstarch therapy in Type I glycogen-storage disease. *New England Journal of Medicine*, **310**, 171–175

CLOTHIER, C. M. and DAVIDSON, D. C. (1983) Galactosaemia workshop. *Human Nutrition: Applied Nutrition*, **37A**, 483–490

FRANCIS, D. E. M. (1987) *Diets for Sick Children*, 4th edn. Oxford: Blackwell Scientific

HOLTZMAN, M. A., KRONMAL, R. A., IAN DOORNOCK, W., AZEN, C. and KOCH, R. (1986) Effect of age at loss of dietary control on intellectual performance and behaviour of children with phenylketonuria. *New England Journal of Medicine,* **314,** 593–598

LLOYD, J. K. (1984) Plasma lipid disorders. *Chemical Pathology and the Sick Child,* edited by B. E. Clayton and J. M. Round, pp. 245–264. Oxford: Blackwell Scientific

ROBINSON, B. H. (1985) The lacticacidaemias. *Genetic and Metabolic Disease in Pediatrics,* edited by J. K. Lloyd and C. Scriver, pp. 111–139. London: Butterworths

SCHWENK, W. F. and HAYMOND, M. W. (1986) Optimal rate of enteral glucose administration in children with glycogen storage disease type I. *New England Journal of Medicine,* **314,** 682–685

SMITH, I. (1985) The hyperphenylalaninaemias. *Genetic and Metabolic Disease in Pediatrics,* edited by J. K. Lloyd and C. R. Scriver, pp. 166–210. London: Butterworths

SMITH, I., LOBASCHER, M. E., STEVENSON, J. E., *et al.* (1978) Effect of stopping low phenylalanine diet: intellectual progress of children with phenylketonuria. *British Medical Journal,* **ii,** 723–726

THOMPSON, G. R. (1985) The hyperlipidaemias. *Genetic and Metabolic Disease in Pediatrics,* edited by J. K. Lloyd and C. Scriver, pp. 211–233. London: Butterworths

WILLIAMS, J. C. (1986) Nutritional goals in glycogen storage disease. *New England Journal of Medicine,* **314,** 709–710

Chapter 14
Intolerant reactions to food

Intolerant responses to food may occur through a variety of mechanisms, and the range of food substances that can cause effects in this way is wide. Well-defined food intolerances giving rise to definite clinical entities (disaccharide, cows' milk protein and gluten intolerance and the inborn errors of metabolism) are discussed elsewhere in this book (*see* Chapters 13 and 15).

Food intolerance, particularly 'food allergy', is a currently fashionable problem and is probably grossly over-diagnosed, frequently without any medical suggestion that this is the nature of the problem. Too often diagnosis is made on whim rather than substantial evidence. This can be dangerous since wrong diagnosis may result in delay in diagnosing the real cause for symptoms and thus delay in initiating appropriate management. Wrong diagnosis may also lead to unnecessarily restricted diets and nutritional deficiencies.

Contrary to popular opinion, many abnormal reactions to food have a 'non-allergic' or 'non immunologic' basis. *Table 14.1* outlines types of allergic and non-allergic adverse reactions to food.

Diagnosis of food intolerance, other than those with biochemical abnormality accounting for the intolerance, should be made only if symptoms occur with a particular food, disappear if that food is withdrawn and recur with reintroduction of the food. Ideally, such a procedure should be carried out three times under

Table 14.1 Intolerant reactions to food*

Psychological	
Food avoidance:	Dislike of taste, texture or connotations.
Psychogenic reactions:	Conditioned reflexes; Meadow's syndrome (Munchausen by proxy)
Pathological	
Inborn errors of metabolism:	Fructose intolerance, glucose-6-phosphate-dehydrogenase deficiency
Digestive enzyme deficiency:	Lactose intolerance
Pharmacological effect:	Tyramine, caffeine
Direct histamine releasing effect:	Shellfish, strawberries
Immunological or allergic responses:	Local; anaphylactoid; delayed hypersensitivity
IgE mediated – like acute response:	Tartrazine, quinoline yellow

* Examples, not complete lists, are given.

'double-blind' circumstances to be truly convincing, since emotional responses can confuse the findings (Goldman *et al.*, 1963). This is not always practical (*see below*). An outline procedure for 'double-blind' food challenge is outlined:

1. Child, parent and observer should be unaware of whether challenge or blind substance being administered.
2. Children with anticipated immediate (<60 minute) responses should be skin tested before oral challenge. A small extract of allergen (or blind) should be injected intradermally.
3. Oral challenge should only follow positive skin test if very low allergen dose used (1% solution or less).
4. Foods for oral challenge should be prepared as solution (50–100 ml of 10% solution of allergen usually), capsule or tablet indistinguishable in appearance and taste from 'blind' challenge.
5. Where an immediate response is expected, food or blind need only be administered once before observing response. Where a delayed response is expected, food or blind may have to be administered regularly for some days before presence or absence of response can be assessed.
6. Responses should be documented as objectively as possible. Responses vary with individuals but are usually rashes, oedema, stridor, wheezing, tachycardia, change in blood pressure, vomiting, abdominal pain, diarrhoea, behavioural change or headache.

When foods appear to produce acute, profound and dangerous reactions, challenge procedures must be waived and a presumptive diagnosis made. When reactions to foods are delayed for days after eating the food, it may be impossible to establish cause and effect for particular foods. It is this latter type of late reaction that leads to the greatest proportion of assumed, but unsubstantiated food 'allergy' diagnoses.

Psychogenic responses

Reactions to food may be psychogenic and inspired by previous experience (or parental experience) with particular foods. Pseudo food allergy syndrome and Munchausen's syndrome by proxy (Meadow's syndrome) are also included amongst psychogenic responses. In this syndrome, children are described by a parent as suffering symptoms in relation to food ingestion but the symptoms are eventually recognized as fabricated by the parent or fictitious.

Separation of purely psychogenic situations from those with a definite pathological origin may be difficult since true allergic phenomena may themselves be exaggerated by anxiety or fear over the possible consequences of contact with a food. In purely psychogenic situations, conditioned or suggested reflexes or hyperreactivity to normal autonomic nervous system activation by emotion precipitate the symptoms. Such psychogenic reactions to food are not necessarily part of a wider psychological disturbance, but when manifest as Munchausen's by proxy (Warner and Hathaway, 1984) they usually indicate seriously disturbed mother–child interaction requiring psychiatric help.

Allergic responses

Acute or immediate allergic reactions to food are probably the easiest to recognize. Radioallergoabsorbent tests (RAST) on blood for the specific food are often positive, and serum IgE levels may be raised. Skin-prick tests to food extracts may also be positive.

Symptoms of acute reactions may be vomiting, profuse diarrhoea, wheezing, an urticarial-like eruption, or angioneurotic oedema with swelling of face, tongue, neck and stridor or major respiratory obstruction. If an acute response is suspected, testing with the suspect foods should occur only under close medical supervision with steroids, adrenaline and other resuscitative measures immediately available (David, 1984).

Many food intolerances presenting in early life and mediated through IgE mechanisms resolve within the first 3 years of life (Wood, 1986). It is thus worth attempting supervised introduction of previously allergenic food at 3 years old since persisting with dietary restrictions can be very inconvenient – particularly if no longer necessary.

Delayed hypersensitivity responses to food lead to much more confusion. Confirmation that the food is cause of the symptoms is normally made by withdrawing the food and curing the symptoms. It may be difficult to demonstrate definite relationship between reintroducing the food and recurrence of the symptoms because of a considerable time lag. Thus the diagnosis of delayed hypersensitivity response to food is susceptible to a lot of subjective interpretation. The diagnosis is further complicated by the attribution of food allergy to explain chronic gastrointestinal conditions such as Crohn's disease, ulcerative colitis and irritable bowel syndrome. Relief of symptoms with withdrawal of foods in these chronic gastrointestinal conditions does not necessarily mean that the foods are causing the conditions.

Food intolerances are commonly sought as explanations for chronic conditions such as atopic eczema and asthma. Cows'-milk protein is the most commonly blamed food, and it may be necessary to exclude this from the mother's diet in breast-fed infants with an atopic family history (Cant et al., 1986). The evidence that exclusion of cows' milk protein from the diet of all infants aged under 6 months with an atopic family history makes a significant difference to the incidence of eczema in these children is controversial (Atherton et al., 1978; van Asperen, Kemp and Mellis, 1984). Nevertheless, it seems wise to recommend mothers of infants with a strong family history of atopy to breast feed and to avoid, if possible, introducing other foods, particularly cows' milk and egg protein, before 6 months of age. Almost certainly some infants are helped by allergen avoidance, but not all. Maximum benefit is probably gained in the first 3 months of life when the gut is most permeable to foreign proteins. Breast milk protects against allergy by allowing avoidance of foreign proteins and by sIgA coating the gastrointestinal mucosa and protecting against absorption of antigens (Atherton, 1983). It is not wise to insist on pursuing a 'breast milk only' diet if mother's milk is insufficient to meet the infant's needs for normal growth. Close monitoring of all diets recommended for present and potential food allergy must include regular assessments of nutrition and growth.

Elimination diets

Elimination diets – diets that initially exclude all except a few hypoallergenic foods – are widely used to try to define food causes for severe eczema, migraine and a number of other conditions. Belief in the importance of food allergy for development or exacerbation of these conditions is not necessarily based on scientific justification. Initial attitudes readily colour the interpretation of results. Double-blind controlled studies of very careful design are needed to prove the place of food intolerance in these conditions. Where reactions to foods are delayed, such studies are extremely difficult to perform to a cynic's satisfaction. When elimination diets have been used with success, great dedication and discipline by child, family and paediatrician is necessary to complete the elimination programme. Elimination diets should not be introduced without significant symptomatology and a clearly defined elimination procedure.

It is unwise for parents to try to find out their children's allergies through gradual elimination of foods without medical and dietary supervision. The procedure requires hospital supervision, if not admission, in order to ensure that nutrition is not disadvantaged. Such diets must be approached in conjunction with paediatric dietetic departments where nutrient intake can be assessed and the child's overall nutritional status closely monitored. To find out which foods precipitate eczema, for example, the child is managed in hospital on an elemental diet until the skin clears. The elemental diet consists of simple carbohydrate sources, medium-chain triglycerides, essential amino acid mixtures, vitamins and minerals, and spring or distilled water. Products such as Elemental 028 diets (Scientific Hospital Supplies) and Vivonex (Norwich Eaton), with vitamins (Ketovite liquid and tablets; Paines & Byrne) and minerals (Metabolic Mineral Mixture; Scientific Hospital Supplies) may be used in children aged over 1 year (Francis, 1987). Following resolution of the skin problems the child is gradually introduced to different foods. Initial foods are often pears and chicken since these seem amongst the least allergenic foods. No additives must be used. One new food is introduced each day and signs and symptoms closely monitored. Any food associated with signs or symptoms is excluded. Once a reasonable diet is established, the child is discharged from hospital and encouraged to continue on the diet. Mineral and vitamin supplements usually remain necessary if more than the occasional food is eliminated. Despite such supplements many of these diets end up deficient in calcium (David, Waddington and Stanton, 1984).

Food elimination procedures are quite widely and successfully used in the management of severe eczema and less frequently in the investigation of migraine and various gastrointestinal symptoms. Most conditions for which they are used follow a relapsing course, frequently respond to hospital admission alone and are strongly influenced by emotion. Often too the response to an 'allergen' is not immediate. For these reasons it is difficult to judge the real value of these complicated procedures and to estimate what proportion of children will be benefited (Carter, Egger and Soothill, 1985).

Food additives

This is a difficult topic since the practice of some paediatricians and nutritionists is heavily committed to belief in the importance of food additives in the symptomatology of both childhood and adult life. The activity of parents over providing what they believe to be best for their children may be misdirected into obsessive additive avoidance, sometimes to the children's nutritional disadvantage (Warner and Hathaway, 1984).

Many will disagree with our views on food additives and food allergy. Attitudes on these matters are so strongly polarized that we seem bound to offend some, if not all, our readers. Yet it is always wise to look critically at the scientific evidence for practices that invoke such heightened emotions (David, 1987).

What are food additives? These are substances – and there are a great many of them – added to food as preservatives, colourants or taste enhancers. Taken in the widest sense, additives must include substances such as whey or wheat starch, used as thickeners or emulsifiers and to which those who are intolerant of milk or gluten may react. Substances such as ascorbic acid, often used as a preservative in canning or to replace natural vitamin C lost in processing, are essential nutrients. Ascorbic acid is food additive E300. Riboflavin – also an essential nutrient – is E101 (*see below*).

Without additives, many of the processed and packaged proprietary products that make life so much easier for housewives and mothers could not exist. Not included in the additive list but important if the overall contribution of food to allergic disease is considered are the hormones and antibiotics fed to animals and the pesticides and fertilizers that may be present in small quantities of 'raw' foods. Other additives, for example fluoride, occur in the drinking water supply.

In principle, it would seem advisable that no food should have substances that do not class as foodstuffs added simply to make that food look more attractive or have a more attractive taste. This should apply particularly to food colourants since the chemical studies of colourants and dyes suggest many colourants have chemical structures known to be poorly accepted by the body. On the same principle, all 'treatment' given to plants or animals to increase yield, financial gain for stock, etc., should be reviewed so that unnecessary substances are not introduced into foods.

Thus there is a burden on modern food manufacturers to review all forms of food additives and reduce their use. The potential risk to the population will then diminish.

But what are the risks? As already mentioned, many so-called 'additives' are nutrients or food substances in themselves. The 'E' numbers indicate their European Community authorization (which does not necessarily permit their use throughout all the Member States). Addition of no more than the levels available in many foods of substances such as ascorbic acid is unlikely to cause anyone harm. By contrast, substances such as tartrazine (E102) and quinoline yellow (E104) are used basically as colourants. They do seem unnecessary nutritionally although they may make foods look – according to conventional views – more appetizing. Acute reactions presenting as similar to, but not due to, IgE associated allergic responses develop in some individuals when they ingest these colourants. It would seem reasonable that their use should cease.

What about the effect of food additives on children's behaviour? Diets that are basically additive free have been developed (the Feingold Diet) for the treatment of hyperactive children. Some studies purport to show a definite improvement in behaviour with additive-free diets. Most of these studies can be criticized for lack of proper control studies, and controversy rages between exponents and debasers of these diets.

One of the problems in studying the effect of these diets is that of defining hyperactivity as well as food allergy. A hyperactive child is not just one who is exhausting to his or her parents – most children are this at some period in their lives – but a child who has no other effect on parents. Hyperactivity is 'a long term childhood pattern characterized by excessive restlessness and inattentiveness' and 'a persistent pattern of excessive activity in situations requiring motor inhibition' (Gadow, 1986).

Most studies suggest that the majority of hyperactive children are no different on additive-free diets. Where there is improvement it may be related more to the strong discipline imposed in order to maintain the diet in behaviourally disturbed children than to specific effects of the diet. Very few children show response confirmed in double-blind controlled studies. Thus there seems little point in subjecting children if benefit is unlikely. Parents should certainly be discouraged from introducing these dietary regimens without medical guidance since the possibilities for nutritional deficiency are great. How clinicians cope with parents who insist on pursuing additive-free diets despite advice is a decision dependent on individual circumstances. It may be wiser to accept a child for an additive-free regimen rather than to antagonize the parents so that the child is subjected to unsupervised dietary restriction or to the vagaries of an untrained or unprincipled nutritional counsellor. The clinician should be aware, however, that obsessive pursuit of an additive-free diet may reflect abnormal mother–child interaction amounting to a bizarre form of child abuse (Warner and Hathaway, 1984; David, 1985).

References

ATHERTON, D. J. (1983) Breast feeding and atopic eczema. *British Medical Journal*, **287**, 775–776

ATHERTON, D. J., SEWELL, M., SOOTHILL, J. F., WELLS, R. S. and CHILVERS, C. E. D. (1978) A double blind controlled crossover trial of an antigen avoidance diet in atopic eczema. *Lancet*, **i**, 401–403

CANT, A. J., BAILES, J. A., MARSDEN, R. A. and HEWITT, D. (1986) Effect of maternal dietary exclusion on breast fed infants with eczema: two controlled studies. *British Medical Journal*, **293**, 231–233

CARTER, C. M., EGGER, J. and SOOTHILL, J. F. (1985) A dietary management of severe childhood migraine. *Human Nutrition: Applied Nutrition*, **39A**, 294–303

DAVID, T. J. (1984) Anaphylactic shock during elimination diets for severe atopic eczema. *Archives of Disease in Childhood*, **59**, 983–986

DAVID, T. J. (1985) The overworked or fraudulent diagnosis of food allergy and food intolerance in children. *Journal of Royal Society of Medicine*, **78**, Suppl. 5, 21–31

DAVID, T. J. (1987) Reactions to dietary tartrazine. *Archives of Disease in Childhood*, **62**, 119–122

DAVID, T. J., WADDINGTON, E. and STANTON, R. H. J. (1984) Nutritional hazards of elimination diets in children. *Archives of Disease in Childhood*, **59**, 323–325

FRANCIS, D. E. M. (1987) *Diets for Sick Children*, 4th edn., p. 89. Oxford: Blackwell Scientific

GOLDMAN, A. S., ANDERSON, D. W. J., SELLERS, W. A., SAPERSTEIN, S., KNIKER, W. T. and HALPERN, S. R. (1963) Milk allergy 1. Oral challenge with milk and isolated milk proteins in allergic children. *Pediatrics*, **32**, 425–443

GADOW, K. D. (1986) *Children on Medication. Volume I. Hyperactivity, Learning Disorders and Mental Retardation*, p. 33. London: Taylor & Francis

Van ASPEREN, P. P., KEMP, A. J. and MELLIS, C. M. (1984) Relationship of diet in the development of atopy in infancy. *Clinical Allergy*, **14**, 525–532

WARNER, J. O. and HATHAWAY, M. J. (1984) Allergic form of Meadow's syndrome (Munchausen by proxy). *Archives of Disease in Childhood*, **59**, 151–156

WOOD, C. B. S. (1986) How common is food allergy? *Acta Paediatrica Scandinavica*, **Suppl. 323**, 76–83

Chapter 15
Gastrointestinal disorders

Acute diarrhoea

Acute diarrhoea is probably the commonest antecedent of childhood malnutrition both in developed and in developing countries. Single episodes of diarrhoea if severe and prolonged may result in malnutrition, but recurrent episodes of diarrhoea with little time for recovery in between episodes are particularly likely to lead to progressive nutritional deterioration (Rowland, Cole and Whitehead, 1977; Mata, 1985). Management of diarrhoea must therefore be geared to mimimizing the malnourishing effects.

By far the commonest cause of acute malnourishing diarrhoea is infection – bacterial, viral or parasitic – but food intolerances such as lactose or cows' milk protein intolerance following these episodes of infection and prolonging the diarrhoea commonly contribute to failure to thrive and to malnutrition (Walker-Smith, 1986).

The use of oral rehydration therapy (ORT) solutions has revolutionized management and prognosis for children with acute diarrhoea. Sodium absorption linked to glucose or amino acid transport mechanisms is unaffected by acute diarrhoea even in secretory states such as cholera. Water is transported passively with the other molecules. Thus, provided sodium salts are supplied in the presence of glucose or amino acids, water absorption occurs both between and through cells, and this continues even though water and sodium are being excreted by other mechanisms (Mahalanabis, 1985). ORT has enabled children and adults to be rehydrated orally in situations where previously intravenous therapy was necessary. This has meant effective home management, fewer hospital admissions and fewer deaths from acute diarrhoea.

The aim of oral rehydration is to maximize absorption of salt and water without leaving unabsorbed solutes – saline or glucose – in the small intestine since these encourage osmotic diarrhoea in the large intestine. The optimal concentration of glucose for sodium–water absorption appears to be a 2% solution. Where sucrose is used instead of glucose, twice this amount of sucrose is necessary for optimal sodium absorption, and treatment failure rates are slightly higher owing to the slower rates of absorption of fructose.

Table 15.1 outlines the composition of various solutions used for ORT. Some ORT solutions contain only glucose and saline. Others contain bicarbonate and potassium as well. Bicarbonate facilitates sodium absorption even without glucose. Bicarbonate or citrate also avoid the need to provide chloride in excess of

Table 15.1 Composition (in mmol/l) of some preparations used in oral replacement therapy

Solution	Sodium	Potassium	Chloride	Bicarbonate	Glucose
WHO recommended formula*	90	20	80	30	111
Sodium chloride and glucose oral powder (BNF)†	35	20	37	18	200
Dioralyte (Armour)‡	35	20	37	18	200
'Dextrose–saline' (sodium chloride 0.18%, glucose 4% solution)§	30	–	30	–	222

* Distributed by UNICEF as Oral Rehydration Salts. One packet dilutes to 1 litre.
† Sachets to be diluted to 500 ml (standard size) or 200 ml (small size).
‡ Sachets to be diluted to 200 ml.
§ Only available as fluid, therefore bulky.

anticipated needs. Potassium is sometimes included since diarrhoea may readily give rise to potassium deficiency states. There is a slight risk in giving potassium to children whose renal function is uncertain because of dehydration. In Britain, potassium can easily be added to the solutions by flavouring them with fruit juices once the children start to pass urine well or when potassium is seen to be falling on measuring electrolytes. ORT preparations used in paediatrics are often made lower in sodium concentration than those used for adults because of the occasional presentation of hypernatraemic dehydration with diarrhoea in infancy. Where there is secretory diarrhoea such as in cholera, full-strength solutions should be used. ORT preparations can be presented in the form in which they are to be drunk but they will be bulky for transport from clinic to home. Several powdered forms are available which require dilution in variable quantities of clean boiled (and cooled) water (*Table 15.1*). *Boiled* water is probably unnecessary after infancy if drinking-water sources are *clean* piped water.

In the developing world where ORT has made such a difference to the outlook for sick children, recipes have been devised for making up the ORT solutions from appropriate amounts of domestic constituents and measures. One such recipe would be five cupfuls of boiled water, eight level teaspoons of sugar and one level teaspoon of salt. It is obviously important that advice given to mothers in disadvantaged circumstances is practical, simple, and free from risk or confusion. Even if only community-health workers are taught the procedure and encouraged to use ORT, the management of sick dehydrated children will be greatly improved and, since diarrhoea is such a common antecedent of malnutrition, overall nutrition should be improved as well.

Children presenting with significant diarrhoea should be taken off all food except breast milk and provided with ORT solution equivalent to daily fluid requirements plus calculated fluid deficit plus any ensuing fluid losses in diarrhoea (*Table 15.2*). Where breast feeding is continuing, ORT should be provided in quantities sufficient to correct dehydration and account for abnormal losses such as diarrhoea stools and vomit. Fluids should be given so as to provide half the expected requirements in the first 8 hours and the rest over the next 16 hours. Even where the child has been vomiting, it is worth trying ORT (unless the child is *in extremis*) since frequent (hourly or more frequently) administration of ORT may be tolerated where feeding other fluids, or larger volumes of fluid less frequently, have not been tolerated.

Table 15.2 Example of fluid requirements for dehydrated weaned child of 1 year (volumes apply to oral or intravenous fluids)

Weight of child	≃ 10 kg
Severe dehydration	≃ 10% loss body weight
Therefore fluid loss	≃ 1000 ml
Daily fluid requirements	≃ 100 ml/kg
Therefore requirements over next 24 hours	= 2000 ml
given as 1000 ml in 8 hours	at 125 ml/hour
1000 ml over 16 hours at	63 ml/hour

Plus calculated fluid losses in vomit and stools measured by collecting liquid or weighing clean and dirty nappies

Where the child is breast fed, the excellent absorption of breast milk plus its anti-infective properties are beneficial for the infant, and breast feeding should continue if possible. Studies from Burma suggest that infants given breast milk and ORT had fewer, smaller stools than those on ORT alone (Khin-Maung et al., 1985).

The usual practice for non-breast-fed children is to restrict intake to ORT solution until diarrhoea stops and then gradually 'regrade' feeds. 'Regrading' means introducing dilute (usually quarter-strength) milk for the next 24 hours and gradually increasing the strength of feeds over the next few days. Many children, although perhaps not infants less than 9 months, are able to tolerate full-strength milk once diarrhoea has settled and 'regrading' is unnecessary. If immediate introduction of full-strength milk is possible, children have shorter periods of weight loss and suffer less debilitating malnutrition (Placzek and Walker-Smith, 1984; McDowell and Evans-Jones, 1985). Consequently they are less at risk of succumbing to further diarrhoea than those who are regraded gradually.

How long should ORT continue? Although extremely effective in the management of diarrhoea, ORT provides little energy, and children fed ORT solution alone will be in negative nitrogen and energy balance. Where children are already malnourished, this is worrying since the diarrhoea may have been exacerbated by their previous poor nutrition. ORT should be continued for as short a time as possible and for not more than 24 hours without other food source, except under medical supervision. It can be given in association with other bland foods if diarrhoea persists and hydration remains at risk, although ORT is less effective in settling diarrhoea if food is being given as well. Severely malnourished children should be tried on some food (preferably small quantities frequently) after 12 hours of ORT – or considered as candidates for parenteral nutrition.

One of the common causes for continued diarrhoea and progressive malnutrition in children with initially an acute gastrointestinal infection is food intolerance. This may be disaccharide, particularly lactose, intolerance or alternatively cows' milk protein intolerance.

Disaccharide intolerance

Intolerance of disaccharides, particularly lactose, is a common problem. It usually occurs during or following gastrointestinal insults such as gastroenteritis, untreated coeliac disease, gastrointestinal surgery or malnutrition or other severe illness. Very rarely it presents as a primary, genetically determined, deficiency – alactasia.

Lactase is present in the brush border of the mucosal cells of the small intestine. Concentrations peak around birth but lactose concentrations are never greatly in excess of those required for digestion of a milk diet. Unlike most other enzymes, concentrations seem to some extent determined by dietary lactose content. Thus traces of lactose may be found in the stools of infants at a few days of age, but these traces gradually disappear by a week, presumably secondary to increases in gastrointestinal lactase production. Man is unusual compared with other mammals in that he keeps his lactase activity into post weaning life. However, in those races who do not drink milk traditionally (especially Bantu African and Asian) there is a particular tendency for lactase levels to decline significantly with age. Lactose intolerance is thus common in healthy, well-nourished older children and adults from these races. Lactase activity is also very sensitive to any damage affecting the gastrointestinal mucosa.

Lactose intolerance usually presents as diarrhoea with the explosive passage of frothy, yellow stools. Undigested lactose is subjected to bacterial digestion in the large bowel with the production of hydrogen (detectable in breath assays) and organic acids. Hyperosmolality of gastrointestinal contents due to undigested lactose leads to intestinal hurry, abdominal distension, discomfort secondary to large amounts of gas in the large intestine and perianal excoriation due to the passage of frequent acid stools which burn the perianal skin. Because sugars are malabsorbed, the wasting in predominantly milk fed infants is often marked.

Diagnosis of lactose intolerance is by collecting fresh liquid stool and demonstrating an acid pH (pH<5.5) and the presence of reducing substances (five drops of liquid or emulsified stool: ten drops of water and a Clinitest tablet (Ames): positive response = >¼% reducing substances). Stools tested for lactose must be fresh since bacterial digestion of lactose to organic acids rapidly destroys reducing activity in the stool. If the stools are very liquid they should be collected with the infant lying on a plastic sheet. Lactose is very soluble and rapidly absorbed into cotton sheets or napkins. Lactase levels in the jejunum can be measured if jejunal juice is aspirated.

Treatment of lactose intolerance is by exclusion of lactose from the diet until gastrointestinal function appears normal (usually indicated by return to normal weight for height). Since many children with symptoms of lactose intolerance are infants still consuming predominantly milk diets, it is usually necessary to provide them with lactose-free formula. *Table 15.3* indicates the composition of some commonly used lactose-free formulas.

Occasionally, damage to the gastrointestinal tract results in intolerance to other disaccharides as well as lactose. Symptoms are similar with acid stools but when sucrose intolerance is present, reducing substances are not demonstrable in the stools since sucrose is not a reducing sugar. Sugar electrophoresis of the stools demonstrates significant amounts of the relevant disaccharides. Again, management is by provision of disaccharide-free diet using one of the sucrose–lactose free milks indicated in *Table 15.3*.

It is important that children should only be put on specialized milks and diets such as those described above when there are clear indications. To use more commonplace terms, these diets should be used only under medical supervision. It is not uncommon to find children with gastrointestinal or other symptoms who have been changed onto specialized formula and lactose- or milk-free diets for rather

Table 15.3 Basic composition of some lactose-free formulas

Formula	Manufacturer	Carbohydrate source	Protein source	Fat source
Galactomin 17*	Cow & Gate	Dextrose, maltose and glucose syrup solids. Trace of lactose	Cows' milk protein	Coconut and maize oils
Formula S	Cow & Gate	Glucose syrup	Soya protein isolate + 1-methionine	Vegetable oil
Isomil	Abbott	Corn syrup solids and sucrose	Soya protein isolate + 1-methionine	Corn and coconut oils
Nutramigen	Mead Johnson	Modified starch and sucrose	Casein hydrolysate	Corn oil
Pregestimil	Mead Johnson	Modified starch	Casein hydrolysate	Corn oil and MCT
Prosobee	Mead Johnson	Glucose syrup solids	Soya protein isolate + 1-methionine	Coconut and soya oil
Wysoy	Wyeth	Sucrose, corn syrup solids	Soya protein isolate + 1-methionine	Animal and vegetable oils

* Requires added vitamins and minerals.

nebulous reasons. Confusion may then arise when the symptoms persist or recur and appropriate investigation of the symptoms may be delayed whilst the effect of another specialized milk is tried.

There is a tendency – for reasons of profit, presumably – for milk marketing firms to devise formulas suitable for an ever-increasing variety of clinical circumstances. This author can see no place for the low-carbohydrate, low-fat, high-protein formulas currently marketed for use in the convalescent period after diarrhoea, particularly since such formulas tend to be low in total energy content – a particularly undesirable feature for children recovering from periods of diarrhoea and oral rehydration therapy. If children really cannot tolerate fat and at least non-disaccharide carbohydrate, they require close paediatric dietetic supervision to ensure that formula and solid foods are free of disaccharides, but adequate in energy content.

Disaccharide intolerance usually resolves once normal nutritional status is restored and gastrointestinal infection resolved. Small quantities of disaccharide containing dilute feed (¼ strength) should be offered as one feed 1 or 2 months after loss of symptoms and restoration of normal weight for length. If this feed has no adverse effects, one feed a day should be gradually built up to a full-strength milk feed and then other feeds of normal formula or cows' milk (depending on the child's age) introduced as required.

Cows' milk protein intolerance (CMPI)

CMPI commonly develops secondary to gastrointestinal insult such as infection, malnutrition or surgery. Under such circumstances, CMPI usually causes gastrointestinal disturbance with vomiting, diarrhoea or gastrointestinal blood loss. Rarely, CMPI develops acutely in otherwise healthy previously breast-fed infants introduced to cows' milk protein containing foods.

The problem with CMPI is that it presents no specific clinical features and cannot be proven in the same way as lactose intolerance. Diagnosis is therefore by suspicion and loss of symptoms on exclusion of cows' milk protein. If lactose intolerance has been excluded, symptoms of CMPI resolve rapidly after stopping cows' milk or formula ingestion and should recur within a day or so of introducing full-strength milk again. As with other exclusion diets, stringent criteria for diagnosis should be applied since many infants are unjustifiably labelled CMPI on slim and inadequate grounds. Incorrect diagnosis can cause a lot of unnecessary anxiety for parents over their children's diets and may even result in time-wasting before symptoms are correctly diagnosed.

CMPI may present as either an acute or a chronic condition. *Table 15.4* lists some of the ways in which CMPI may present. The acute response to cows' milk protein feeding may be very dramatic with anaphylactic collapse in response to only small amounts of ingested cows' milk protein. Alternatively oedema (often of lips and tongue), wheezing and urticaria may present over a matter of hours. Infants presenting in an acute and dramatic way often have increased levels of serum IgE and elevated milk specific antibodies demonstrable by skin-prick tests and RAST responses. IgG, IgA and IgM milk antibodies are usually low. Frequently the children presenting with anaphylactic responses to cows' milk are not those with preceding illness. Some are infants who have been introduced to cows' milk or formula having previously been breast fed. Presumably such infants have been sensitized through cows' milk antigens crossing the placenta or into the breast milk and being ingested by the infants.

Table 15.4 Presentations of cows' milk protein intolerance

Related to gastrointestinal pathology

Vomiting
Diarrhoea – acute or chronic
Abdominal pain
Intestinal blood loss:
  Massive
  Insidious
Weight loss secondary to enteropathy
Iron-deficiency anaemia

Systemic response

Anaphylaxis
Angioneurotic oedema
Urticaria
Asthma
Eczema

A more typical pattern than the acute anaphylactic response of CMPI occurs as a delayed response in infants following gastrointestinal insult. These children develop vomiting, diarrhoea, failure to thrive, abdominal pain and occult or overt rectal bleeding. Where CMPI induces haemorrhagic colitis (with marked eosinophilic infiltration of colonic mucosa), small bowel mucosa is often normal. Conversely, abnormal small bowel histology is usually associated with normal colonic histology. Small bowel biopsy may demonstrate a moderate enteropathy often with dense accumulations of fat in the epithelium. The enteropathy is patchy, and the transient nature of CMPI may make it difficult to prove the diagnosis by withdrawing CMPI, restoring histology to normal, and then demonstrating deterioration with reintroduction of CMPI. Gastrointestinal challenge with cows' milk protein to confirm CMPI (*see below*) should be done extremely cautiously and in hospital since these children occasionally show dramatic anaphylactoid responses (Walker-Smith, 1985).

Recovery from cows' milk protein intolerance is usually slower than that from lactose intolerance, and it is advisable to keep affected infants on cows' milk protein free diets until after the age of 1 year and then to challenge these infants very carefully: 5 ml cows' milk are given on one day and the child is observed very closely for evidence of shock, angioneurotic oedema, urticaria or diarrhoea. If all is well, one feed of quarter-strength milk is offered the next day. If the child remains symptom free, one feed a day can be gradually built up to full-strength milk. Once the child is tolerating one feed of full-strength cows' milk per day it is probably reasonable to allow the child home and explain to the parents to increase full-strength milk feeds at the rate of one feed per day provided there are no suggestive symptoms.

CMPI can be treated with soya-based formulas (intolerance to soya is probably as common as CMPI); formulas containing non-allergic casein hydrolysate (*see Table 15.3*); or comminuted chicken protein combined with carbohydrate and fat sources and supplemented with vitamins and minerals. Soya-based formulas are probably better avoided in early management of CMPI since the gastrointestinal damage caused by CMPI may make the infant more liable to soy protein intolerance (Committee on Nutrition, 1983).

Malabsorption syndromes

The potential list of causes of malabsorption in childhood is huge. *Table 15.5* outlines some causes of malabsorption in childhood giving a few specific examples. Malabsorption of major nutrients is generally manifest by frequency of stools and failure to thrive. Where malabsorption of fat predominates, stools are often bulky,

Table 15.5 Some causes of malabsorption syndrome in childhood

Pancreatic enzyme deficiency:
   Congenital: Cystic fibrosis, Schwachman syndrome
   Acquired: Chronic pancreatitis

Hepatic:
  Congenital biliary atresia
  Neonatal hepatitis syndrome
  Cirrhosis:
    Congenital, e.g. Wilson's disease
    Acquired, e.g. post hepatitis

Enteropathic: Gluten sensitive, CMPI

Infections and infestations: Giardiasis, Ascariasis

CMPI = Cows' milk protein intolerance.

pale, greasy and may be difficult to flush in the toilet owing to their tendency to float. Where protein absorption (as in cystic fibrosis) is particularly poor, stools may also be exceptionally smelly owing to bacterial breakdown of undigested protein. Carbohydrate malabsorption tends to lead to formation of organic acids and hydrogen by bacterial fermentation in the large bowel and causes a lot of skin excoriation secondary to the acid stools. Malabsorption of other nutrients may be manifest by clinical features of the specific nutrient deficiency.

Coeliac disease (gluten-sensitive enteropathy; GSE)

This is a relatively common problem affecting perhaps 1 in 2000 individuals in UK but in certain areas it may be much more common (e.g. 1 in 300 in Western Eire). Coeliac disease occurs as a result of gastrointestinal intolerance to gluten and only occurs when infants have been weaned onto gluten-containing solids. Symptoms do not necessarily present with first introduction to gluten and may only develop late in life. There is a strong familial tendency to gluten-sensitive enteropathy which can be followed by HLA typing since certain HLA patterns (particularly HLA B8, which is linked into a number of diseases with abnormalities of immune function), are associated with gluten-sensitive enteropathy more commonly than they are distributed in the general population (Bullen, 1985; McNicholl, 1986). The incidence of coeliac disease in first-degree relatives of cases is 5–19%.

Gluten is present in wheat, flour, oats and rye. It is the insoluble portion of wheat flour and is a mixture of proteins. It appears to have a toxic effect on the mucosal cells of susceptible individuals, but the specific factor in gluten that causes this toxic effect and the way in which it exerts this effect is ill understood. Attempts to fractionate gluten to produce a toxic fraction have not been very successful. Gliadin, the alcohol-soluble fraction, is usually considered the most damaging component but other fractions also have cytotoxic effects.

Children with coeliac disease present with the symptoms of malabsorption frequently a few months to a year after weaning (*Table 15.6*). However, coeliac disease may present at any age. Where nutrient demands are high – such as during infancy, adolescence, pregnancy, lactation and, possibly, old age where maintenance of adequate bone mineralization may be difficult – the malabsorption resulting from gluten damage to the gastrointestinal tract is sufficient to produce clinical effects and symptomatic nutritional deficiency. Often, however, children

Table 15.6 Presentation of coeliac disease

Infant and young child

History:	thrived until weaning, failure to thrive or weight loss, misery and apathy, motor delay, anorexia, vomiting, abdominal pain, frequent loose bulky stools (occasionally constipation if severely anorexic), may be short or prolonged history
Clinical features:	underweight, wasted (muscle and fat loss), abdominal distension with doughy feel to abdomen, iron-deficiency anaemia, angular stomatitis, rickets, mild oedema

Older child

Any, all, or more or less none, of above signs.
May present as persistent, unexplained anaemia, especially iron-deficient anaemia.
May present as short stature with no other signs or symptoms.
Dermatitis herpetiformis

with gluten-sensitive enteropathy have minimal symptoms but are short and may have refractory iron-deficiency anaemia. Some appear to have no clinical signs whatsoever despite abnormal jejunal histology.

The diagnosis of coeliac disease is suspected from history and clinical signs. It is supported by evidence suggesting malabsorption (iron-deficiency anaemia; low serum folate or red cell folate levels; low albumin; low serum calcium and high alkaline phosphatase, etc.) and by screening tests such as xylose absorption. In the xylose absorption test xylose 5 g is fed rapidly and blood is collected for measurement of xylose levels exactly 1 hour later. The normal blood xylose should be greater than 1.7 µmol/l (25 mg/dl). Alternatively, more than 20% of the ingested dose should be excreted in the urine in 5 hours, but timed urine collections are not easy in the age group usually being studied. Blood xylose test is quite useful as a screening test in infants and children under about 10 kg but not helpful in older children.

There is only one way of confirming suspected coeliac disease and that is by finding total or sub-total villous atrophy on jejunal biopsy (Tripp and Candy, 1985). Children should not be started on gluten-free diets without this confirmation. There is loss of the normal villus pattern, often obvious with binocular microscopy of a fresh jejunal specimen; hypertrophy of the crypts of Lieberkühn; cuboid abnormal surface epithelium (usually columnar); lymphocytic infiltration of the epithelium and plasma cell infiltration of the lamina propria. On electron microscopy there is damage to the brush border and the presence of immature cells and increased cell loss. Often there is evidence of inadequate epithelial cell function with low lactase activity in the jejunum.

Once diagnosed convincingly as having the condition, children must remain on a gluten-free diet for life. In 1969 the European Society for Paediatric Gastroenterology listed criteria for making the definitive diagnosis of gluten-sensitive enteropathy using a minimum of three jejunal biopsies (Meeuwisse, 1970; McNeish et al., 1979). These are as follows:

1. A flat jejunal mucosa with histological evidence of total villous atrophy.
2. Restoration to normal jejunal mucosa following removal of gluten from the diet.
3. Recurrence of total villous atrophy subsequent to re-introduction of gluten.

In some ways these criteria are a counsel of perfection. *Transient* gluten intolerance quite frequently follows severe diarrhoea or malnutrition in young children and so it is important that the criteria are fulfilled if possible, and particularly for children under a year. The first two jejunal biopsies present little controversy for diagnosis and it is not usually necessary to argue the need for them to parents. It is, however, frequently very difficult to persuade parents of the need to re-introduce gluten and allow recurrence of symptoms or at least deterioration in gastrointestinal function to prove the diagnosis. Moreover, if the children are introduced to gluten in normal foods, it may be difficult to get them back onto the gluten-free diet for a second time. It is probably easier to introduce a specific quantity of gluten (10 g/day) as powder sprinkled on the food rather than to re-introduce gluten-containing foods such as biscuits and normal bread. Usually the second biopsy is obtained about a year after recovery on gluten-free diet. If 2 years then lapse on gluten without symptoms or deterioration in biopsy, coeliac disease is usually considered ruled out. In view of occasional cases where *many* years lapse before deterioration occurs, decisions that coeliac disease has been excluded should be circumspect (Kuitunen, Savilahti and Verkasalo, 1986).

In theory, management of gluten-sensitive enteropathy is simple. Gluten is all that need be excluded from the diet. In practice, the management of a gluten-free diet in childhood is quite difficult. Many children eat a lot of biscuits, bread and wheat-flour-containing foods such as wheat-based breakfast cereals, cakes and pastry. These must be excluded, but in addition so must many other foods where wheat starch is added as a thickener or filler. As with so many other diets it is necessary for these mothers to wander round supermarkets reading small print on manufactured foods or to rely on the lists of acceptable and unacceptable foods produced by the Coeliac Society and other interested groups. (For addresses, *see* Appendix.)

The immediate management of the acutely ill child with coeliac disease requires cessation of all gluten in the diet, supplementation with vitamins (Ketovite liquid and tablets; Paines & Byrne) and oral iron therapy. Mildly affected children may show no obvious evidence of nutritional deficiency, but their nutrient requirements must increase if they are to show catch-up growth and therefore vitamin and iron supplementation are advisable until gastrointestinal function and nutritional status have been restored to normal.

Occasionally children present in acute 'coeliac crisis' and are unable to tolerate any food. Such children are at risk of hypoglycaemia. Small frequent nasogastric feeds may be tolerated or the children may respond to short courses of high-dose corticosteroids. Children who are severely ill may have secondary lactose and/or CMPI. Sick children with the diagnosis of coeliac disease should be started on lactose and cows' milk protein free, as well as gluten-free, diets.

Once these children begin to recover, catch-up growth may be extremely rapid and appetite impressive. After the recovery period, iron and vitamin supplementation should be unnecessary. Lactose and cows' milk protein can be introduced gradually. Annual or more frequent assessments of growth, general health and haemoglobin level are probably advisable until adult life.

Where response to gluten-free diet is unimpressive, other malabsorptive states or food intolerances may be occurring secondary to the severe enteropathy. In the long term, however, a poor response is usually due to one of two causes: either the diagnosis is incorrect or the child is not on a strict gluten-free diet. If the former cause is suspected, careful reassessment of history and clinical findings is necessary and possibly supervised reintroduction to gluten if diagnostic criteria have not been fulfilled. If the latter cause is suspected, a sympathetic approach to the problem of maintaining a coeliac diet is advisable. The typical British diet contains a lot of wheat flour. It may be difficult to get young children to co-operate with dieting. With older children the need to participate in peer-group activities together with a desire to be 'normal' may interfere with adherence to strict diets. Whilst occasional dietary lapses usually have few immediate symptoms, less than *totally* gluten-free diets have minor effects on intestinal function, nutrition and growth (McNicholl, 1986). More concerning, perhaps, is the association of small bowel neoplasms, especially lymphomas, in patients with coeliac disease. It is not absolutely certain whether avoidance of gluten reduces the prevalence of small bowel malignancy in coeliac disease, but it would seem a reasonable assumption that it might do so and therefore dietary adherence is advisable.

Cystic fibrosis

This is an autosomal recessive condition affecting about 1 in 2000 children. The exact defect in cystic fibrosis is not known but it results in abnormal exocrine gland secretion and produces a wide variety of symptoms and signs (*Table 15.7*). Nevertheless, although the presentation of cystic fibrosis is varied, there are usually symptoms both of gastrointestinal and of respiratory tract involvement. Occasionally there is a family history of the condition but diagnosis is usually suspected from clinical features. Confirmation is by demonstration of high sweat electrolytes (sodium >60 mmol/l; chloride >60 mmol/l) on a collection of at least 100 mg of sweat. If there is still doubt about the diagnosis, aspiration of duodenal juice should show small volumes of duodenal juice and low enzyme and bicarbonate concentrations after appropriate stimulation procedures (Goodchild and Dodge, 1985). Under the age of 2 months, sweat tests often yield insufficient sweat. Duodenal aspiration at that age is also difficult. Serum immunoreactive trypsin levels may be high in early infancy and can lend support to a clinical diagnosis of cystic fibrosis in young infants.

Table 15.7 Presentations and complications of cystic fibrosis

Newborn and infant:
　Slightly low birth weight
　Meconium ileus; meconium peritonitis
　Neonatal cholestatic jaundice
　Failure to thrive (often despite large appetite)
　Hypoproteinaemic oedema
　Hyponatraemia
　Recurrent or persistent lower respiratory tract symptoms
　Diarrhoea with frequent bulky stools; rectal prolapse
　Abdominal distension
　Tasting salty when kissed!

Older children:
　Wheezing; recurrent lower respiratory tract infection
　Short stature; underweight
　Chronic diarrhoea
　Nasal polyps
　Heat prostration
　Subacute intestinal obstruction 'meconium ileus equivalent'

Problems usually delayed until adolescence:
　Biliary cirrhosis and portal hypertension
　Diabetes mellitus
　Cor pulmonale
　Chronic respiratory failure
　Hypogonadism and poor secondary sexual development in males
　Sterility in males

Management of cystic fibrosis centres around treatment of the respiratory condition and management of the malabsorption which results from pancreatic enzymatic deficiency. Social and psychological support for these children and their families is also extremely important for normal emotional development of the children.

We do not intend to discuss the respiratory management of cystic fibrosis in detail here. Physiotherapy, antibiotics and sometimes bronchodilators and mucolytics are the mainstays of treatment for the chest problems. Although in early life infants with cystic fibrosis may fail to thrive due to the effects of malabsorption, in later childhood the anorexia and energy deficit between intake and expenditure secondary to chronic chest infection and extra respiratory and cardiac effort in respiratory failure probably play a more important part in contributing to poor growth, poor physical development and general wasting than do the effects of malabsorption.

The nutritional management of children with cystic fibrosis should be tailored to the individual's capacity to cope with dietary fat and protein. Deficiency of pancreatic lipase and pancreatic trypsin lead to diminished absorption of fat and protein. Absorption of fat-soluble vitamins is likely to be deficient. The presence of salivary amylase and intestinal amylase means that starches and carbohydrates are absorbed fairly well. These children therefore require high energy intakes, perhaps 125% normal requirements for age, to allow for inadequate absorption even in the presence of pancreatic supplements. Carbohydrate intake should be high since there are fewer problems absorbing carbohydrates than other major nutrients. Low-fat diets used to be recommended for children with cystic fibrosis since deficiency of pancreatic lipase led to fat malabsorption. However, some children always tolerated normal diets even without pancreatic supplements. Great improvements in pancreatic enzyme preparations have enabled even those with significant malabsorption to tolerate normal fat intakes. This makes it much easier to provide high total energy intakes and reduces the risk of vitamin and essential fatty acid deficiencies.

The protein content of the diet should be normal, but the protein supplied must be high quality so that potential deficiencies of essential amino acids secondary to malabsorption are minimized. Vitamins, particularly fat-soluble vitamins, should be provided in double the routine dose and preferably as water-soluble preparations. Ketovite (Paines & Byrne) liquid 5 ml together with Ketovite tablets (3 tablets daily) are a commonly prescribed vitamin preparation but less expensive preparations providing vitamins A, C, D and thiamine, riboflavin, pyridoxine and nicotinamide (e.g. Dalivit, Paines & Byrne; Abidec, Warner-Lambert) are probably adequate in children who are maintaining satisfactory nutrition and growth.

Extra vitamin E (10 mg in infants, 25 mg in young children, 50 mg in older children, or a standard dose of 50 mg to all children, and 200 mg in adults) is advisable since neurological degeneration similar to that associated with abetalipoproteinaemia (*see below*), has been described in adolescents and adults with cystic fibrosis (Elias, Muller and Scott, 1981). Neurological degeneration is not a feature commonly associated with cystic fibrosis, probably because survival of these children is limited by their respiratory problems. However, the outlook for cystic fibrosis children is improving: 50% now survive to 20 years (Goodchild and Dodge, 1985) so it is likely that neurological disease will become more common unless effectively prevented.

In order to obtain high energy and protein intakes in cystic fibrosis, it is usually necessary to provide children with three good quality main meals and then to provide supplementary carbohydrate snacks in between the main meals. All meals and snacks must be accompanied by enzyme supplements with smaller doses of enzymes for snacks than for meals.

Table 15.8 lists points relevant to the use of pancreatic enzyme supplements. Some commonly used preparations are listed in *Table 15.9*. Enzymes mixed with fluid should not be allowed to stand more than 30 minutes before swallowing. Enzymes should not be sprinkled on food since digestion starts before the food has

Table 15.8 Relevant points in the use of pancreatic enzyme supplements

Titrate dose against individual response
Take at the beginning of all meals and (smaller dose) snacks
Swallow preparations with a little food or liquid but do not chew
Do not mix with very hot food or drink
Do not sprinkle on food
Enteric-coated granular preparations (Pancrease: Ortho-Cilag; Creon: Duphar) are most satisfactory and give best protein and fat absorption*
Imagination may be needed to devise methods of disguising unpleasant taste of non-coated preparations

* Gow, Broadbear and Francis, 1981

Table 15.9 Some commonly used pancreatic enzyme supplements

Product (manufacturer)	Enzyme content (BP units)/capsule			Dose (capsules)	Comments
	Amylase	Lipase	Protease		
Suitable for infants:					
Cotazym (Organon)	10 000	14 000	500	½–1/feed	Dose stated is for infants <9 months. Open capsules and mix contents with a little milk and give at beginning of feed
Pancrex V capsules (Paines & Byrne)	9000	8000	430	1–2/feed	
Suitable for older children:					
Creon (Duphar)	9000	8000	210	½–1 for young children 1–4 at meals for older children 1 at snacks	Enteric-coated granules have largely superceded other preparations. Capsules swallowed whole or opened and mixed with a little food or drink. Can be fed before or during meal.
Pancrease (Ortho-Cilag)	2900	5000	330	1–2 for young children 2–5 at meals for older children 1 at snacks	Do NOT chew granules

been ingested, and the subsequent smell of partially digested food may make the meal unacceptable.

Specific nutritional problems in cystic fibrosis
Nutritional supplementation may be necessary to enable small or sick children to increase their energy intake sufficiently to allow adequate absorption and improved growth. *Table 15.10* outlines some suitable supplements. Infancy is a particularly difficult period for these children since nutrient demands are high and coughing, and sometimes breathlessness, can make it difficult for infants to take in sufficient milk to maintain adequate nutrition despite enzyme supplements. Failure to thrive is very common. A milk formula which contains medium-chain triglycerides (MCT) and cows' milk protein hydrolysate may facilitate absorption both of fat and of proteins (e.g. Pregestimil; Bristol-Myers) and is recommended. Nenatal (Cow & Gate) which contains some MCT oil and has high energy content may also be

helpful in young infants. It has the disadvantage of only being available as prepacked liquid feed supplied through hospitals. Vitamin supplements are essential.

Infants should be encouraged to take more than the usually recommended volumes of milk and many at this stage show considerable hunger and, if not unwell with respiratory infection, feed voraciously. If infants are having difficulty consuming adequate volumes of milk because of respiratory problems or sheer inability to ingest the volume, early weaning may enable a greater energy intake without increased bulk or volume to the diet.

Table 15.10 Carbohydrate nutritional supplements useful in cystic fibrosis and other malabsorptions*

Name	Contents	Manufacturers
Caloreen	Water-soluble dextrins mostly 5 glucose molecule polymers 1674 kJ/100 g (398 kcal/100 g)	Roussel
Polycal	Glucose, maltose and polysaccharides 1610 kJ/100 g (380 kcal/100 g)	Cow & Gate
Polycose†	Glucose polymers 1610 kJ/100 g (380 kcal/100 g)	Abbott
Maxijul†	Glucose polymers 1570 kJ/100 g (375 kcal/100 g)	Scientific Hospital Supplies

* Electrolyte low powders: add to liquid to increase carbohydrate energy content.
† Liquid versions also available.

Newborn infants with cystic fibrosis can present with acute intestinal obstruction secondary to meconium ileus. These infants may require parenteral nutrition to tide them over early weeks after surgery. Older children sometimes present with clinical features of sub-acute intestinal obstruction or colicky abdominal pain and vomiting. This is the 'meconium ileus equivalent'. Viscid mucus and partially digested gastrointestinal contents cause subacute intestinal obstruction. The symptoms may be relieved by increasing pancreatic enzyme supplements and by oral ingestion of n-acetyl cysteine (200 mg granule sachets dissolved in water): one sachet daily in children aged 1–2 years, one twice daily for those aged 2–6 years and one sachet 3–4 times daily in older children and adults. This should be continued on a long-term basis. Adequate hydration is also important in avoiding meconium ileus equivalent. Occasionally hospital medical management of acute intestinal obstruction is indicated for severe cases.

Children with cystic fibrosis lose a lot of salt in their sweat. This means that they often take extra salt on their food voluntarily, and this should be encouraged. Occasionally infants with cystic fibrosis present with hyponatraemia secondary to salt loss in the sweat and the low salt content of modern formula milks. In hot countries collapse due to salt deficiency is not uncommon.

Poor weight gain and poor linear growth despite enzyme and nutritional supplementation have led to the development of complicated dietary regimens which attempt to increase the efficiency of utilization of food. It was suggested that poor respiratory function in children with cystic fibrosis was exacerbated by deficiencies of essential fatty acids and infusions of fat such as Intralipid (KabiVitrum) were used, but with little benefit. This procedure has been abandoned. Some paediatricians treated children with major malabsorption or growth retardation by elemental diets (The 'Allan' diet: Allan, Mason and Moss, 1973). Here the essential needs of the diet were supplied as peptides or amino acids, glucose and medium-chain triglyceride oil. The diet made pancreatic enzymes unnecessary. Great claims were made for these diets, and some children did seem to improve on them. For most children and their parents, however, the unpleasantness of the diets outweighed possible advantages since children refused to accept the diet for more than short periods of time. The nutritional advantages of these diets, if any, are slight (Yassa, Prosser and Dodge, 1978). If elemental diets are used, it is vital that they contain adequate vitamin and mineral supplementation and that nutrient intakes of children on them are closely monitored. There seem few, if any, indications for subjecting children with cystic fibrosis – who have enough problems anyway – to these unpleasant diets.

Children with cystic fibrosis should be assessed nutritionally whenever they are seen in clinics. Weight and height are measured routinely. Mid-upper arm circumference and skinfold thickness may be useful indicators of muscle and fat development. Poor weight gain is often a major problem with young infants, but after infancy when nutrient needs /kg/day decline, these children may gain weight better and show a steady increase in stature. Once chronic respiratory infection or respiratory failure develop, growth rates decline and the children become wasted with loss of subcutaneous fat and anorexia. Chronic ill health and poor nutrition contribute to delayed pubertal development which exacerbates the small size of these children in relation to their peers. Unexplained intrauterine growth retardation (mean birth weight 2.9 kg) is another factor contributing to overall small size, particularly in infancy (Boyer, 1955).

In general terms the outlook for girls with cystic fibrosis seems to be less good than for boys. Girls often show steady deterioration in respiratory function in their teens. Possibly greater growth in height and, with this, the lungs for boys at puberty helps counteract the preceding lung damage. Trying to improve girls' nutrition in the prepubertal years may protect against some of the nutritional and respiratory problems of adolescence.

Cystic fibrosis causes progressive fibrosis and destruction of the pancreas so that eventually the endocrine pancreas is damaged and diabetes results. Many children with cystic fibrosis show abnormal glucose tolerance long before overt diabetes develops. Initially, the diabetes may respond to oral hypoglycaemic agents, perhaps suggesting that insulin is produced but release is ineffective. Insulin is usually required eventually. The combination of a high-carbohydrate diet, uncertain protein and fat absorption and frequent respiratory tract infection confuses normal diabetic management. The emotional effects of having yet another problem to cope with in a disabled adolescent also makes good control and positive management extremely difficult.

Biliary cirrhosis is a late complication of cystic fibrosis. It is usually suspected by the presence of an enlarged spleen but generally causes no symptoms until it erupts as haematemesis or melaena secondary to bleeding varices. If there are symptoms of poor fat tolerance a low-fat diet may be useful now but it is essential that these children receive adequate vitamin K. Daily oral supplements of 0.5–1 mg or weekly supplements of 5–10 mg oral vitamin K are recommended (Lloyd-Still, 1983). In acute bleeding episodes intravenous administration is advisable.

Chronic cholestatic jaundice

Severe liver disease is unusual in childhood. Acute hepatitis is usually a mild, short-lived illness where nutritional management resolves around maintaining hydration and persuading the vomiting, anorexic child to take some food. Chronic liver failure is the end point of a wide variety of conditions some of which are at least partly reversible (e.g. Wilson's disease) provided liver disease is not far advanced. For others, liver transplantation provides the only hope of cure and hopefully transplant will be available before the complications of end stage liver failure are well established. However, for infants with extrahepatic biliary atresia in whom the Kasai operation has failed to re-establish bile flow, there will, almost certainly, be a prolonged period between establishing the diagnosis of incurable liver and biliary tract disease and reaching a body weight (>10 kg) at which liver transplant a feasible possibility. During that prolonged period nutritional state should be maintained as normal as possible if the child is to survive, and ultimately benefit from, transplant.

Absence of bile in the intestine leads to profound fat malabsorption and to malabsorption of fat-soluble vitamins and some minerals. Maintenance of an adequate energy intake (exacerbated by the anorexia of chronic illness) is a major problem in these infants. Medium-chain triglycerides are likely to be absorbed better than long-chain triglycerides since they are less dependent on the formation of bile-acid containing micelles for absorption. Pregestimil (Mead Johnson) is probably the most suitable infant formula and may have to be used to supplement breast-fed infants who are gaining weight poorly. Portagen (Mead Johnson) contains less of the essential fatty acids, linolenic and linoleic acids, and is not suitable since poor fat absorption may result in inadequate essential fatty acid absorption. Supplementation of formula with carbohydrate calories (*Table 15.10*) may enhance energy intakes in infants who are gaining weight poorly. However, the infants should be fed by mouth or by gavage to the limits of tolerance (unless oedematous when fluid restriction may become necessary) in order to improve protein as well as energy intakes.

Fat-soluble vitamin supplementation of these infants is essential. Vitamin K can be given by mouth as 2.5–5 mg water-soluble menadiol (Synkavit, Roche) but prothrombin times and partial thromboplastin times should be checked regularly. Otherwise vitamin K is given by intramuscular injection phytomenadione (Konakion, Roche) 1 mg weekly. Vitamin E can also be given by mouth and the dose should probably be monitored against plasma levels (normal 5–15 mg/l). Normal therapeutic doses of 10–50 mg may have to be greatly exceeded to achieve this blood level. Vitamin A can be provided in a water-miscible product Ro-A-Vit (Roche). Doses required to achieve blood levels of 400–500 µg/l may be 1550–5000 RE (5000–15 000 IU/day) but the preparation will have to be made up specially to provide these intakes in liquid form.

Vitamin D nutrition presents a much greater problem. Not only is the vitamin likely to be poorly absorbed (a situation that can be obviated by adequate sunlight exposure), but 25-hydroxylation in the liver is likely to be defective. Poor calcium absorption increases the need for the active hormone 1-25$(OH)_2$ D. Bone disease with pathological fractures is a common complication of biliary atresia. Ideally these children should be given either 25 OH D or 1-25 $(OH)_2$ D. In practice this is difficult since the preparations available are in capsular form and not easily presented in the small doses (15–30 ng/kg/day of calcitriol (Rocaltrop; Roche);

5–7 μg/kg/day of 25 OH D) required by these underweight infants. It is usually possible for the pharmacy to make up special preparations and it is probably essential that they should do so. Serum calcium must be closely monitored. The uncertain absorption and delayed effects of vitamin D itself makes vitamin D an impractical drug for this condition.

The main nutritional problem these infants encounter apart from severe failure to thrive is bone disease. The changes of rickets are present but in addition there is usually gross osteoporosis and spontaneous fractures are likely. Whilst the infant is on a formula diet, calcium intake may be satisfactory even though calcium is precipitated in the gut bound to fat as insoluble soaps. Once a weaning diet is started calcium intake should be maintained by encouraging retention of a high medium-chain triglyceride formula intake. The infants may also present with iron and zinc deficiencies although these minerals should not be given routinely if there is clinical suggestion of deficiency.

The success of nutritional management of biliary atresia should be evaluated against clinical and biochemical criteria since different degrees of severity of intestinal deficiency of bile determine the need for therapy. Gain in weight and length will indicate overall nutritional adequacy particularly for energy and protein intakes.

Biochemical parameters will indicate adequacy of supplementation of most vitamins. Because of biliary obstruction, alkaline phosphatase activities are not useful in determining the onset of bone disease unless the bone component of alkaline phosphatase can be measured separately. Moreover, *healing* rickets may be accompanied by a further rise in alkaline phosphatase activity. Radiology of bones only gives crude measurement of the presence or absence of adequate mineralization or evidence of definite rickets. Yet measurement of the relevant metabolities – 25 OH D, 1–25 $(OH)_2 D$, or both – is not a routine procedure in most laboratories.

This is a difficult condition to manage nutritionally and one that taxes therapeutic ingenuity in provision of the necessary nutrients in forms and quantities that will be effectively absorbed (Kaufman *et al.*, 1987).

Other malabsorptions

There are a wide variety of inborn errors of metabolism which influence gut absorption of various nutrients. Some of these conditions are described elsewhere (e.g. Chapters 9, 10 and 13). Neither the scope of this book nor our experience permit a description of most of these conditions in detail here. Three conditions, however – acrodermatitis enteropathica, abetalipoproteinaemia and intestinal lymphangiectasia – deserve mention because of particular points in their nutritional management.

Acrodermatitis enteropathica

This is a rare autosomal recessive disorder where intestinal zinc absorption is defective (*see Table 9.5*). The symptoms are those of severe zinc deficiency. Children present – usually at weaning if previously breast fed – with chronic diarrhoea, failure to thrive and severe mucocutaneous rash affecting mouth and perianal areas. Symmetrical vesicobullous and eczematous lesions also develop on cheeks, elbows, knees, fingers and toes. With time these lesions become dry, hyperkeratotic and psoriaform. Hair is sparse and reddish or absent. There may be conjunctivitis and corneal dystrophy. Resistance to infection is reduced, and if left untreated these children die.

Diagnosis is from clinical presentation and demonstration of low plasma zinc and alkaline phosphatase (a zinc-dependent enzyme) levels and low leucocyte zinc levels.

Before the importance of zinc in this condition was recognized, the protective effects of breast milk were known. Treatment used to be with breast milk and di-iodohydroxyquin. Barnes and Moynahan (1973) demonstrated resolution of symptoms and signs with zinc supplementation but the exact defect in zinc metabolism is still uncertain. Jejunal mucosa from these children shows defective zinc absorption. Zinc-binding molecules in the mucosa or zinc-binding ligands in gastrointestinal secretions may be absent or abnormal. The zinc-binding ligands in breast milk presumably obviate the need for the infant's own binding proteins in absorption and protect against zinc malabsorption.

Management of acrodermatitis enteropathica is with zinc supplementation which should be continued for life. Zinc sulphate heptahydrate 50–150 mg daily in infancy is the usual treatment but doses should be titrated against plasma zinc levels. Zinc therapy usually results in rapid, total resolution of symptoms and signs and normal growth and development thereafter.

Abetalipoproteinemia

In this condition, which is transmitted as an autosomal recessive condition, there is complete absence of serum β lipoproteins. This leads to absence of β lipoprotein containing lipoproteins such as chylomicrons, very low density lipoproteins (VLDL) and low density lipoproteins (LDL). Fat absorption is grossly deficient and children present with steatorrhoea initially. Later, between 2 and 17 years, neurological symptoms develop with demyelination and neuronal loss in brain and spinal cord. There is progressive weakness, ataxia and loss of proprioception and sometimes loss of other peripheral sensory nerve function. About one-third of the children are mentally retarded. Retinal degeneration and cardiomyopathy may occur. Blood film shows acanthocytosis and there is plasma hypocholesterolaemia.

Recent evidence suggests that the neurological damage occurs as a result of vitamin E deficiency secondary to fat malabsorption. Serum vitamin E and A levels are very low. Vitamin E deficiency may allow free radical damage of myelin phospholipids. The red blood cells in abetalipoproteinaemia have decreased linoleic acid content and abnormal phospholipid distribution. Oral supplementation of the diet with high doses of vitamin E (50–200 mg daily) seems sufficient to prevent neurological and retinal degeneration. Other fat-soluble vitamins should also be provided as in cystic fibrosis.

Intestinal lymphangectasia

Here small intestinal lymph vessels are dilated either over a segment or over the whole small intestine. This appears to be a congenital abnormality, and children with this condition may have lymphatic abnormalities elsewhere.

The children present with severe intestinal loss of protein and lymphocytes. Hypoalbuminaemia, ascites and pleural effusions develop. Transport proteins in the blood are low and there is absolute lymphopenia. Diarrhoea is mild, but

Table 15.11 Fat supplements of use in cystic fibrosis and other malabsorptions*

Name	Contents	Manufacturers	Use
Long-chain fatty acids			
Calogen	50% arachis oil Osmolality 83 mosmol/kg 1700 kJ/100 g (400 kcal/100 g)	Scientific Hospital Supplies	Liquid MUST be diluted and mixed with other foods. Introduce gradually because high osmolar load may give nausea and vomiting initially
Prosparol	50% arachis oil Osmolality 77 mosmol/kg 1880 kJ/100 g (450 kcal/100 g)	Duncan Flockhart	
Medium-chain triglycerides			
Liquigen	MCT 52% 1700 kJ/100 g (400 kcal/100 g)	Scientific Hospital Supplies	Liquid. Useful where problems with fat absorption. Introduce to diet gradually
MCT Oil	3490 kJ/100 g (830 kcal/100 g)	Cow & Gate	
Alembicol D	C_8 and C_{10} triglycerides	Alembic	

* All these preparations are electrolyte low.

steatorrhoea is usually present. Diagnosis is by small intestinal biopsy or Cr^{51} labelled albumin studies.

Absorption of long-chain fatty acids distends the lacteals and exacerbates this condition. Medium-chain triglycerides are largely transported by the portal vein. Dietary management is thus to restrict fat intake (5–15 g/day) and to allow medium-chain triglyceride fat only (*Table 15.11*). Vitamin supplements, especially fat-soluble vitamins (A, D, E and K) are essential.

Chronic inflammatory bowel disease

Crohn's disease

Crohn's disease appears to be increasing in prevalence in childhood. Certainly it is being diagnosed more frequently. It is only proposed to outline the nutritional problems of Crohn's disease and their management here, since the manifestations of this disease are protean and nutritional support should probably be designed to cope with individual symptoms and signs. Although aspects of the diet have been suggested as causative in Crohn's disease, there is no conclusive evidence that diet is the cause of the condition.

Table 15.12 lists nutritional problems that may present or occur in Crohn's disease. Poor linear growth often pre-empts other symptoms and signs by many years. Why poor growth in otherwise symptom-free individuals should be so marked is not clear. It seems probable that there is a complex aetiology to the growth retardation (Motil and Grand, 1985).

Dietary management is only part of the treatment of Crohn's disease but it is important in encouraging normal growth and restoration of nutrition in order to reduce susceptibility to infection. It may also have some effect in controlling the overall inflammatory condition. Dietary regimens follow one or several of four

Table 15.12 Nutritional problems of Crohn's disease

Problem	Possible explanations
Failure to thrive	Anorexia
Weight loss	Malabsorption: 　Enteropathy 　Resections 　Fistulae 　Protein-losing enteropathy 　Bile acid losses 　Secondary bacterial overgrowth
Short stature	Energy, mineral and vitamin deficiencies. Chronic inflammation and infection
Anaemia	Iron deficiency: hypochromic anaemia Folate deficiency: macrocytic anaemia Vitamin B_{12} deficiency: megaloblastic macrocytic Chronic inflammation: normochromic normocytic
Hypoproteinaemic oedema	Anorexia, malabsorption, protein-losing enteropathy
Vitamin deficiency	Anorexia, restricted inappropriate diets, fat malabsorption, bile salt malabsorption
Mineral deficiency	Anorexia, restricted inappropriate diets, secondary bacterial colonization, losses in diarrhoea

patterns: diets low in fat but high in total energy content; elemental diets; elimination diets, and parenteral nutrition.

High-energy diets
Here the aim is to increase the total energy intake and thus encourage growth and weight gain by counteracting the effects of poor absorption. Diets rich in good-quality protein and high in carbohydrate should be provided together with vitamin supplementation (Ketovite tablets and liquid; Paines & Byrne), iron and folic acid, with vitamin B_{12} if the terminal ileum is affected. Increased fat should be avoided since long-chain triglycerides may be poorly absorbed. Energy and protein supplements as used in cystic fibrosis may be helpful (*Table 15.10*). If it is impossible to achieve increased energy intakes by carbohydrate supplementation, medium-chain triglyceride supplementation can be used (*Table 15.11*).

This sort of diet is probably only appropriate where gastrointestinal symptoms are minimal. If anorexia is a problem, it seems unlikely that the goal of increased energy intake will be achieved. The diet may be given in liquid form by nasogastric tube overnight but it may be more appropriate to provide an elemental diet if tube feeding is being used.

Elemental diets
This is reminiscent of the Allan diet in cystic fibrosis. The only diet provided is in the form of amino acids, glucose, fatty acids, vitamins and minerals provided to meet daily requirements and the needs of catch-up growth. The diet is usually made up by the manufacturers (Scientific Hospital Supplies) and administered in distilled or spring water. Spring or distilled water is also allowed freely, but no other foods

or substances are taken by mouth. The diet is not particularly pleasant to take, and co-operation with the regimen is a major problem. It may have to be administered by continuous or intermittent nasogastric infusion. The success of the regimen is closely related to the enthusiasm with which it is propagated. In many patients it does induce remission of symptoms and weight gain. Sadly, symptoms often recur as the diet is normalized.

Elimination diets
Here the implicit understanding is that some, at least, of the symptoms and signs of Crohn's disease are precipitated by food intolerance (Hunter, 1985). Children are put onto an elemental diet until there is remission and then foods are gradually introduced with one new food per day until there is some evidence of relapse. The food most recently introduced is then withdrawn. Foods are introduced in an order thought to represent the least likelihood of provoking intolerance. Initially a diet of chicken, pears and rice is instituted. Units following these regimens usually provide the children with the foods to be introduced listed in the order least likely to induce early intolerance. Responsible families can cope with gradually introducing foods at home once the procedure has been established in hospital and an adequate intake devised.

If recurrence of symptoms occurs with a wide variety of foods or at an early stage of working through the list, it is likely that the child will be unable to maintain an adequate intake with an elimination diet. This child should go back onto a normal diet eating only sparingly those foods known to cause symptoms. Otherwise, elemental diets must be pursued in association with the search for food intolerances until adequate nutrient intakes from whole foods are achieved. The development of elimination diets is only practical where children have definite symptoms such as diarrhoea or abdominal pain which can be recognized and related to recent food intake. Elimination diets cannot be developed for children whose main symptom is poor growth as response will be too slow and indefinite.

Food intolerance is a fashionable subject. Not all those involved in the treatment of chronic inflammatory bowel disease find dietary exclusion effective in inducing remission in Crohn's disease. That Crohn's disease sometimes responds to the elimination of certain foods does not prove the condition is caused by these foods but may only indicate acquired food intolerance due to gastrointestinal damage.

Total parenteral nutrition
Where gastrointestinal symptoms are severe, the only satisfactory way of inducing remission in Crohn's disease may be through total parenteral nutrition. The decision to rest the gut by stopping enteral nutrition should not be taken lightly since total parenteral nutrition is invasive, expensive and carries its own risks, particularly for infection. However, it does allow opportunity to rest the gut and improve overall nutrition. Energy intakes should be calculated in relation to expected requirements, but with a bonus (perhaps 10% energy increase) to allow for the effects of inflammation and to stimulate catch-up growth. Remission usually occurs within 14 days. Four weeks' total parenteral nutrition would seem a reasonable length of time before the gradual reintroduction of normal or elemental diet.

Ulcerative colitis

Ulcerative colitis is not common in childhood, but affects children in increasing numbers as they reach adolescence. Like Crohn's disease it is a variable condition, the progress of which is largely unaffected by dietary management. Anorexia, weight loss secondary to inflammatory bowel disease, blood and protein loss, all cause nutritional deterioration. Thus a balanced high-energy, high-protein diet with supplementary vitamins and minerals is advisable. Foods that appear to exacerbate symptoms should probably be avoided, but there is no satisfactory evidence that bland diets affect symptoms or outcome. In acute attacks it may be appropriate to reduce the fibre intake.

Malabsorption secondary to gastrointestinal resection

Volvulus in the newborn, intestinal vascular accidents, severe necrotizing enterocolitis with perforation or stricture, Crohn's disease or abdominal trauma can precipitate extensive bowel resections. When this happens, and particularly when there is loss of the ileocaecal valve, problems with food absorption and nutrition are likely (*Table 15.13*). The most serious problems of 'short bowel

Table 15.13 Causes of diarrhoea and malabsorption in short-gut syndrome

Inadequate mucosa for absorption of fluids and nutrients

Inadequate mucosa for reabsorption of digestive secretions

Gastric acid hypersecretion (associated with increased gastrin):
  Peptic ulceration
  Acid diarrhoea
  Pancreatic digestive enzyme hypofunction due to acid in jejunum

Secondary small intestinal colonization by bacteria (especially if ileocaecal valve resection) leading to steatorrhoea

Bile acid malabsorption:
  Bile salts entering colon and causing diarrhoea
  Steatorrhoea secondary to reduced bile acid pool

Other hormonal disturbances affecting motility due to abnormal intestinal function

Failure to absorb vitamin B_{12} when terminal ileum resected

syndrome' are due to inadequacy of the bowel remnant to absorb sufficient nutrients or to absorb digestive secretions, but other problems can complicate even adequate lengths of gut. With most large resections a prolonged period of supportive parenteral nutrition is necessary to maintain adequate nutrition during the period of profuse diarrhoea and malabsorption which follows recovery from postoperative paralytic ileus. Considerable intestinal adaptation takes place with time, provided nutrition is maintained. Mucosal hyperplasia and increased cell count per unit length of intestine occur gradually. Adaptation is a response to increased concentrations of nutrients within the lumen and to hormonal influences as well. Thus it is important to stimulate adaptation by introducing some enteral feeding as soon as practical. Small feeds of breast milk may – through their hormonal content – facilitate maturation and development in infancy. Mucosal adaptation is usually greater in the ileum than in the jejunal or colon.

Although the main intestinal adaptation takes place in the first 2 months after resection so that considerable oral nutrition is usually possible after that, adaptation continues for much longer. Tolerance of fairly normal diet is usual by 6–12 months and, with time, children who have survived resections in early infancy may have almost normal absorptive capacity (Rickham, Irving and Schmerling, 1977). In the early stages of adaptation, however, complicating illness such as infective diarrhoea may once more put the child's nutritional state at risk.

It is in infancy – which is often when the massive resections occur – that the problems of short gut syndrome are greatest. It has been estimated that the area of neonatal small intestine available to absorb 1 kcal (4.2 kJ) of energy requirement, if energy requirements are to be met, is $2\,cm^2$. In adults an equivalent area would be $3.5\,cm^2$. There is therefore greater 'intestinal reserve capacity' in adults than in infants and young children and massive resections are consequently better tolerated in adults (Klish, 1985). However, the normal neonatal intestine is 200 cm in length and that in the adult is 700–800 cm so, with time, growth will help short-gut problems in young infants.

As a result of massive resection specific problems arise independent of the problems of diminished area for absorption. These are described below.

Gastric hypersecretion, apparently due to increased circulating gastrin, follows resection. This may be due to lack of gastrin-degrading tissue or gastrin inhibitors. With time, the hypersecretion subsides. The possible effects of hypersecretion include peptic ulceration, diarrhoea secondary to highly acid bowel contents and poor pancreatic enzyme function due to low intestinal pH. Cimetidine 20–40 mg/kg/day may be helpful in controlling hypersecretion.

Ileal resection presents more problems than jejunal resection since the ileum usually compensates quite well for loss of jejunum but some specific functions of the ileum are not replaced by jejunal activity. If the terminal ileum is resected, absorption of vitamin B_{12} will be impaired. Provided the problem is recognized this is easily managed by three monthly intramuscular injections of vitamin B_{12} – for life.

The distal ileum is also involved in absorption of bile salts. Bile salt secreting capacity is limited and loss of bile salts due to ileal resections leads to impaired fat absorption. Bile salts in the colon may be deconjugated by bacteria, and these together with unabsorbed fatty acids may interfere with colonic absorption of water and sodium, thus exacerbating the diarrhoea. Cholestyramine resin, 0.5–1 g four times daily, binds bile acids and reduces the diarrhoea. Cholestyramine can cause folate malabsorption.

Resections of the distal ileum may have included removal of the ileocaecal valve. This region is normally effective in reducing colonization of the small intestine by colonic bacteria. Overgrowth of bacteria in the small bowel causes increased bile salt deconjugation leading to fat malabsorption and free bile acids, with the problems discussed above. Bacterial overgrowth may also interfere with absorption of other nutrients, particularly B_{12} and folate, by utilizing nutrients in metabolism. Antibiotics (ampicillin or co-trimoxazole) may be helpful in reducing small intestinal contamination.

Dietary management should aim to provide adequate nutrition – which may mean providing much more than expected requirements due to anticipated losses – in forms likely to be absorbed effectively. Fat absorption is most likely to be inefficient. Initially diets should be low in fat and the fat content of the diet 'titrated' against fat-absorbing capacity. Medium-chain triglyceride (MCT) fat is partly water soluble and does not require bile acids for solubility. Because of relative solubility, MCT oil can be digested by brush-border lipases as well as intraluminal pancreatic lipase. Some MCT preparations have been listed in *Table 15.11*. MCT preparations do not contain essential fatty acids. Introduction of long-chain fatty acid preparations should therefore be attempted as soon as possible or in combination with MCT preparations.

Protein absorption is likely to be affected in short-gut syndrome due to decreased absorptive surface area and, frequently, decreased pancreatic flow and altered intestinal pH. Intakes need to be proportionately greater than normal requirements, especially for essential amino acids. Protein is less efficiently absorbed and metabolized than peptides or amino acids. Short-chain peptides seem better absorbed than free amino acids – perhaps because this is the form in which protein is normally presented to the brush border for hydrolysation and absorption. Comminuted chicken meat (CCM; Cow & Gate) is an aqueous protein hydrolysate which has proved very useful in these circumstances. It is NOT a complete food and must only be used with sources of energy and vitamins and minerals (*see below*). Often it is appropriate to match up diets based on comminuted chicken meat to individually tolerated recipes. If intestinal function is less fragile it may be possible to try nutritionally complete proprietary mixtures such as those described in *Table 16.1* or the Pepdite range (Scientific Hospital Supplies) in older children, or a fomula milk containing peptides and MCT oil (Pregestimil; Mead Johnson) in infants.

In short-gut syndrome the quality and quantity of the dietary carbohydrate is very important for intestinal symptoms and function. Glucose is usually well absorbed but in significant quantities the osmolality of high concentrations of glucose leads to hypertonic feeds which are inadequately diluted by small intestinal fluids in the short gut. Fluid and solute are still incompletely absorbed by the time they reach the large bowel, and osmotic diarrhoea results.

Lactose is not a suitable carbohydrate for use in formulas or feed preparations for short gut syndrome. Lactose-absorbing capacity is always close to requirements and in the short gut will almost certainly be inadequate. Sucrose also has rather poor absorption and is better avoided. Maltodextrins and synthetic glucose polymers (*see Table 15.10*) are useful since they are hydrolysed by maltase which has more efficient intestinal activity than lactase or sucrase. Moreover, they have lower osmolality relative to their energy content than glucose or disaccharides.

Vitamin supplements (Ketovite; Paines & Byrne) MUST be provided in adequate or increased quantities. Mineral supplements (Metabolic Mineral Mixture, Scientific Hospital Supplies) should be given. For Metabolic Mineral Mixture the daily intake should be 1.5 g/kg body weight to a maximum of 8 g/day. The mixture is made up in a paste with warm water, oil or glucose polymer and given in distilled water with each of the main meals.

A possible regimen for introduction of enteral feeding after parenteral feeding is outlined below.

Feeds are gradually built up using low concentration protein, carbohydrate and fat and adjusting to tolerance. Intravenous feeds are reduced when there is a substantial intake from oral feeds:

1. Comminuted Chicken Mix 10% solution: 1 ml/hour. Increase concentration to 50% solution by 10% increase/day. Watch blood urea for intolerance of protein in young infants. Increase volume of this and associated nutrients at rate of 5–10% requirements/day.
2. Include carbohydrate as glucose polymer at 1 g/100 ml feed. Monitor stools for

carbohydrate: if insignificant, increase carbohydrate daily by 1 g/100 ml to maximum of 12 g/100 ml feed.
3. Add fat as long- or medium-chain triglycerides initially as 1 ml (=0.5 g fat)/100 ml feed. If fat tolerated, increase by 1 ml/100 ml daily to maximum of 6 ml/100 ml feed.
4. Metabolic Mineral Mixture (Scientific Hospital Supplies). 1 g/100 ml feed when total daily volume of feed over 100 ml (to a maximum of 1.5 g/kg/day or 8 ml total). Ketovite (Paines & Byrne) liquid 5 ml/day and tablets one three times daily.

Once a regimen is well tolerated, feeds such as Pregestimil (Mead Johnson) or, in older children, Nutrauxil (KabiVitrum) can be introduced gradually. Vitamin and mineral supplementation will probably still be required to bring the content of the feeds up to the needs of young children with poor absorptive capacity and catch-up growth.

Toddler diarrhoea

Many young children pass frequent unformed stools. Owing to the natural incontinence of young children this presents major nuisance and worry to parents. These children generally thrive and seem undisturbed by their 'toddler diarrhoea' except to the extent of developing occasional mild napkin dermatitis.

It may be difficult to distinguish toddler diarrhoea from other causes of diarrhoea in early childhood. It is always important to exclude conditions such as *rotavirus* infection or *Giardia* infestation which may cause persisting symptoms following acute episodes of gastroenteritis. Clinical judgement should be used to decide how much to investigate the diarrhoea. Toddlers with diarrhoea who thrive do not suggest the need for extensive investigation.

Toddler diarrhoea is difficult to treat since the aetiology is not definite and management is not clear. The toddler age group is a particularly temperamental one liable to fussy eating habits and determined to show independence, so dietary changes are difficult to impose. Some toddlers have diarrhoea secondary to diets containing high-sugar, high-refined carbohydrate and low-fat and low-fibre content. Sweetened fruit juices, sweets and added sugars should be discouraged and more fats and particularly fibrous foods in the form of wholemeal bread and whole vegetables introduced to the diet. The presence of tomato skins and bean husks in stools, so often mentioned with concern by parents as 'undigested food', should not be regarded as indication that there is malabsorption or poor digestion. These food remnants are normally passed in stools but are unnoticed or ignored when the stools are formed.

Toddler diarrhoea usually resolves with time and as the children acquire continence. To the parent, toddler diarrhoea is a major, messy problem. To the clinician its importance is as an entity which has to be distinguished from major gastrointestinal pathology but in itself it is not clinically very important. Thus management must be directed towards explanation, guidance and support for parents.

Constipation

Constipation in small babies usually resolves by feeding small quantities of boiled water (cooled!) with one teaspoonful (5 g) of sugar and 1–2 oz (30–60 ml) of water).

Brown sugar is usually suggested, although there seems no reason why white sugar should not be equally successful. Constipation in older children – characteristically in those of pre-school and early school years – is an annoying management problem in which diet has a place in treatment. Chronic constipation with overflow must be distinguished from encopresis – inappropriate bowel action – which is a troublesome behavioural problem usually requiring expert management by a child psychiatrist or other appropriately trained person.

Chronic constipation is rarely due to an underlying medical problem (hypothyroidism; Hirschsprung's disease). Occasionally acute illness with dehydration or an anal fissure leads to reduce defaecation or pain, and thus reluctance, with defaecation so the normal urge to open the bowels is ignored. Commonly, however, the condition reflects a disordered household where the child is not encouraged to go to the toilet after meals or on any other regular basis; toilets may be remote from the place of play and therefore inertia prevents the child going regularly, or the toilets are too cold or unattractive (e.g. across school yards) to encourage the child to visit them. All these factors may cause children to ignore normal urges to have their bowels open. Constipation then develops.

Training requires re-training the child in bowel function through facilitating bowel action with laxatives (Elixir Senokot; Reckitt and Colman, 2.5–5 ml at night; or lactulose solution, 3.35 g/ml, 2.5 ml under 1 year, 5 ml from 1–5 years, 10 ml twice daily for 6–12 years). Regular toilet visits after meals when gastro-colic reflex is induced and a diet that encourages regular bowel action are also important aspects of management. Dietary manipulation is perhaps the most difficult since these children are usually of an age and environment where fruit and vegetables are eaten little and wholemeal bread not at all. Bran-containing cereals may be encouraged (Weetabix; Branflakes; All Bran; Wheatflakes) successfully, but it is often difficult to change these children's diets substantially in other ways. Often a combination of a tendency to constipation goes with a negative, obstinate, encopretic personality, thus frustrating management further. Patience, persistence and frequent review are necessary.

References

ALLAN, J. D., MASON, A. and MOSS, A. D. (1973) Nutritional supplementation in treatment of cystic fibrosis of the pancreas. *American Journal of Diseases of Children*, **126**, 22–26

BARNES, P. M. and MOYNAHAN, E. J. (1973) Zinc deficiency in acrodermatitis enteropathica: multiple dietary intolerances treated with a synthetic diet. *Proceedings of Royal Society of Medicine*, **66**, 327–329

BOYER, R. H. (1955) Low birth weight in fibrocystic disease of the pancreas. *Pediatrics*, **16**, 778–781

BULLEN, A. (1985) Mechanisms of gluten toxicity of coeliac disease. In *Food and the Gut*, edited by in J. O. Hunter and V. Alun Jones, pp. 187–207. London: Balliere-Tindall

COMMITTEE ON NUTRITION (1983) Soy-protein formula: recommendations for use in infant feeding. *Pediatrics*, **72**, 359–363

ELIAS, E., MULLER, D. P. R. and SCOTT, J. (1981) Association of spinocerebellar disorders in cystic fibrosis and chronic childhood cholestasis and very low serum vitamin E. *Lancet*, **ii**, 1319–1321

GOODCHILD, M. N. and DODGE, J. A. (1985) *Cystic Fibrosis*, 2nd edn. Eastbourne: Balliere Tindall

GOW, R., BROADBEAR, R. and FRANCIS, P. (1981) Comparative study of varying regimens to improve steatorrhoea and creatorrhoea in cystic fibrosis: effectiveness of an enteric-coated preparation with and without antacids and cimetidine. *Lancet*, **ii**, 1971–1974

HUNTER, J. O. (1985) The dietary management of Crohn's disease. In *Food and the Gut*, edited by J. O. Hunter and V. Alun Jones, pp. 221–237. London: Balliere Tindall

KAUFMAN, S. S., MURRAY, N. D., WOOD, P., SHAW, B. W. and VANDERHOOF, J. A. (1987) Nutritional support for the infant with extra hepatic biliary atresia. *Journal of Paediatrics,* **110,** 679–686

KHIN-MAUNG, U., NYUNT NYUNT WAI, MYO-KIN, MU MU KHIN, TIN U. and THANE TOE (1985) Effect on clinical outcome of breast feeding during acute diarrhoea. *British Medical Journal,* **290,** 587–591

KLISH, W. J. (1985) The short gut. In *Nutrition in Pediatrics: Basic Science and Clinical Applications,* edited by W. A. Walker and J. B. Watkins, pp. 561–568. Boston: Little Brown

KUITUNEN, P., SAVILAHTI, E. and VERKASALO, M. (1986) Late mucosal relapse in a boy with coeliac disease and cows' milk allergy. *Acta Paediatrica Scandinavica,* **75,** 340–342

LLOYD-STILL, J. D. (1983) *Textbook of Cystic Fibrosis,* p. 277. Bristol: John Wright

McDOWELL, H. P. and EVANS-JONES, G. (1985) Is gradual reintroduction of milk feeds after gastroenteritis necessary? *Lancet,* **i,** 690

McNEISH, A. S., HARMS, H. K., REY, J., SCHMERLING, D. H., VISAKORPI, J. K. and WALKER-SMITH, J. A. (1979) The diagnosis of coeliac disease. *Archives of Disease in Childhood,* **54,** 783–786

McNICHOLL, B. (1986) Coeliac disease: ecology, life history and management. *Human Nutrition: Applied Nutrition,* **40A,** Suppl. 1, 55–59

MAHALANABIS, D. (1985) Oral rehydration therapy – physiological basis. In *Diarrhoeal Disease and Malnutrition,* edited by M. Gracey, pp. 145–157. Edinburgh: Churchill-Livingstone

MATA, L. (1985) Global importance of diarrhoeal disease and malnutrition. In *Diarrhoeal Disease and Malnutrition,* edited by M. Gracey, pp. 1–14. Edinburgh: Churchill-Livingstone

MEEUWISSE, G. W. (1970) Round table discussion. Diagnostic criteria in coeliac disease. *Acta Paediatrica Scandinavica,* **59,** 461–463

MOTIL, K. J. and GRAND, R. J. (1985) Inflammatory bowel disease. In *Nutrition in Pediatrics: Basic Science and Clinical Applications,* edited by W. A. Walker and J. B. Watkins, pp. 445–462. Boston: Little Brown

PLACZEK, M. and WALKER-SMITH, J. A. (1984) A comparison of two feeding regimens following acute gastroenteritis in infancy. *Journal of Pediatric Gastroenterology and Nutrition,* **3,** 245–249

RICKHAM, P. P., IRVING, I. and SCHMERLING, D. H. (1977) Longterm results following extensive small intestinal resection in the neonatal period. *Progress in Pediatric Surgery,* **10,** 65–76

ROWLAND, M. G. M., COLE, T. J. and WHITEHEAD, R. G. (1977) A quantitative study into the role of infection in determining nutritional status in Gambian village children. *British Journal of Nutrition,* **37,** 441–450

TRIPP, J. A. and CANDY, D. C. A. (1985) *Manual of Paediatric Gastroenterology.* Edinburgh: Churchill Livingstone

WALKER-SMITH, J. A. (1985) Cows' milk intolerance and other related problems in infancy. In *Food and the Gut,* edited by J. O. Hunter and V. Alun Jones, pp. 166–186. London: Balliere Tindall

WALKER-SMITH, J. A. (1986) Nutritional management of acute gastroenteritis – rehydration and realimentation. *Human Nutrition: Applied Nutrition,* **40A, Suppl. 1,** 39–43

YASSA, J. G., PROSSER, R. and DODGE, J. A. (1978) Effects of an artificial diet on growth of patients with cystic fibrosis. *Archives of Disease in Childhood,* **53,** 777–783

Chapter 16

Parenteral nutrition – intravenous feeding (IVF)

The development of successful methods of providing parenteral feeding has revolutionized the management of VLBW infants and children with severe intractable diarrhoea, major gastrointestinal resections and short gut syndrome. Parenteral feeding is, however, a hazardous procedure and should be undertaken only with clear indications that it is necessary and only practised where there are appropriate care and support services. Ward staff must be familiar with the techniques. Laboratory and pharmacy staff must be able to provide efficient back-up services. Wherever possible a nutrition team should be involved with children who have evidence of serious nutritional problems *before* intravenous feeding becomes inevitable since with appropriate management some children can be prevented from reaching the state of poor nutrition and intolerant gastrointestinal tract that makes parenteral nutrition unavoidable. *Table 16.1* outlines some of the feeding regimens that may make it possible to avoid IVF in children with chronic and developing problems.

Table 16.2 lists conditions in which intravenous feeding may be necessary. Intravenous feeding should not be started unnecessarily but delaying the start of

Table 16.1 Alternative feeds for children intolerant of normal diet

Feed		Outline composition	Problems
Hypoallergenic formula:			
Soya milks	Wysoy (Wyeth), Prosobee (Mead Johnson), Formula S (Cow & Gate)	Soya protein with added methionine. No lactose	Soya protein intolerance quite common
Cow's milk protein hydrolysates	Nutramigen (Mead Johnson) Pregestimil (Mead Johnson)	Sucrose Maltodextrins	Intolerance of sucrose may be significant
Elemental diets	Vivonex (Norwich Eaton) Flexical (Mead Johnson)	Sucrose	Unpleasant. Not suitable for infants. Deficient in trace elements. Vivonex deficient in essential fatty acids.
	Comminuted Chicken Meat (Cow & Gate)	Chicken protein, fat and few minerals	Not suitable as food alone. Requires carbohydrate, fat, mineral and vitamin sources as well

Table 16.2 Indications for IVF in childhood

More or less obligate situations:
- Neonates: major gastrointestinal surgery, necrotizing enterocolitis, severe hyaline membrane disease
- Older children: major gut resections where small intestine remnant thought adequate to support life after a period of adaptation; chronic diarrhoea with intolerance of hypoallergenic diet; severe burns

Situations where IVF may be nutrition of choice: extreme immaturity; chronic inflammatory bowel disease requiring a period of bowel rest; acute renal failure

---

intravenous feeding when it is needed can result in deterioration of nutrition to a state where the chances of resumption of normal gastrointestinal activity and normal nutrition become even more remote. There is downward progression of poor nutrition, poor gut structure and function, deteriorating resistance to infection and further deterioration in nutrition. IVF is introduced to intercept this process when other methods have failed.

Parenteral feeding regimens designed for use with adults cannot be translated directly to paediatric practice. Children need more amino acids/kg body weight than adults in order to restore nutrition and achieve catch-up growth. Yet young infants may be unable to cope with the metabolic load of amino acids, fat and carbohydrate necessary to achieve this growth. Regimens must be introduced slowly and cautiously. Initial biochemical monitoring must be frequent.

Growth does not begin as soon as IVF begins as it is usually some time before children are established on regimens that provide sufficient energy for growth. Even when energy intakes are sufficient, weight may remain static for a few days before the growth response appears. This is a common feature of nutritional recovery in many conditions and not only those treated with IVF. The explanation is not clear but may relate to correction of the metabolic changes that result from malnutrition and stress before tissue is laid down.

How?

IVF can be supplied through a catheter placed either peripherally or centrally. It is easier to set up a peripheral line but thrombotic blockage due to the hypertonic solutions infused is common. Drips have to be re-sited frequently and, if IVF is prolonged, potential drip sites may be exhausted. Routine regular re-siting, however, may preserve veins and enable peripheral IVF to be continued for long periods. Usually, if IVF is prolonged a central venous line is necessary at some stage. Central venous lines are introduced into the superior vena cava via external or internal jugular vein burrowing under the skin to provide a point of exit for the catheter remote from the site of entry to the vein. Or they can be introduced through cannulas placed in peripheral veins such as the subclavian or median cubital veins. Broviac silastic catheters are now commonly used. These have advantages from their strength, Luer lock connections, and Dacron cuff which anchors the catheter by encouraging adhesions.

IVF solutions should be made up to suit individual needs since the infusion bag must allow the infant or child to receive, in a predetermined volume of fluid, calculated requirements of nutrients. Solutions must be made up under strictest aseptic techniques, preferably in laminar flow chambers to diminish the risks of bacteria getting into the solutions. In the past it was customary to provide IVF solutions in two bags, one containing glucose, amino acid and vitamin mixture and one glucose and additional minerals. Because of compatibility problems with calcium and phosphate, these minerals were often supplied on alternate days. Many units seem to have solved the problems of non-miscibility of nutrients by careful selection of mineral and amino acid preparations and, particularly where volumes are not grossly restricted, it is often possible to introduce all nutrients except the fat solution into one IVF bag. It is sometimes even possible to incorporate the lipid solution into the one bag with preparations for older children. This reduces the practical complications of IVF.

Computer programs can be designed to calculate children's daily needs from weight, plasma biochemistry and general state. Programming for the composition of IVF solutions eases the burden of calculating feeds and equivalent chemical composition of intravenous infusions whilst still adjusting for nutrient losses in urine or stools and increased requirements (MacMahon, 1984).

A team approach is important in successful management of IVF. The IVF team should represent medical, surgical and nursing staff, dietetics (or nutrition) and pharmacy departments. Members of the departments of microbiology and biochemistry should be available for consultation, and these departments must be prepared to provide efficient laboratory services for IVF patients so that nutrient needs can be calculated on the day's biochemical profile and so that infective episodes can be managed aggressively. If children are on either prolonged IVF, or planned for home IVF eventually, social work and health visitor representatives should be included in the team. All members of the team have critical roles in management of these children but one person should take on the role of leader and organizer. Training other staff in IVF procedures is important. There are considerable resource implications to IVF programmes which often require difficult decisions and management. Ideally the team should be a 'Nutritional Support Team' rather than simply an IVF Team, so that it can be consulted about all children with major nutritional problems before IVF becomes absolutely necessary.

When to start

IVF should not begin in a child who is in significant electrolyte imbalance, acutely ill with infection, or in an immediately post-surgical or traumatic catabolic state. Infection should be controlled, electrolyte and fluid balance restored to normal and postoperative recovery begun before IVF is implemented. Thus IVF is not an emergency procedure set up in the middle of the night or at weekends by untrained junior staff. It is a planned procedure which starts at a time acceptable to the facilities and staff available. There must be some urgency in initiating IVF in children with severe burns, major trauma and neonates after surgery where catabolism may be intense and other methods of feeding impossible.

What is given?

IVF may be total nutrition or supplemental to enteral feeding. Wherever possible, some enteral feeding should continue so as to avoid excessive atrophy of gastrointestinal function. Total IVF must provide all nutrients needed not only for maintenance but for normal and even catch-up growth. *Table 16.3* outlines the components of IVF regimens.

Table 16.3 Preparations used in IVF solutions

Nitrogen source:	
Vamin 9 glucose (KabiVitrum)	Essential and non-essential L-amino acids; some glucose, some electrolytes
Energy source:	
Dextrose solution	Dextrose, water only
Intralipid (KabiVitrum)	Essential fatty acids, lecithin, phosphate and vitamin E
Minerals/trace elements:	
Sodium and potassium solutions	
Ped-el (KabiVitrum)	Mixed minerals
Addamel – for older children (KabiVitrum)	Mixed minerals but no phosphate
Vitamins:	
Solivito (KabiVitrum)	Water soluble
Vitlipid (KabiVitrum)	Fat-soluble vitamins
Multibionta (Merck)	Mixed vitamins but no vitamin D or folic acid
Multiple Vitamin solution (MVS: International Medications)	Mixed vitamins including D but no K, folic acid nor B_{12}

Carbohydrate

Glucose is virtually the only carbohydrate source used now although a variety of other carbohydrate sources have been used in the past. Glucose has the advantage of being immediately available for metabolism. It needs to be given in high concentrations to provide adequate energy for the high-energy needs of growing children since volumes of fluid infused are usually low. High concentrations of glucose are apt to thrombose peripheral veins so drip sites require frequent changes. If extravasation into subcutaneous tissues occurs there may be unsightly sloughing of skin and permanent scarring. Infusion sites need close observation and should be covered with transparent dressings.

High concentrations of glucose stimulate hyperglycaemia unless concentrations are built up slowly when hyperinsulinaemia develops to compensate for the glucose load. It is sometimes, but not often, necessary to give small doses of insulin to control hyperglycaemia. Hyperinsulinaemia resulting from high rates of glucose infusion with or without insulin infusion may precipitate dangerous hypoglycaemia if the infusion stops suddenly. Thus when a drip site obstructs or the drip has to be removed for other reasons, children must be watched very closely for reactive hypoglycaemia. Re-siting the drip is urgent. Glucose infusion strengths should be reduced gradually as IVF is being withdrawn.

Protein source

Amino acid solutions and protein hydrolysates used in IVF preparations for adults are not all suitable for IVF in children. Cysteine is an essential amino acid in young children, and the proportion of essential to non-essential amino acids required for growth by children is much higher than in adults. The preparation usually used in Britain is Vamin 9 Glucose (KabiVitrum). This contains a high proportion of branch-chain amino acids as well as glucose and some electrolytes (*Table 16.4*). As with glucose infusions, concentrations of amino acid solutions must be built up slowly. Hyperammonaemia, hyperaminoacidaemia and acidosis develop in infection or catabolism when infused amino acids are not being utilized in growth. The cholestatic jaundice that develops occasionally with prolonged IVF has been attributed to the amino acid infusion. Whether or not this is the mechanism whereby cholestatic jaundice develops is not certain.

Table 16.4 Composition per litre of Vamin 9 Glucose (KabiVitrum)*

Amino acids	70.2 g
(Nitrogen	9.4 g equivalent to about 60 g of first-class protein)
Glucose	100 g
Sodium	50 mmol
Potassium	20 mmol
Calcium	2.5 mmol
Magnesium	1.5 mmol
Chloride	55 mmol
Osmolality	1350 mosmol/kg water
Energy content	2.7 MJ (650 kcal)

* Vamin 9 without glucose but otherwise identical composition is also available

Fat

Energy can be provided from lipids as well as carbohydrate. If IVF is providing total nutrition some source of essential fatty acids is necessary if IVF is for more than 2 weeks' duration. The advantages of a fat source such as Intralipid (KabiVitrum) are that the energy density is greater than that of the carbohydrate solutions. The volume of fluid that needs to be given is less. Essential fatty acids and some phosphate are also provided. However, Intralipid has many problems. It is usually given separate to the other infused fluids or through a Y junction close to the entry point of the catheter since otherwise the lipid emulsion may be denatured. It cannot be infused through a 0.2 µm filter. It should not be given if there is sepsis, uraemia or jaundice (serum bilirubin >120 µmol/l). If it is incompletely utilized fat may be deposited in small capillaries in lungs, kidney, liver and brain (Levene, Wigglesworth and Desai, 1980). The plasma should be checked regularly for lipaemia and the plasma triglycerides measured 4–6 hours after Intralipid infusions are stopped to check that there is clearing of the fat from the blood. The presence of lipaemia interferes with measurement of other blood biochemistry.

Vitamins

Vitamins are essential in total parenteral nutrition but can often be given by mouth if IVF is only supplementary. Several intravenous preparations are available. They require protection from light to prevent denaturation during administration so infusates should be covered. If there are increased requirements for particular vitamins, for example vitamin D, this should be provided as a separate preparation given possibly by separate infusion since a generalized increase in concentration of mixed vitamin preparation in the infusate may result in dangerous intakes of some vitamins, most notably vitamin A. Multibionta (Merck) is deficient in vitamin D and folic acid. All vitamin preparations probably fail to meet full requirements and additional folic acid 5 mg, vitamin K 1 mg, B_{12} 100 µg weekly are advisable in prolonged intravenous nutrition (*Table 16.5*).

Table 16.5 Composition *per ml* of vitamin preparations used in IVF

Preparation		Solivito (KabiVitrum)	Vitlipid (KabiVitrum)	Multibionta (Merck)	MVS (MVI Pediatric) (International Medications)
Vial size		Made up to 10 ml	1 ml	10 ml	10 ml
Dose/kg/day		1 ml (maximum 10 ml)	1 ml (maximum 4 ml)	0.15 (maximum 2 ml)	5 ml/l infusion fluid
Thiamine B_1	mg	0.12	–	5.0	0.24
Riboflavin B_2	mg	0.18	–	1.0	0.3
Nicotinamide	mg	1.0	–	10	3.4
Pyridoxine B_6	mg	0.2	–	1.5	0.2
Pantothenic acid	mg	1.0	–	2.5	1.0
Biotin	µg	30	–	–	4.0
Folic acid	mg	0.02	–	–	0.14
Vitamin B_{12}	µg	0.2	–	–	1.0
Vitamin C	mg	3.4	–	50	80
Retinol A	µg	–	100	300	150
Calciferol D	µg	–	2.5	–	10
Phytomenandione K	µg	–	50	–	40
Tocopherol E	mg	–	–	0.5	0.5

Minerals

Minerals should be administered initially according to outline recommendations in *Table 16.6*. The quantities given are then adjusted according to losses in urine and other fluids and to plasma biochemistry. Calcium and phosphate administration presents many problems since needs for these minerals in growing children are high but the minerals are relatively insoluble and tend to precipitate out in solution

Table 16.6 Guidelines for electrolyte requirements in IVF*

	VLBW (mmol/kg/day)	Newborn (mmol/kg/day)	Older children (mmol/100 kcal 'feed')
Sodium	2–3	2–4	3
Potassium	2–3	2–4	2
Chloride	2–3	2–4	2
Calcium		0.5–1.0	
Phosphate		0.6–1.2	
Magnesium	0.25–0.5	0.25–0.3	0.3–0.5

* Wheeler, 1984; Roberton, 1986.

when mixed together. One approach is to administer calcium in the infusion every other day and phosphate on the alternate days, administering twice the normal daily requirements of each at a time. Another approach is to give calcium into the glucose electrolyte mixture and to administer phosphate with the amino acid vitamin mixture. In many cases, however, careful preparation of intravenous feeding infusates allows all the intravenous nutrients to be put into one bag. The fluid requirements of a child are often critical to whether this is possible, since low fluid requirements demand higher concentrations of nutrients and greater likelihood of precipitation of some components.

It is very difficult to estimate trace element needs for children (or even adults). Many children on IVF have had prolonged periods of diarrhoea and poor nutrition before beginning IVF. Trace elements may be deficient. Needs should be met by the mineral mixtures Ped-el (KabiVitrum) for infants and Addamel (KabiVitrum) for older children (*Table 16.7*). Weekly infusions of fresh blood or plasma reduce the need for trace elements in the infusate but do not meet needs.

Table 16.8 outlines a programme for build-up to a full IVF regimen. Neonatal regimens are outlined in Chapter 5.

Table 16.7 Composition per ml of mineral supplements used in IVF

Mineral mixture:	Ped-el (KabiVitrum)	Addamel (KabiVitrum)
Dose	4 ml/kg/day (max 40 ml/day)	0.2 ml/kg/day (max 10 ml/day)
	µmol	µmol
Calcium	150	500
Magnesium	25	150
Iron	0.5	5
Zinc	0.15	2
Manganese	0.25	4
Copper	0.075	0.5
Fluoride	0.75	5
Iodine	0.01	0.1
Phosphate	75	–
Chloride	350	1130
Potassium	<1.0	<100

What are the complications of IVF?

Children on IVF require close supervision, particularly in the early stages when metabolic response to the infusion is uncertain. *Table 16.9* outlines particular clinical and biochemical points that should be watched.

Infection

The most important and commonest major complication of IVF is infection. There are a variety of reasons why infection is so common in these children. Children on IVF have either undergone a period of stress or poor nutrition and normal defences

Table 16.8 Outline for IVF Programme*

	Day 1	Day 5
Fluid intake	Maintenance volumes	
Amino acids (g/kg/day)†	0.5–1.0	2.0–2.5
Glucose (g/kg/day)	10	15–20
Fat (g/kg/day)‡	–	2–3
Ped-el§		4 ml/kg/day
or Addamel§		0.2 ml/kg/day if >10 kg
Solvito§		0.5 ml/kg/day‖
Vitilipid§		1 ml/kg/day (maximum 4 ml)

* Electrolytes additional to those in amino acid and fat solutions in *Table 16.6*.
† Lower levels of amino acids for infants on Day 1. Higher levels for infants by Day 5.
‡ Fat should not be introduced before Day 2. Level of administration determined by whether fat being cleared from circulation. Should not exceed 2 g/kg/day in VLBW.
§ KabiVitrum.
‖ Folic acid administered 1–5 mg weekly; vitamin K 1 mg weekly; iron by injection weekly; vitamin B_{12} injection 100 μg monthly.

Table 16.9 Monitoring child on IVF

Check frequently for pyrexia.
Observe entry site of infusion: stop infusion if evidence of extravasation or sepsis.
Weigh daily.
Record all fluid input and output.
Check urine specimens for sugar, protein, ketones.
Daily urea, electrolytes, including calcium, phosphate and magnesium until regimen stabilized.
Check for clearance of lipid from plasma 4–6 hours after stopping lipid infusion.
Weekly:
    Liver function tests
    Prothrombin time
    Partial thromboplastin time
    Alkaline phosphatase
    Serum iron
Monthly trace elements in plasma.

against infection are depressed (*see* Chapter 8), or they are very immature infants with poor resistance to infection. The fluid administered in IVF infusates is nutritious and encourages growth of bacteria. Sterilization of the infusate after preparation is not possible since this denatures nutrients but a 0.2 μm filter effectively prevents bacteria entering the circulation via the infusate. Where a central line is being used, there is a portal of entry for bacteria to the circulation and a foreign body in the ciculation encouraging bacterial vegetation and persistence of the infection. The nutrients infused may also affect host resistance to infection. Intralipid (KabiVitrum) reduces chemotaxis and bacteriocidal and phagocytic actions of white blood cells.

Infection may be obvious with pyrexia, toxicity, shock, breathlessness and localizing symptoms. Alternatively, it may be shown by poor growth, low-grade fever, non-specific malaise, disturbed metabolism with hyperglycaemia, hyperlipidaemia, rising blood urea and low plasma sodium, or by falling haemoglobin, evidence of haemolysis and altered white blood count. Suspected infection indicates urgent need for a 'septic screen' with blood cultures, urine culture, possibly lumbar puncture and swabs from catheter entry point, nose, throat and any other possible site of infection. If blood cultures are positive there is little alternative but to remove the catheter and stop IVF until the infection has been treated. If this seems very undesirable it is possible to try to treat infection with the catheter still *in situ* using a prolonged course of bacteriocidal drugs. This latter procedure is often ineffective and usually only delays the time when the catheter has to be removed to allow the infection to clear. The catheter tip should always be examined and cultured after removal to check for evidence of infection.

Because these children are sick and frail they are susceptible to infection by organisms not usually responsible for systemic illness. Systemic candidiasis is relatively common. Pneumonia with organisms such as *Pneumocystis carinii* is another possibility. This is why it is important to have efficient microbiological support for the IVF team since considerable skill may be required to isolate the relevant organisms.

Jaundice

Cholestatic jaundice is not unusual in children on prolonged IVF especially in VLBW infants. The cause of the jaundice is not known but it usually resolves slowly once IVF ceases. Intralipid should not be infused in children with bilirubin levels over about 120 μmol/l since the lipid will be incompletely metabolized. Theoretically at least, lipid may also displace bilirubin from albumin binding and, in LBW infants, increase the risk of kernicterus for a particular bilirubin level.

Nutrient deficiencies

One of the common problems following IVF is that the child does not gain weight as expected. In children in whom weight remains static for long periods there are various possible causes:

1. The child may have an infection and should be investigated for this.
2. The energy intake may be insufficient for this child due perhaps to high losses (with burns, for example).
3. Energy intake may be adequate but other nutrients may be deficient and restricting growth.
4. The child has some other conditions preventing normal growth, e.g. some VLBW infants who have had severe, prolonged intrauterine growth retardation and who will remain small.

Essential fatty acid (EFA) deficiency

EFA deficiency presents with reduced growth rates, eczematous skin changes and hypotonia. If it continues there will be degeneration in renal, lung and liver function. Platelet aggregation is increased. EFA deficiency can be avoided by giving fat preparations. EFA deficiency takes 4 weeks to present with obvious symptoms although lowered plasma EFA levels can be demonstrated after only 48 hours' inadequate intake. Clinical signs are thus only likely to develop after prolonged IVF. Attempts have been made to replace EFAs by rubbing the child's skin with oils containing EFA but the effect of these methods is uncertain.

Intralipid contains 54% linoleic acid and should enable deficiencies of EFA to resolve rapidly. As little as 0.5 ml Intralipid (KabiVitrum) kg/day will prevent EFA deficiency.

Hypophosphataemia

This may occur as growth begins due to sudden utilization of phosphate for protein synthesis and growth. Regular monitoring of electrolytes should enable extra phosphate to be given before levels fall significantly. It is more common in VLBW infants than in older children owing to the rapid rates of growth and bone deposition in VLBW.

Hypoalbuminaemia

Hypoalbuminaemia is sometimes responsible for the development of oedema. It is particularly likely in children who have had a prolonged period of poor nutrition prior to IVF and in LBW infants where albumin levels are normally low. Levels of albumin below 25 g/l (20 g/l in neonates) should probably be managed with infusions of plasma protein fractions, fresh frozen plasma or blood transfusion if there is accompanying anaemia.

Carnitine deficiency

Newborn infants are capable of synthesizing carnitine but carnitine is present in breast milk (13 μmol/kg/day), and it may be that newborns have difficulty synthesizing sufficient for needs. It is essential for normal fatty acid oxidation. Carnitine deficiency presenting as myopathy and failure to thrive has been described after prolonged IVF (Schmidt-Sommerfield, Penn and Wolff, 1982).

Trace nutrient deficiency

IVF infusates should contain trace elements but the 'trace' nature of these elements makes determination of individual needs difficult. IVF has been associated with deficiency syndromes for a variety of trace elements. Usual presentation is with inexplicably poor growth, often poor tone and non-specific malaise. Infusions of fresh plasma or blood may provide the missing element even if the exact causative substance has not been established. Other nutrients such as biotin may also become deficient under the artificial circumstances of prolonged IVF. Failure to thrive on IVF may be due to deficiency of some previously ignored nutrient (Zlotkin, Stallings and Pencharz, 1985).

Anaemia

Anaemia is not uncommon in children on IVF. There are a multitude of possible explanations including both infection and blood loss secondary to over-enthusiastic investigation of small children with low blood volumes. Folic acid deficiency, iron deficiency and, in prolonged cases, vitamin B_{12} deficiency may be causative. If no obvious deficiency is found treatment should be with transfusion of fresh blood or fresh packed cells, depending on the fluid balance of the child and the possible need for other nutrients from the blood. Iron supplements are usually needed for children on prolonged IVF except with the newborn. The normal drop in the high haemoglobin levels of the neonate facilitates iron balance in early life.

Home IVF

Most children receive IVF for short periods only. Occasionally children with short bowel syndrome or severe Crohn's disease spend prolonged periods on full or supplementary IVF. Hospital admission seriously disrupts normal family life, the child's social development and schooling, as well as being stressful to both child and family. It is also expensive. Where the child has a supportive family and IVF is stable but likely to continue for months, it is sometimes possible to continue IVF at home. Solutions should be made up as previously and given to the family fully prepared. Regular checks of biochemistry and growth must continue but home management does allow greater freedom to child and family.

Home management is not cheap, but it is almost invariably cheaper than hospital maintenance and, if successful, emotionally much more satisfying to all concerned.

Reintroduction of enteral feeding

This must be done gradually. Initial oral feeding should be with a hypoallergenic preparation given in small quantities and gradually increased. If IVF has been the child's sole nutrition, intestinal function is likely to be suppressed and the mucosa atrophied. It will take time for normal function to be resumed. As more food is given by mouth the volumes and concentrations of intravenous feeds can be decreased.

A common preparation used in reintroduction of feeds is Comminuted Chicken Meat – CCM (Cow & Gate). This contains a protein hydrolysate only and must be used with a carbohydrate and fat source as well as vitamins and minerals. The build up to full nutrition on CCM has been described in the previous chapter. The preparation is introduced as a one in ten dilution of the aqueous solution and concentration gradually increased to half strength. A glucose polymer source (Maxijul, Scientific Hospital Supplies; Polycal, Cow & Gate; Caloreen, Roussel) is introduced initially with CCM in low concentration and gradually increased. Monosaccharides added to CCM will increase the osmolality of the feed and encourage diarrhoea. Long-chain fatty acids (Prosparol, Duncan Flockhart) can also be introduced as initial feeding is established. When volumes are about half expected feed volume vitamin and mineral preparations are introduced and corresponding intravenous intake reduced. When it is clear that the child tolerates fortified CCM well, the change to a protein hydrolysate, disaccharide free milk such as Pregestimil (Mead Johnson) should be introduced since this is much easier to prepare and will allow the child to be sent home.

References

LEVENE, M. I., WIGGLESWORTH, J. S. and DESAI, R. (1980) Pulmonary fat accumulation after Intralipid infusion in the preterm infant. *Lancet*, ii, 815–819

MacMAHON, P. (1984) Prescribing and formulating neonatal intravenous feeding solutions by microcomputer. *Archives of Disease in Childhood*, 59, 548–552

ROBERTON, N. R. C. (1986) *A Manual of Neonatal Intensive Care,* p. 34. London: Edward Arnold
SCHMIDT-SOMMERFELD, E., PENN, D. and WOLFF, H. (1982) Carnitine deficiency in premature infants receiving TPN: effect of 1-carnitine supplementation. *Journal of Pediatrics,* **102,** 921–925
TRIPP, J. and CANDY, D. C. A. (1985) *Manual of Paediatric Gastroenterology.* Edinburgh: Churchill-Livingstone
WHEELER, N. (1984) Parenteral nutrition. *Manual of Pediatric Nutrition,* edited by D. G. Kelts and E. G. Jones, pp. 151–165. Boston: Little Brown
ZLOTKIN, S. H., STALLINGS, V. A. and PENCHARZ, P. B. (1985) Total parenteral nutrition in children. *Pediatric Clinics of North America,* **32,** 381–400

Chapter 17

Renal problems

The role of the kidney in helping maintain the 'milieu interieur' of the body – clearing excess nitrogenous products, minerals, hydrogen ions and water – means that renal failure can affect growth and nutrition profoundly. Nutrition can also influence the degree to which normal metabolism is maintained despite abnormal renal function (Richards and Ell, 1982). In acute renal failure the need for metabolic control may be dramatic but there is hope for complete resolution. In chronic renal failure, resolution is unlikely but long-term problems may be modified by attention to nutritional aspects of metabolic control.

Acute renal failure (ARF) results from prerenal, renal or post-renal causes. In prerenal failure, glomerular and tubular integrity is intact. There is poor renal perfusion and low urine flow. Plasma urea level rises more rapidly than plasma creatinine level since urea diffuses passively back into the blood from high concentrations in the renal tubules. Creatinine is not reabsorbed in the tubules and is filtered and excreted at normal rates during mild hypoperfusion. Urine osmolality is high (>400 mosmol/l). Urine:plasma urea ratio and creatinine levels are high (>10 and >20 respectively). Sodium is retained. Correction of hypovolaemia and hypoperfusion with intravenous fluids, blood or plasma transfusion restores renal function if hypoperfusion is not prolonged. Prolonged hypoperfusion will lead to acute tubular necrosis and failure due to renal causes.

In renal failure there is renal tissue damage. Neither urea nor creatinine is adequately filtered and excreted. Plasma levels of both are high. Urine:plasma urea ratio and creatinine level are low, urine osmolality is low, and there is usually sodium loss in the urine. In post-renal failure (i.e. urinary tract obstruction) back-pressure on the kidneys usually results in renal tissue damage with tubular function and water, pH and mineral balance particularly affected.

In the newborn, and especially in premature infants, renal retention of sodium is less effective and sodium losses are high both in prerenal and in renal failure. Distinction between the types of renal failure is difficult.

ARF of renal origin in childhood is usually due to either acute tubular necrosis secondary to shock, haemorrhage, severe anoxia, trauma, or to haemolytic–uraemic syndrome or, rarely, to acute glomerulonephritis secondary to streptococcal infection or Henoch–Schönlein syndrome.

The severity of ARF in childhood varies with the cause, but mortality remains high in established ARF. Outlook is poor when ARF develops following cardiac surgery but quite good in haemolytic uraemic syndrome. The initial phase of low urine output and retention of urea, creatinine and potassium is followed by a diuretic phase for which correct management is just as important as management in the oliguric phase (Renvall, 1984). Nowadays, peritoneal or haemodialysis usually prevent the crises that assailed prolonged ARF in the past.

The principles of nutritional and related management of ARF are outlined below. Where the child is conscious and eating voluntarily severe anorexia may prevent ideal nutritional management.

During the oliguric phase

1. Weigh.
2. Consider setting up central venous line to monitor central venous pressure.
3. Restrict fluid intake to previous day's urine output + losses in vomit, stools, exudate and estimated insensible loss (*Table 17.1*). Greater restriction may be necessary if there has been fluid overload.
4. No salt added to food; avoid high potassium containing foods (fruit, fruit squash, milk, etc.). Daily requirements should be anticipated as sodium, 2 mmol/kg/day; potassium, 2 mmol/kg/day; phosphate, 13 mmol (400 mg)/m^2 body surface area/day. Further requirements are based on urine output, losses in vomit, stools, etc., and plasma electrolyte levels.
5. When hypertension is present, provide a low-sodium diet (about 10 mmol sodium/day). (Diuretics may produce some increase in renal sodium output but can also induce undesirable changes in fluid compartments.)
6. Measure plasma urea and electrolytes at least daily in acute oliguric phase.
7. Save all urine to measure electrolyte output.
8. Provide as high-energy intake as practical in order to diminish catabolism and urea synthesis. Aim for 240–420 kJ (50–100 kcal)/kg/day. Concentrated carbohydrate preparations (*see Table 15.10*) may be helpful in supplementing the diet because of the restrictions on fluid intake.
9. Limit protein intake: initially 0.5 g/kg/day (1.5 g/kg/day in infants) of first-class protein (meat, eggs, milk).

Table 17.1 Guidelines for estimating insensible fluid losses in children (Insley, 1986; Fleming, Spiedel and Dunn, 1986)

	Weight (kg)	*Fluid loss*
Infants*†	<1.5	1.0–3.0 ml/kg/hr
	>1.5–2.5	1.0 ml/kg/hr
	Term >2.5	0.6 ml/kg/hr (15 ml/kg/day)
Children*†§	>10	300 ml/m^2 BSA/day

* About 50% insensible loss is via lungs. Requirements reduced by 50% in infants and children on ventilators.
† Requirements increased by about 50% in infants receiving phototherapy.
‡ Requirements increased in pyrexia: about 10% for every 1°C rise in body temperature.
§ BSA = body surface area: $\frac{(\text{weight (kg)} \times 4) + 7}{\text{weight (kg)} + 90}$ m^2 or determined from nomograms (Insley, 1986).

Peritoneal dialysis may be required for hyperkalaemia, severe fluid overload or severe hyponatraemia and/or acidosis. Dialysis increases protein requirements through losses in the dialysate. Protein intakes should then be at least 2 g/kg/day. Children on dialysis should be able to resume normal diet and fluid intake.

During diuretic phase

1. Watch blood pressure, pulse, central venous pressure closely.
2. Correct hypovolaemia with plasma or other intravenous plasma expander.
3. Maintain adequate fluid intake.
4. Correct hyponatraemia or hypokalaemia, preferably by oral supplements.

The diuretic phase is dangerous, particularly when there is gross oedema. In contrast to the oliguric phase, fluid intake should be liberal since the kidneys are unable to concentrate urine and hypovolaemia readily ensues. Prerenal failure may follow hypovolaemia secondary to rapid diuresis and is managed by restoration of blood volume with either oral fluids, if the condition is not severe, or intravenous plasma. Losses of sodium and potassium may be dramatic. Children's weights, blood pressure, urea and electrolytes must be monitored closely, possibly several times a day.

Nephrotic syndrome

In this condition there is heavy proteinuria, hypoproteinaemia, hyperlipidaemia and gross oedema. Protein losses in the urine are commonly 5–10 g/day but may exceed 30 g/day. There are many precipitating causes although the most common form in childhood is steroid-responsive minimal change nephrotic syndrome. If the condition is rapidly responsive to treatment, and particularly to steroids, nutritional management, although important, is less important than in relatively unresponsive cases where prolonged heavy protein loss in the urine and hypoproteinaemia make nutritional management one of the few effects countering the gross disturbance of metabolism that occurs. Unfortunately, anorexia often prevents the high protein and energy intakes required by these children.

In steroid-responsive nephrotic syndrome, growth may be hindered owing to the high doses of steroids required initially to induce remission. Obesity may develop due to steroid therapy. Thus whilst a high energy and protein intake is advisable before steroids induce remission, total calorie intake whilst in remission on steroids should be low. It may be advisable to avoid fried foods, sweetened drinks and snacks in-between meals to reduce steroid-induced obesity. In steroid-unresponsive conditions, even if the ineffective doses of steroids are not prolonged, growth is likely to be retarded due to gross inadequacy of protein and energy intake compared with the energy and nitrogen losses in the urine.

Heavy proteinuria leads to intense protein loss from the body and mobilization of protein from muscles to restore serum albumin. The loss of protein from muscles requires energy for resynthesis of more protein and there is both fat and protein wasting. One of the aims of nutritional management is to replace as much of the protein loss in the urine by a high intake of first-class protein. A high-energy diet minimizes protein catabolism. The diet is, however, rarely adequate to keep up with the protein losses in severe nephrotic syndrome since most of the affected children refuse the high-protein diets, and many are anorexic. The aetiology of oedema in the nephrotic syndrome is complex but salt retention is a significant factor in the development of oedema. Thus there are conflicting objectives in nutritional management of these children. Salt should be restricted but diets need to be palatable. Dietary measures to achieve the first may defeat the second objective. Children with nephrotic syndrome should have 'no added salt' diets. Protein-containing foods are often fairly salty and very severe restrictions on salt intake yet with high protein intake can lead to restricted and bizarre diets without careful planning (Francis, 1987).

The usefulness of high-protein diets in the management of nephrotic syndrome is questioned, although logically they seem appropriate therapy. In practice, it is extremely difficult to get children to take such diets. A high-energy intake so as to conserve protein as much as possible may be all that can be achieved. More important perhaps is to restore nutrition to normal as rapidly as possible once remission occurs. When diuresis does take place, these children require a good convalescent diet with high energy and first-class protein supplies to restore the fat and muscle loss as soon as possible and to allow catch-up growth.

In nephrotic syndrome, hypovolaemia and hyponatraemia occurring despite fluid and salt overload in the body may stimulate secondary hyperaldosteronism and further fluid retention. Antialdosterone diuretics should be included in management. Salt and water losses in the diuretic phase may lead to dangerous hypovolaemia and prerenal failure.

Chronic renal failure

Children with severe chronic renal problems fail to thrive. Anorexia is a main contributing factor. Why so many of these children show profound anorexia as blood urea rises and renal function deteriorates is unexplained. The clinical picture of loss of taste, poor growth and anorexia is similar to that of zinc deficiency. Many of these children do show low plasma zinc levels, but administration of zinc or other trace elements is not associated with consistent improvement in growth or appetite. The effects of hospitalization, chronic ill health, anxiety for the future, and the accompanying psychosocial response to being small in relation to peer age group can exacerbate poor appetite. Psychosocial support for these children and their families is sometimes helpful in encouraging children to eat even when their appetite is poor.

Failure to thrive in children with chronic renal failure may or may not be accompanied by low height for age (Betts, Magrath and White, 1977). Older children with fairly recent onset of chronic renal failure often show relatively normal height for age, although pubertal growth is likely to be delayed. Deficits in weight and in weight for height are the main features in these children. Younger children, in whom renal failure has been present since early life, usually show profound deficits in both height for age and weight for age. Weight for height may be less affected. The onset of renal rickets causes further deterioration in height for age due to the effects of abnormal bone mineralization and deformity on linear growth (Chesney and Friedman, 1984).

In the past, diets for renal failure aimed to maintain acceptable metabolism for as long as possible with the implicit understanding that there would be gradual deterioration in renal function and no long-term prospect of resolution. Now, peritoneal dialysis, haemodialysis and renal transplantation have improved the outlook for children with chronic renal failure enormously. Diets should therefore aim to maintain normal growth as long as possible since non-dietary methods of management can be introduced as renal function deteriorates. However, adequate growth is not necessarily achieved by maintenance of adequate energy intake. Betts, Magrath and White (1977) could not improve growth rates in chronic renal failure despite 8.4% increase in energy intake by affected children. Other factors such as acidosis may inhibit growth more than dietary inadequacy.

The advent of successful chronic dialysis programmes and transplantation have meant that no specific diet (excluding the proviso on protein intake discussed below) is advised for children in chronic renal failure since dietary needs must be related to present management of the renal failure.

The principles of dietary management in chronic renal failure are as outlined below:

1. Aim for palatability. Most diets fail to achieve their aims simply because children are unable or unwilling to tolerate them.
2. Avoid starvation: feed frequently; renal function deteriorates and blood urea levels rise rapidly owing to tissue breakdown under conditions of starvation.
3. Avoid excessive intakes of carbohydrates: hyperglycaemia with hyperinsulinaemia is a feature of chronic renal failure. Hypertriglyceridaemia has also been reported. Energy provided predominantly as fat may reduce the hyperglycaemia.
4. Correct acidosis.
5. Maintain adequate protein intake for growth. Protein should be good quality, but there is little evidence that providing protein only as essential amino acids and providing keto acids as skeleton for utilization of waste nitrogen to form non-essential amino acids, has any benefit. Again, palatability is probably the most important aspect of ensuring that a diet achieves its aims. High-quality protein supplements may be necessary to increase protein content of the diet the children accept. In the absence of adequate energy intakes such supplements are wasted (*Table 17.2*).

Table 17.2 Protein preparations suitable for supplementing diets in chronic renal failure

Preparation	*Manufacturer*	*Composition*
Casilan	Boots/Farley	90% calcium caseinate. Electrolyte low; glucose free
Maxipro	Scientific Hospital Supplies	88% whey protein. Low salt

The optimum level of protein intake for children with chronic renal failure is controversial (Attman, 1986; Brouhard, 1986). Work in animals suggests that low protein intakes protect the kidney so slowing the rate of deterioration in renal function. There is some evidence that this may also be the case in man. In mild renal failure restricting protein may create more problems, through risking growth inhibition, than it creates benefits. Once renal function has deteriorated to less than 50% glomerular filtration rate, protein restriction may be beneficial. It is essential, however, that protein intakes are adequate for growth and that energy intakes are sufficient for maximum utilization of protein in anabolism. Tube feeding in infancy and perhaps overnight with older children may be necessary to achieve this.

If dietary protein is restricted, children over 1 year should receive diets containing about 1.5 g protein/420 kJ (100 kcal) energy (0.5–1.0 g/kg body

Table 17.3 Management of problems in chronic renal failure

Problem	Explanation	Possible management
Failure to thrive, especially stunting	Anorexia	Provide energy-dense appetizing diet. Carbohydrate and fat supplements (see Tables 15.10 and 15.11) may be useful. Polyunsaturated fats should be used where practical to reduce hypertriglyceridaemia. Maintain adequate protein intake for growth. Correct acidosis and 1-25(OH)$_2$D deficiency
Impaired sodium retention. Impaired sodium excretion	Failing renal function	Restrict salt intake only if hypertension or oedema; avoid adding salt and avoid obviously salty foods
Impaired potassium, magnesium, phosphate and acid excretion	Failing renal function	Avoiding protein intake in excess of needs reduces acid load. Avoid high phosphate and high potassium foods in end-stage renal disease. Aluminium hydroxide gel binds phosphate in gut but risks aluminium toxicity. Calcium carbonate is now more commonly used. If tolerated, a high-fibre diet may also be effective. Sodium bicarbonate 2 mmol/kg/day, increasing as necessary, may help acidosis
Impaired water regulation	Failing renal function	Probably controlled by thirst until end-stage renal disease, when intake = previous day's urine output + estimated insensible loss (see Table 17.1) (total usually 600–1000 ml/day depending on child's size)
Inability to excrete nitrogenous waste	Failing renal function	Restrict protein intake to recommended minimum requirements for growth
Essential amino acid deficiencies	Impaired intracellular metabolism	Histidine and possibly tyrosine and serine may be deficient owing to unexplained impaired metabolism. Supplementary individual amino acids may be helpful, but essential amino acid supplementation can also lead to hyperaminoacidaemia
Vitamin deficiencies	Poor appetite. Loss in dialysate	Ketovite liquid 5 ml daily. Ketovite tablets 1 tds
Failure to synthesize 1-25(OH)$_2$D 'Renal rickets'	Loss of renal tissue	Alfacalcidol (One-Alpha; Leo) in daily dose determined by response (initial dose 0.05 µg/kg/day in infants; 1 µg/day for children >20 kg)
Anaemia	Chronic illness. Loss of blood in haemodialysis. Reduced erythropoetin synthesis	Treat for symptomatic anaemia with blood transfusion. Iron therapy is contraindicated. Serum iron levels do not give a good indication of iron stores but ferritin levels are usually high indicating adequate bone marrow iron
Hyperglycaemia	Insulin resistance	Reduce carbohydrate intake and supply more energy as fat.
Hypertriglyceridaemia	Secondary to high carbohydrate intake	Energy intake from fat should not exceed energy intake from carbohydrate as this risks ketosis

weight/day). In infancy, requirements for protein are greater (1.5 g/kg body weight/day). Fomon, Thomas and Filer (1971) demonstrated equal growth rates in normal healthy infants fed formula containing 6.4% of total energy as protein when compared with infants on formula of higher protein content. Below 6.4% total energy as protein, growth rates were slower. Thus feed recommendations for infants with chronic renal failure are usually suggested as about 8% total energy as protein and a low phosphate content with a calcium:phosphorus ratio of more than 2.0. (Breast milk contains about 6% total energy as protein but the protein is very efficiently utilized and calcium:phosphorus ratio is approximately 2.4.)

Chronic renal failure is associated with many specific nutritional and metabolic problems (Grupe, 1985). Management of some of these are outlined in *Table 17.3*.

Dialysis, particularly peritoneal dialysis, causes protein loss and carbohydrate gain from the glucose in the dialysate solution. Lee (1978) has quoted losses of 20–30 g protein and 13–15 g amino acids in 40 litre dialysates in adults. Losses in children, where the dialysis volume is smaller, are less and usually 4–8 g protein/day (*Table 17.4*).

Table 17.4 Losses (gains) of nutrients during dialysis

Peritoneal dialysis. Approximately:
　0.16 g protein/kg/day lost
　7.5 kcal/kg/day gained by absorption of glucose from dialysate
　Loss of water-soluble vitamins
　Loss of minerals

Haemodialysis:
　Some loss of protein
　Loss of blood in dialysing machine
　Loss of vitamins
　Loss of minerals

Protein needs are altered and children on peritoneal dialysis require at least 2 g protein/kg/day. Adults on haemodialysis may lose 2–3 g amino acids/hour. Again, losses in children are smaller but significant. In both forms of dialysis there is a loss of water-soluble vitamins and trace elements. Thus children with chronic renal failure must have vitamin supplements (Ketovite liquid and tablets; Paines & Byrne). Mineral supplements should be given only when deficiency is apparent since the kidney is unable to excrete mineral loads. Trace element deficiency is most appropriately prevented by encouraging a liberal, varied diet which is possible when the children are on regular dialysis.

Renal rickets

One hydroxylation of 25(OH)D normally occurs in the mitochondria of renal tissue. Since 1–25 $(OH)_2D$ is the active metabolite of vitamin D, one of the causes of renal rickets is shortage of the active form of vitamin D. Inadequate normally functioning renal tissue reduces conversion of 25(OH)D to 1–25$(OH)_2D$. Other aspects of renal failure contribute to the development of renal rickets. Phosphate retention leads to an alteration in the balance between calcium and phosphate in the blood and causes serum calcium levels to fall. Secondary hyperparathyroidism due to the fall in serum calcium level leads to bone mineral reabsorption and the low calcium:phosphate product inhibits bone mineral deposition. Ineffective anabolism due to chronic renal failure probably also affects development of the protein matrix for bone mineral deposition. Thus features of renal rickets are more complex than those of vitamin D deficiency rickets.

The clinical manifestations of renal rickets are similar to those of nutritional rickets (see Chapter 10). Clinical features are often a late development when radiological abnormalities are gross. These children have short stature, bone pain and deformity. Muscular hypotonia may not be as marked as in nutritional, vitamin D deficient rickets.

Radiology shows changes of rickets with widened epiphyseal plates and frayed metaphyses but also localized areas of bone resorption. Bone resorption occurs particularly under the terminal phalanges of the fingers due to secondary hyperparathyroidism. Hyperphosphataemia contributes to areas of excess mineralization in bone. Deficient protein metabolism may be responsible for the generalized osteoporosis. X-rays show splayed shaggy metaphyseal plates with areas of both increased bone density and gross osteoporosis with lytic lesions.

Anaemia

The anaemia of chronic renal failure may be due to inadequate bone marrow stimulation secondary to low levels of erythropoietin. The blood picture is usually of a normochromic, normocytic anaemia. Other factors contributing to anaemia are anorexia and poor nutrient intake, depression of the bone marrow due to toxic effects of products retained in renal failure, blood loss due to frequent haemodialysis, and frequent venepuncture in small children. Blood transfusion is the only effective way of treating the anaemia but the effects of blood transfusion on haemoglobin levels are shortlived and have little effect on growth. A past history of blood transfusion does, however, seem to improve the chances of a kidney transplant being accepted, perhaps due to induced tolerance to a variety of foreign antigens.

Monitoring children with chronic renal failure

These children should be seen regularly. They should be weighed, their heights measured and growth velocity assessed each time they are seen. Their nutritional needs will be judged to some extent by their response to various dietary intakes and by their particular metabolic problems. Serum alkaline phosphatase activity should be measured regularly as rising levels may be one of the more useful methods of demonstrating the onset of the bone changes of renal failure. Regular hand X-rays may demonstrate lytic lesions resulting from secondary hyperparathyroidism. Haemoglobin should be checked regularly. Blood transfusion should be used to maintain haemoglobin over 5 g/dl. Once the anaemia is symptomatic or signs of cardiac failure secondary to anaemia develop (e.g. breathlessness and hepatomegaly) blood transfusion risks causing a critical increase in the high venous pressure and intractable cardiac failure.

Maintenance of growth and nutrition as close to normal as possible is important for these children since the outlook in chronic renal failure has improved greatly with the introduction of peritoneal and haemodialysis and renal transplant. If the child has had a successful renal transplant it is sad if their return to relative normality is hampered by being nutritionally dwarfed. Some catch-up growth can occur during chronic renal failure if efforts are made to correct dietary and metabolic problems as described.

Catch-up growth should occur more dramatically after successful transplant but the extent to which this occurs depends on the growth-suppressing effects of drugs (e.g. steroids) used in post-transplant immunosuppression, the degree of growth retardation, the duration of the growth retardation and the maturity of the child. The use of cyclosporin A seems to have improved post-transplant catch-up growth possibly because it allows a reduction in the steroid dose soon after transplant (Mehls et al., 1986). Children close to puberty are unlikely to have complete catch-up growth since bone age impairment is commonly less than height age impairment. Epiphyseal fusion is likely before height has caught up completely.

References

ATTMAN, P. O. (1986) Recent advances in feeding during renal failure. In *Proceedings of XIII International Congress of Nutrition*, edited by J. G. Taylor and N. K. Jenkins, pp. 666–668. London: John Libbey

BETTS, P. R., MAGRATH, G. and WHITE, R. H. R. (1977) Role of dietary energy supplementation in growth of children with chronic renal insufficiency. *British Medical Journal*, **1**, 416–418

BROUHARD, B. H. (1986) The role of dietary protein in progressive renal disease. *American Journal of Diseases of Children*, **140**, 630–637

CHESNEY, R. W. and FRIEDMAN, A. L. (1984) The medical management of chronic renal failure. *Pediatric Nephrology. Contemporary Issues in Nephrology*, No. 12, edited by B. M. Tune and S. A. Mendoza, pp. 321–342. New York: Churchill Livingstone

FLEMING, P. J., SPIEDEL, B. D. and DUNN, P. M. (1986) *A Neonatal Vade Mecum*, pp. 212–215. London: Lloyd Luke

FOMON, S. J., THOMAS, L. H. and FILER, L. J. (1971) Food composition and growth of normal infants fed milk based formulas. *Acta Paediatrica Scandinavica*, **Suppl. 223**, 1–7

FRANCIS, D. E. M. (1987) *Diets for Sick Children*, 4th edn. Oxford: Blackwells

GRUPE, W. E. (1985) Persistent Renal Disease. In *Nutrition in Paediatrics: Basic Science and Clinical Application*, edited by W. A. Walker and J. B. Watkins, pp. 423–444. Boston: Little Brown

INSLEY, J. (ed.) (1986) *A Paediatric Vade-Mecum*, 11th edn., p. 6. London: Lloyd Luke

LEE, H. A. (1978) The nutritional management of renal disease. In *Nutrition in the Clinical Management of Disease*, edited by J. W. T. Dickerson and H. A. Lee, pp. 210–235. London: Edward Arnold

MEHLS, O., HEINRICH, U., GILLI, G. and SCHARER, K. (1986) Growth in children with chronic renal failure. *World Pediatrics and Child Care*, **1**, 113–122

RENVALL, M. (1984) Renal disease. In *Manual of Pediatric Nutrition*, edited by D. G. Kelts, pp. 244–247. Boston: Little, Brown

RICHARDS, P. and ELL, S. (1982) Nutrition in renal disease. *Human Nutrition: Clinical Nutrition*, **36C**, 103–113

Chapter 18
Diabetes

With few exceptions, diabetes in childhood is type I, insulin dependent diabetes mellitus (IDDM), sometimes described as juvenile diabetes. Rarely, grossly obese children, usually teenagers, present with type II diabetes or non-insulin-dependent diabetes. The majority of type II diabetes are overweight, and the principal course of management is to reduce weight and increase activity in order to increase the insulin sensitivity of tissues and normalize blood sugar. Type II children of normal weight should consume energy intakes only sufficient to maintain normal weight for height. Type II diabetes only affects 2% of childhood diabetics and in 80% has a dominant family history (maturity-onset diabetes of youth: MODY).

A wide variety of factors relevant to childhood make management of diabetes more complicated than in adult life (*Table 18.1*). Management essentially revolves around administration of insulin and regulation of the diet in order to restore normoglycaemia and normal lipid metabolism; to allow normal growth, development and lifestyle; and to prevent, or at least reduce, the late complications of diabetes.

In normal physiological circumstances the body balances the secretion of insulin against changes in blood glucose that arise from ingested food and metabolic events. In diabetes, glucose provided by the diet has to be balanced against a steady release of injected insulin. Although novel methods of giving insulin by insulin pump have modified management for some individuals, the majority of

Table 18.1 Factors complicating management of diabetes in childhood

Diet	Young children eat variably and choosily. Children may eat in appropriate foods when not supervised
Growth	Changing size and effects of changing growth rates necessitate frequent modifications of diet and insulin
Activity	Children's activity is variable and largely unpredictable Small children spend a large part of the 24 hours asleep
Insulin	Small children may not co-operate with injections Older children may cheat over giving injections
Monitoring control	Small children may not pass urine on demand. Children may not co-operate with blood testing
Emotion	Emotional stress and behavioural disturbances lead to difficulties with control, particularly in adolescence

insulin-dependent diabetics are likely to continue on once or twice daily subcutaneous insulin injections for some time to come. Each insulin has its own pattern of release which is influenced by individual circumstances also. Thus food is provided in anticipation of peak insulin levels in the body. *Figure 18.1* illustrates theoretical patterns of peak insulin levels on once daily and twice daily mixtures of long- and short-acting insulins.

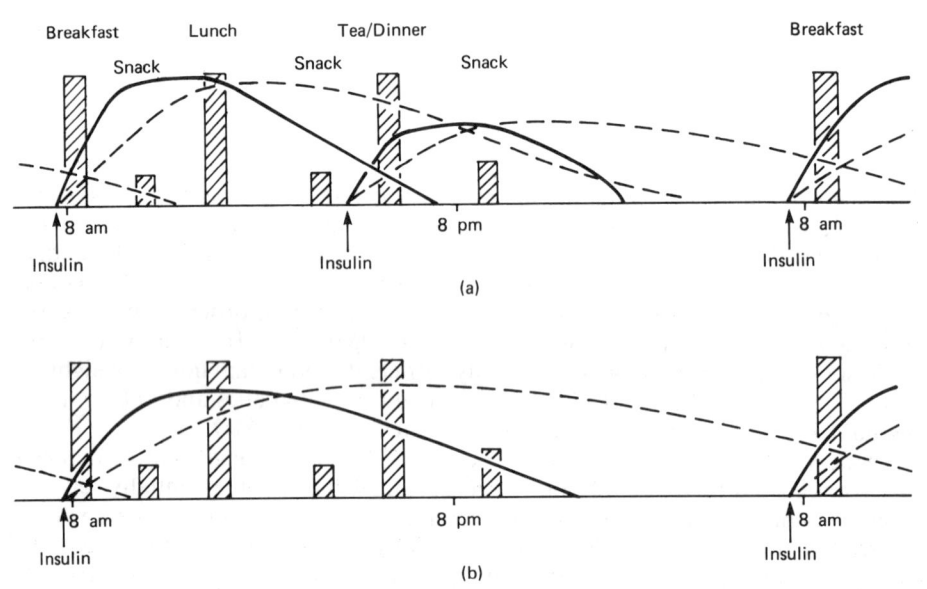

Figure 18.1 Schematic representation of insulin levels and meals using (*a*) twice daily injections of short- (———) and medium-length (- -) action insulins; and (*b*) once-daily regimen of medium- (———) and long-acting (- -) insulins. One mixed insulin zinc suspension may be as effective in (*b*).

Attitudes towards the dietary management of diabetes vary. A few paediatricians feel the restraints the diabetic condition places on children are such that to impose dietary restraint is neither acceptable nor necessary. Such attitudes fail to recognize that if normoglycaemia is facilitated by dietary control, the restraints on children and the interference with their lifestyle due to diabetes are effectively less. Most paediatricians accept that some dietary guidance is essential, but that dietary restraints are inevitably a compromise between practices that achieve ideal control and those that are possible for children and their families.

The development of portable 'pen' syringes containing short-acting human insulin in cartridge form allowsinsulin injections conveniently before the main meals creating a more physiological pattern of insulin release in relation to food. A long-acting insulin is administered by conventional syringe at night. Blood sugar control is potentially greatly improved and many older children find this regimen very acceptable and satisfactory. 'Pen' regimens may become more widely used, and their use means that the timing and even the size of the meals can be varied since timing and size of insulin dose can be modified in relation to the anticipated meal.

Diet

Carbohydrate

Before insulin was available for the treatment of diabetes, the only possible management was through the diet. Some moderately successful diets restricted carbohydrate intake enormously and encouraged exercise to try to maintain low blood sugars. Perhaps for this reason the traditional Western diabetic diet has tended to restrict carbohydrate. However, concern over the later complications of microvascular disease and particularly atherosclerosis in which dietary fat may have a part, has changed attitudes more towards restricting the dietary fat intake in diabetes. Since there is no indication for an abnormally high protein intake in diabetes, fat reduction means that more energy must be obtained from carbohydrate. Provided weight is normal for height and age, there is no evidence that high-carbohydrate diets adversely affect the management of diabetes. The opposite is probably the case (Brunzell et al., 1971; Simpson et al., 1979). Present-day diets for childhood diabetics recommend a minimum of 50% total energy from carbohydrates (and probably more), with no more than 30% total energy from fat and about 15% of total energy from protein (Pittler and Kretchner, 1975; Wolfsdorf, 1985). In areas where traditional diets are low in protein, growth and development in diabetics are not adversely affected by lower protein intakes than those described above but clearly the proportion of carbohydrate will increase relatively if fat is not excessive.

Carbohydrate may be regulated through the provision of lists of equivalent portions of carbohydrate-containing foods and even of other foods so that meal planning occurs through a series of exchanges. It is probably more educative to provide advice on the relevant carbohydrate content of foods by the provision of lists of the weight of foods which contain 10 g portions of carbohydrate, thus allowing children and families to design meals with carbohydrate content according to the number of 10 g portions recommended at each meal. Protein can then be taken freely. The fat content of the diet seems irrelevant to the immediate management of diabetes, but may be very relevant to prevention of long-term complications (*see below*).

Total energy requirements of children can be estimated roughly as 1000 kcal daily (4.2 MJ) at 1 year and an additional 100 kcal (0.42 MJ) per day for each subsequent year of life. The logical simplicity of this formula has been upset by the change to SI units and joules instead of calories! With girls over 9 years old this energy intake should probably be modified according to weight for age and height since many girls, whether or not diabetic, tend to put on excessive weight in their adolescent years and become obese. Obesity reduces sensitivity to insulin and greatly inhibits good diabetic management as well as providing a further risk factor for later cardiovascular disease. Boys in their teenage years may have very high energy needs during their peak growth velocity. A 15-year-old boy at peak growth velocity needs approximately 14.7 MJ/day (3500 kcal) – considerably in excess of that suggested by the guidelines provided above. Some may need – and consume – much more. With adolescence and greater evening interest and activities there is often a notable increase in food consumption at tea and supper. This may be out of proportion to increases in food intake at other times of day. Insulin regimens may have to be adjusted to cope with this. Frequent discussions and dietary reviews are thus necessary with diabetic children and their families in order to provide diets which meet needs for growth and development appropriately. Appetite and apparent desire for more food should be balanced against changes in relative weight for height.

Table 18.2 indicates some common foods and the weights that contain 10 g carbohydrate portions. Carbohydrate Countdown (BDA, 1982) provides an extensive list of carbohydrate values for proprietary foods. Initially most diabetics require scales and lists of food values to familiarize themselves with the size of portions. Children and families usually become familiar with estimating portion size quite quickly. Obsessional precision is unnecessary, and household utensils can be used sufficiently accurately to gauge portion sizes in most cases.

Table 18.2 Examples of weights of foods containing 10 g carbohydrate

Sugar	2 teaspoonfuls (10 g)
Milk	One glass (180 ml)
White bread, ⅔ slice	20 g
Wholemeal bread, one slice	28 g*
Potato, uncooked (one hen's egg sized)	50 g
Cornflakes, 3 tablespoonfuls	12 g
Apple, whole, one	100 g
Banana, ⅔ average size	50 g
Grapes, whole, 10 grapes	60 g

* Bread is a typical food where the glycaemic index of a particular bread may be more important than absolute carbohydrate content.

Carbohydrate portions should be distributed throughout the day with three large meals and regular snacks (e.g. mid-morning, perhaps mid-afternoon and late evening in older children) if meals are more than 4 hours apart. Other foods can be taken whenever seems appropriate. As far as possible diabetic diets should be linked in with family and school eating practices, although it is important to remember that if the family are delaying meals or lying in bed late at weekends, these habits risk hypoglycaemia in diabetics. Under these circumstances diabetic children must be provided with their meal on time or at least some carbohydrate-containing snack to carry them through until meal time.

Table 18.3 Example menu for 150 g carbohydrate diet

		Weight (g)	*Carbohydrate* (g)
Breakfast	Cornflakes/other cereal	25	20
	Milk	100	5
	Toast, one round – Butter	30	15
Mid-morning	Sugar-free diabetic squash – One digestive biscuit	15	10
Dinner	Meat – Runner beans – Jacket or boiled potato	100	20
	Four cream crackers – Butter/margarine – Cheese	28	20
Mid-afternoon	Packet of crisps, small – Diabetic squash/tea, small amount of milk	20	10
Tea	Meat – Salad – Bread, two rounds	60	30
	Butter/margarine – Apple	120	10
Bedtime	Milk, one glass	180	10

Table 18.3 outlines an example day's menu with indications of portion distribution. Whilst still the most commonly used and practical approach to designing a regulated diet for diabetics, a rather different approach to carbohydrate portions or exchanges is needed in view of current knowledge. In recent years it has become apparent that the effects on blood glucose levels of the same carbohydrate content in different foods are not identical (Mann, 1984). Simple carbohydrates such as sucrose tend to produce an unacceptably rapid rise in blood glucose, often followed by rapid falls as the sugar is utilized, but the insulin injected to balance it remains. Hypoglycaemia may follow.

Neat sugars are therefore not recommended in most diabetic diets, particularly since they contain no other food substance such as vitamins or minerals or protein. Perhaps this exclusion is unnecessary since evidence suggests that when eaten as part of a meal simple sugars such as sucrose do not aggravate postprandial hyperglycaemia. Sucrose and glucose do also form quite high proportions of the carbohydrates in many foods such as bread, biscuits and vegetables. Complex carbohydrates such as natural starches produce more gradual rises in blood sugar and thus reduce postprandial hyperglycaemia (Bantle et al., 1983). Other factors besides the complexity of the carbohydrate influence the effect carbohydrates have on blood sugars. These factors are outlined in *Table 18.4*.

Table 18.4 Possible reasons for variable glycaemic effect of carbohydrates

Rate of digestion of carbohydrate
Rate of absorption of carbohydrate
Preparation of food: whole, puréed, ground, liquidized
Whether food eaten separately or as part of mixed meal
Whether food eaten raw or cooked
Presence of enzyme inhibitors in food
Presence of lecithins, tannins, pectins, fats and proteins

It has been suggested that carbohydrate intake should be regulated according to tables of each food's 'glycaemic index' rather than its carbohydrate content alone. The glycaemic index is the ratio of the area under the curve of blood glucose response when a small amount of food of known carbohydrate content is given, against the area under the blood glucose curve when the same amount of carbohydrate is given as glucose. Because of what we know of the glycaemic effects of food, most clinicians now recommend that diabetics take their carbohydrate in the form of whole foods – cereals, fruits and vegetables – since carbohydrate release and absorption from whole fruit and cereals is relatively slow and thus blood sugar levels have more gradual and sustained rise postprandially. Insulin requirements may thus be less. Products such as guar gum have been used to try to modify postprandial hyperglycaemia but their long-term effects are unknown and eating more whole foods would appear a more rational approach than adding commercially produced fibres and pectins to the diet (Kinmonth and Angus, 1985).

High-fibre diets also carry the possible benefit of lowering serum cholesterol levels. This may be an advantage in the long-term prevention of the complications of diabetes although the interrelationship of cardiovascular disease and cholesterol is a confused and controversial one (*see* Chapter 21).

Fat

The relation of the early microvascular complications of IDDM to fat intake is not certain. Children with IDDM have an increased predisposition to atherosclerosis and cardiovascular problems in adult life, and there is some evidence that these are affected by serum cholesterol (low density lipoprotein cholesterol) levels. Reduction in the cholesterol and saturated fat intake of childhood diabetics is recommended. This follows the general principles currently thought to reduce risk of disease in adult life, namely restriction of dietary fat to no more than 30% of total energy and increasing the polyunsaturated fat intake to 50–60% of total fat intake. In practice, less pork and beef should be eaten; fatty meats should be avoided and preference given to poultry, fish, vegetable proteins and margarines and oils made from unsaturated vegetable fats. The effect of this type of dietary modification remains largely theoretical (Brink, 1988).

Protein

Diabetic children should be provided with diets containing adequate good quality protein but there is no reason either to increase or restrict protein intake compared with non-diabetic children. The nature of the protein is likely to be determined by the other nutrients, particularly fat, with which it is combined. For example, chicken and fish with fat content more appropriate for the policy outlined above and cottage cheese and skimmed milk (not suitable for young children) seem preferable to beef, pork, Cheddar cheese and full-cream milk.

Other dietary factors

Hypertension is more prevalent in populations with high salt intakes than in those with low salt intakes. The importance of the level of dietary salt intake for the development of hypertension is much debated. If there is a possibility that a high dietary salt intake contributes to the development of hypertension in some individuals, it might seem wise to advise diabetics – with their propensity to microvascular disease which would be made worse by hypertension – to avoid adding salt to foods or during cooking.

Specific issues in management

The principles of dietary regulation in diabetes cannot be grasped at one interview. Frequent discussions with children and their families are necessary and dieticians, nutritionists or paediatricians familiar with diabetic management should be the ones who educate the parents. Initially, advice is needed on survival skills especially coping with hypoglycaemia. Instruction on diet is necessary before children leave hospital after diagnosis and such advice must be followed up by further regular meetings on recommendations of changes associated with growth and development in the child and discussions on general problems.

Insulin

The dose of insulin required by individual children is extremely variable and depends on activity levels, growth rates, dietary intake, general health and, to some extent, duration of diabetes in that soon after diagnosis some children have a 'honeymoon period' of relatively low requirements for insulin. In general terms, however, the majority of children with established but controlled diabetes require 0.5–1.0 units/kg/day.

There have been considerable changes in insulin preparation and administration over the past 10–15 years with beneficial reductions in the lipoatrophy that resulted from the less purified insulins of the past. Areas of lipohypertrophy still occur when children are allowed to inject insulin regularly into the same small area of tissue, whether on leg or arm or elsewhere. All children should receive highly purified bovine, pork or 'human' insulin nowadays. All insulin is presented as 'U-100' strength with 100 units/ml. *Table 18.5* lists duration of action of some of the insulins available. It is not proposed to discuss management of insulin therapy in this book but this provides an outline for the likely peaks of action of insulins against which to organize the diet.

Table 18.5 Duration of action of some insulin preparations*

Type		Manufacturer	Subcutaneous injection	
			Peak action (hours)	Duration (hours)
Short acting:				
Neutral insulin	Bovine	Evans	2–6	8–12
Actrapid MC	Porcine	Novo		
Neusulin	Bovine	Wellcome		
Human Actrapid	Human†	Novo	2–4	8
Human Velosulin	Human†	Nordisk Wellcome	1–2	8
Humulin S	Human‡	Lilly		
Intermediate and long acting:				
Isophane	Bovine	Boots	4–8	22
Humulin	Human isophane‡	Lilly	2–6	20
Monotard MC	Porcine insulin zinc suspension	Novo	6–14	24
Human monotard	Human insulin zinc suspension	Novo	6–14	24

* British National Formulary, 1986.
† Modified from porcine.
‡ Biosynthetic.

Particular problems

Infancy

The two ages in childhood which lead to difficulties in management of diabetes most commonly are infancy and adolescence. Management is difficult in infancy due to problems with compliance over diet and with monitoring blood surgar control. Small children have variable appetites which create problems for the provision of regular carbohydrate intake. They spend a large proportion of the 24 hours asleep, which means that control may be difficult during periods when the children are not eating because they are asleep and yet still require small amounts of insulin.

As a result, many paediatricians and parents of diabetic children prefer that children become mildly hyperglycaemic overnight rather than risk the possibility of hypoglycaemia during a period when children may not be closely observed. There is perhaps more concern about hypoglycaemia in early childhood since, if it is more than transient, it runs the risk of damaging a still developing brain. Reassuringly, perhaps, many children who become mildly hypoglycaemic during the night rouse their parents either by crying and distress or by making 'funny noises' as they become semi-comatose, so parents are aware of their situation and can resuscitate them with oral carbohydrate.

It can be helpful to provide parents with a glucagon injection pack to administer to their child if the child is too hypoglycaemic to take food or drink. Glucagon solution for injection (0.5–1.0 mg subcutaneously or intramuscularly) has to be made up immediately prior to use, and some parents find this difficult whilst at the same time coping with a confused hypoglycaemic child.

Monitoring of diabetic control is difficult in early childhood because small children do not pass urine on demand, and there is a natural reluctance on the part of many parents – and paediatricians – to subject these children to regular finger-pricks for blood sampling. Diets are likely to be a compromise.

There are no ideal ways as yet of controlling diabetes in very young children but happily this remains a fairly uncommon problem, although the incidence may be increasing at a greater rate than that of diabetes in older children. Help from paediatric diabetologists and paediatric dieticians is invaluable in the management of very young children.

Adolescence

Management of diabetes in children developing the condition during adolescence is sometimes relatively easy. These children may recognize that control of their diabetes is necessary for well-being as they have recently experienced ill health. They are usually sufficiently mature to understand and manage their own diabetes with minimal parental supervision and the more children take responsibility for managing their diabetes, the more likely control is to be good.

Nevertheless, many adolescents with diabetes do present major management problems. Commonly, these seem to be the children who have been diabetic since early childhood and who have probably forgotten the acute severe illness that precipitated their diagnosis. Adolescent rebellion may be shown by very negative attitudes towards control of their diabetes. They decide that they are not going to be diabetic any more. Diabetes for the adolescent is interfering in lifestyle since diabetics must eat regularly, usually avoiding the junk foods that are important to social activities in adolescence. They must also inject themselves, often at inconvenient times such as at the end of the school day. Evening injections may mean that they either go home after school rather than go out with friends, or have to carry around injection kits. They may get teased by their school friends and peers or accused of being 'junkies'. Poorly controlled longstanding diabetics may well have poor growth and delayed puberty and remain small and rather puny until later than their peers (Jivani and Rayner, 1973). This may again subject them to teasing.

Brittle diabetes

The emotional conflicts common to adolescence contribute to making diabetic management difficult since emotional stress leads to swings in blood sugar even though diet and insulin are apparently fairly well regulated. In its extreme form this diabetic instability takes the form of 'brittle' diabetes where blood sugar ranges rapidly from hypoglycaemia to hyperglycaemia sometimes without obvious fault in insulin treatment or carbohydrate intake. Commonly, however, there is a significant element of non-compliance with management in these children. Injections may be omitted, blood and/or urine test results fabricated, and any dietary regulation ignored. It is not particularly useful to spend time determining what has or has not been occurring at home. More important is to resolve the stresses that lead to non-compliance, and this can be extremely difficult. Brittle diabetics are almost invariably girls. Social, community and psychiatric help may be very useful in analysing these children's problems and thus helping the control and organization of their diabetes. Sometimes reasonable diabetic control can be re-established only by a period away from home in residential school or other stable environment since the frequent episodes of ketoacidosis may be life threatening.

Realistic and knowledgeable recognition of the individual way diabetes interferes with the lives of all these children, not just with brittle diabetics, is useful in trying to minimize the interference and thus maximize confidence, normality of lifestyle and diabetic control. In this respect, the procedure of administration of small doses of short-acting insulin by 'pen' syringe can help normalize life for older children. Insulin can be administered just before a meal with minimum inconvenience. The dose can be adjusted according to the carbohydrate intake anticipated. Night-time normoglycaemia is maintained by an evening dose of long-acting insulin (*Figure 18.2*).

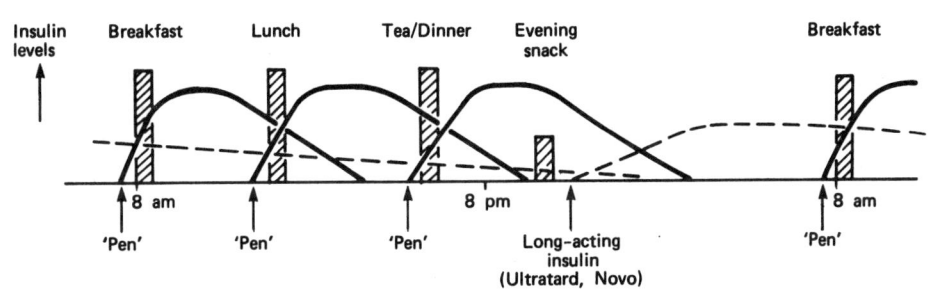

Figure 18.2 Schematic representation of multi-injection 'pen' (short-acting) insulin regimen (———) with night-time long-acting insulin (- - -) in relation to meals (▨). The ease with which size and timing of meals and insulin can be changed is clear.

Hypoglycaemia

Table 18.6 lists factors likely to precipitate hypoglycaemia. Activity in sports is one of the anticipated factors predisposing to hypoglycaemia in otherwise well-controlled diabetic children. An extra 10 g carbohydrate portion before sport for every hour's activity may help prevent hypoglycaemia with activity. Teachers, children and parents should be warned that activity is likely to lead to hypoglycaemia and know how to provide acute resuscitation for the hypoglycaemic

Table 18.6 Situations that predispose to hypoglycaemia in diabetes

Delay of meal
Inadequate carbohydrate intake at previous meal
Unusual or vigorous activity
Overdose of insulin
New bottle of insulin when previous bottle had lost some potency
Anxiety and stress
Drugs
'Brittle' diabetes

diabetic. Hypoglycaemia may be delayed some hours after exercise. Own blood glucose monitoring may help children who understand diabetes to assess whether they need more food following exercise.

Hypoglycaemia presents in many ways (facial pallor, sweating, changes in behaviour such as temper tantrums, drowsiness, vomiting, headache, abdominal pains) but children presenting with one particular pattern of symptoms tend to follow the same pattern on future occasions. Families usually learn to recognize the symptoms readily. If hypoglycaemia is suspected, children should be given some carbohydrate containing food as soon as possible. Ideally this should be a glucose drink or glucose tablets since these will give quick response, but biscuits or a drink of milk or whatever carbohydrate source is available can be used. Schools need to be advised on the recognition and management of hypoglycaemia. They should be provided with 'Lucozade' or dextrose solution to administer by mouth in a crisis.

If the child is comatose, intravenous glucose (50% solution given by rapid injection until recovery of consciousness) should be given as soon as possible. Where there are no facilities for giving intravenous glucose and children are prone to severe hypoglycaemia which cannot be managed by oral carbohydrate, glucagon injections can be provided for emergencies (0.5–1 mg injected subcutaneously, intramuscularly or intravenously, and repeated after 20 minutes if necessary). These may restore consciousness by raising blood glucose so that the children can then be fed from other carbohydrate sources.

Hypoglycaemia should be avoided. If it is prolonged, it may impair brain function permanently and this is a particular fear in infants with IDDM.

Ketoacidosis

Ketoacidosis is usually associated with considerable hyperglycaemia, but the development of symptoms is related more to ketosis and acidosis than the absolute blood glucose level. In MODY ketoacidosis is unusual and blood sugar levels may be extremely high without other major metabolic upset. Clinical symptoms from MODY, when they develop, are secondary to severe hyperosmolality of the blood.

Children with IDDM present much more acutely than adults and the majority show some ketoacidosis at first presentation. Under such circumstances, management is complicated by the need to restore hydration, provide insulin and correct the acidosis. It is not the place of this book to discuss such management in detail. After the initial presentation, ketoacidosis may be precipitated again by a variety of circumstances (*Table 18.7*).

Table 18.7 Situations predisposing to the development of diabetic keotacidosis

Inadequate or no insulin
Major dietary indiscretions
Infection
Adolescent growth spurt
Premenstrually
Reduced activity
Stress, Anxiety
Associated problems: hypothyroidism, Cushing's syndrome
Surgery
Brittle diabetes

The diabetic child who is unwell and vomits presents a difficult problem in management for general practitioners and the child's family. Reasonable advice might be that the family should get in touch with the diabetic team if the child vomits more than once. If ketones are present in the urine, seeking advice is more urgent than if they are not. If the vomiting is recurrent, the child will be unable to take adequate diet and will probably need admitting to hospital. Diabetic children and their families must accept that the children are likely to require hospital admission for otherwise fairly trivial conditions, or minor operations such as dental extractions, since difficulties maintaining adequate carbohydrate intake and the effects of stress on the control of blood sugar commonly lead to failure of normal control. The vomiting, diabetic child still requires insulin to cope with endogenously produced glucose even though no food is eaten. Normal insulin doses (or increased doses if there is reason to feel that the vomiting is secondary to ketoacidosis) should be given and the normal carbohydrate intake met through sweetened drinks, milk, biscuits or acceptable food items. Use of frequent small doses of short-acting insulins may control the situation but most parents will be helped by liaison with their diabetic clinic before adjusting insulin management. Frequent blood or urine testing is necessary to determine whether home management is succeeding.

Assessment of control

The method used to assess day-by-day control depends on the age of the child and the method of daily monitoring. Some children monitor urine and this should be done before breakfast and before the evening meal with occasional tests last thing at night or before lunch. Some children have been taught to test the 'second urine sample' since, if the bladder has been completely emptied first thing in the morning, the urine passed in the second specimen shortly afterwards should give an indication of blood sugar levels around the time of passing, rather than an admixture of blood sugar levels overnight. On the other hand, urine collecting in the bladder over a period of time, such as overnight, can give an overall impression of the amount of sugar passed during that period. Thus both methods of urine testing have advantages, but it is important that whichever method is used, the same method is used each day so that results are comparable.

Blood sampling is the method of choice for monitoring control in many diabetics nowadays. This indicates blood sugar levels at the time of sampling, but does not indicate control in between sampling and cannot demonstrate impending ketoacidosis. Development of a variety of coloured strips has greatly facilitated home blood glucose monitoring. Ideally glood glucose checked before and 1–1½ hours after a meal should be under 10 mmol/l. This is NOT easy to achieve.

Children should be encouraged to test their urine for ketones if blood sugar rises above a certain level, e.g. 20 mmol/l or if they are unwell, particularly with vomiting.

Children must be encouraged to record results of the tests daily, whether blood or urine testing is used, so that clinic visits can be used to assess overall control by examination of the diary of results. *Table 18.8* outlines other parameters of control recorded at clinic visits.

Table 18.8 Clinical parameters of adequacy of diabetic control

History:	Frequency or absence of hypoglycaemia
	Degree of glycosuria and ketonuria recorded on home testing
	General health, activity and school attendance
Examination:	Weight for age
	Height for age
	Pubertal assessment
	(Measurement of subcutaenous fat)
	Liver size
	Hydration
	Evidence of complications:
	Proteinuria
	Blood pressure
	Peripheral pulses
	Fundoscopy
	Peripheral nerve function
Investigations:	Urinary sugar and ketones
	Random blood sugar – series of sugars over day
	Haemoglobin A1c levels in blood
	Lipid profile
	Blood urea and creatinine

Diabeties should be examined thoroughly at least once a year with particular attention given to eyes, blood pressure, presence of all peripheral pulses, peripheral nerve function and presence or absence of proteinuria as well as to growth, nutrition and pubertal development. It is unusual for microangiopathic complications to develop in children who have been diabetic for less than 10 years although there is an increasing prevalence with time after this.

The diabetic who needs to slim

The majority of childhood diabetics are slim or even underweight when they present. Diabetic girls are particularly likely to become significantly obese at or around puberty. Obesity often makes control less satisfactory and exacerbates the cardiovascular risks of diabetes. It is perfectly possible for diabetics to slim satisfactorily but they must be advised sensibly and their control closely monitored. It is unwise to start a sudden strict slimming regimen since this may impair the balance between insulin and carbohydrate intake and lead rapidly to hypoglycaemia. Dietary fat intake should be reduced as the first line of management. Added fats, fried foods, chips, butter on vegetables and other foods should be avoided and low-calorie margarine high in polyunsaturated fatty acids used on bread. Skimmed milk can be used. If it is felt important or necessary to cut down on carbohydrate intake as well – and this will depend on how much fats can be cut down and how obese the child is – one portion of carbohydrate should be reduced at a time, with careful consideration of level of control and reduction of insulin if hypoglycaemia occurs. Hypoglycaemia occurring under these circumstances must be counterbalanced by carbohydrate as an emergency procedure, even if this does not comply with dietary needs, but reduction in insulin dosage should then take place so that the hypoglycaemia does not recur. Diabetics trying to slim should be encouraged to increase their activity and their intake of fibre, whole cereal, fruit and vegetable so that the diet has maximum satiety.

Somogyi effect

This is the hyperglycaemia that sometimes occurs in response to hypoglycaemia. Typically it occurs first thing in the morning. Presumably hormonal responses (catecholamines, glucocorticoids, growth hormone) to hypoglycaemia overswing in restoring blood sugar or antagonize insulin action thus precipitating hyperglycaemia and often ketonuria. The problem must be recognized, since the finding of hyperglycaemia usually indicates the need for more insulin, whereas with the Somogyi response, less insulin is required. Usually these children have a recent history of large increases in total daily insulin. Increasing insulin further (in these children total daily dose usually exceeds 2 units/kg/day) is likely to be followed by more dramatic hyperglycaemia. Any situation where hyperglycaemia is not coming under control with increased insulin levels should be reviewed as a possible Somogyi effect.

Mauriac syndrome (diabetic dwarfism)

Here children are stunted with poor control (both hypo- and hyperglycaemia) and hepatomegaly. There is often a cushingoid appearance with facial obesity and thin limbs. Liver biopsy shows only excessive fat. Inadequate control of diabetes has led to fatty liver, poor nutrition and poor growth and perhaps other hormonal responses to uncontrolled blood sugar levels. Diagnosis of the condition indicates the need for much stricter monitoring and control and usually more insulin. The full-blown condition is rare but elements of the syndrome are not uncommon in poorly controlled children from unsatisfactory home environments.

Long-term complications

Table 18.9 lists the main long-term problems of diabetes. There is a lot of controversy over the importance of management in preventing these complications. It does seem that many of the complications can be delayed by good management in childhood. In adult life the effects of maternal diabetes on the fetus are virtually prevented by rigid maintenance of normoglycaemia during pregnancy.

Table 18.9 Long-term complications of diabetes in childhood

Poor linear growth

Delayed puberty

Complications of pregnancy:
  Increased fetal wastage
  Increased congenital abnormalities
  Increased problems such as toxaemia and hydramnios
  'Infant of diabetic mother' – overweight and immature

Microangiopathic problems:
  Progressive renal disease
  Nephrotic syndrome
  Peripheral vascular disease – infection and gangrene in limbs
  Myocardial ischaemia
  Involvement of the eyes:
    Cataracts
    Retinopathy
    Vitreous haemorrhages
  Peripheral and autonomic neuropathy
  Hypertension:
    Secondary to microvascular disease
    Secondary to renal disease

Lipodystrophy at injection sites

Recent changes in the purity and the type of insulins used for the control of diabetes may have had some effect in reducing the complications. Certainly, they have almost exterminated the unsightly lipoatrophy that used to accompany insulin injections in many individuals although lipohypertrophy does still occur. Since most child diabetics do not begin to show complications until they have had diabetes for at least 10 years, it may be a while before we recognize how effective (or not) these insulins are in preventing complications. Similarly, the effects of better control, achieved by modern methods of monitoring, in the prevention of late microvascular problems will not be apparent for many years. Measurement of glycosylated haemoglobin (HbAlc) is useful in assessing long-term control since HbAlc indicates the occurrence of hyperglycaemia over preceding weeks. Haemoglobin Alc levels amplify the essentially episodic evidence of control provided by occasional urine and blood sugar testing and often show how apparently good control is still far from ideal.

References

BANTLE, J. P., LAINE, D. C., CASTLE, G. W., THOMAS, J. W., HOOGWERF, B. J. and GOETZ, F. C. (1983) Postprandial glucose and insulin responses to meals containing different carbohydrates in normal and diabetic subjects. *New England Journal of Medicine*, **309**, 7–12

BDA (1982) *Carbohydrate Countdown*. London: British Diabetic Association

BRINK, S. J. (1988) (1988) Pediatric, adolescent and young-adult nutrition issues in IDDM. *Diabetes Care*, **11**, 192–200

BRITISH NATIONAL FORMULARY (1986) No. 11, pp. 228–229. London: British Medical Association

BRUNZELL, J. D., LERNER, R. L., HAZZARD, W. R., PORTE, D. and BIERMAN, E. L. (1971) Improved glucose tolerance with high carbohydrate feeding in mild diabetes. *New England Journal of Medicine*, **284**, 521–524

JIVANI, S. K. M. and RAYNER, P. H. W. (1973) Does control influence the growth of diabetic children? *Archives of Disease in Childhood*, **48**, 109–115

KINMONTH, A. L. and ANGUS, R. M. (1985) Dietary management. In *Care of the Child with Diabetes*, edited by J. D. Baum and A. L. Kinmonth, pp. 92–116. Edinburgh: Churchill Livingstone

MANN, J. I. (1984) What carbohydrate foods should diabetics eat? *British Medical Journal*, **288**, 1025–1026

PITTLER, A. and KRETCHMER, N. (1985) Utilization of diet in the treatment of insulin-dependent diabetes (juvenile). In *Pediatric Nutrition*, edited by G. C. Arneil and J. Metcoff, pp. 245–268. London: Butterworths

SIMPSON, R. W., MANN, J. I., EATON, J., CARTER, R. D. and HOCKADAY, T. D. R. (1979) High carbohydrate diets and insulin-dependent diabetes. *British Medical Journal*, **ii**, 523–525

WOLFSDORF, J. I. (1985) Nutrition in diabetes mellitus. In *Nutrition in Pediatrics, Basic Science and Clinical Applications*, edited by W. A. Walker and J. B. Watkins, pp. 517–528. Boston: Little Brown

Chapter 19
Obesity and anorexia nervosa

Definition of obesity

Obesity is by definition an excess of body fat. Measuring body fat accurately is neither easy nor clinically practical. Severe obesity can be recognized by inspection without specific investigation or particular knowledge of nutrition. Distinction of mild cases of obesity from those who are normally fat is extremely difficult.

Because of the difficulties of measuring body fat accurately, obesity is often diagnosed by relative overweight (*Table 19.1*). Weight–height definitions of obesity have a lot of problems, particularly in childhood (Poskitt, 1975; Cole, 1979; Taitz, 1983). Overweight does not define body fatness, although an excess of fat is by far the most likely explanation for severe overweight in childhood.

The proportions of fat and lean tissue in the body can be measured by various experimental procedures such as measurement of density by total body immersion,

Table 19.1 Definitions of obesity from weight–height relations

Relation	Derivation	Comments
% Weight for height*	$\dfrac{\text{Actual weight}}{\text{Mean expected weight for height}\dagger} \cdot 100$	Age independent. Influenced by height for age
% Weight for height for age*	$\dfrac{\text{Actual weight}}{\text{Weight for age at height for age centile}} \cdot 100$	Requires accurate age. Tedious to record
Quetelet's index	$\text{Weight} \div (\text{height})^2$	Varies with age, therefore difficult to judge relative obesity. Widely used with adults
% Quetelet's index for age*	$\dfrac{\text{Weight}}{(\text{Height})^2} \div \left(\dfrac{\text{50th centile W for age}}{(\text{50th centile H for age})^2 \cdot 100}\right)$	Quite useful. Tedious unless 50th centiles for age computerized
Ponderal index	$\text{Weight} \div 3\sqrt{\text{Height}}$	Little use in childhood. Index varies with age

* Underweight, <90%; normal weight, 90–110%; overweight, >110–120%; 'obesity'; >120%.
† WHO, 1983.

measurements of the distribution of heavy water (deuterium oxide) or radioactive inert gases such as xenon and krypton (Garrow, 1971).

Skinfold thickness measured by skinfold calipers (available from Holtain Ltd., Cresswell, Crymmych, Dyfed) are by themselves the most practical way of estimating relative fatness. A fold of fat is pulled up away from muscle at the chosen site (*Table 19.2*), the calipers applied and the handles released so the dial reads the thickness of the fold in millimetres. Several (usually three) readings should be taken at each site since there is considerable variation both with the same observer and more dramatically between observers. Cameron (1974) describes the technique in greater detail.

Table 19.2 Common sites for skinfold measurement*

Triceps:	Arm hanging relaxed. Skinfold measured over triceps midway between tip of acromion and olecranon
Biceps:	As with triceps only over biceps muscle
Subscapular:	At the inferior angle of the scapula. Skinfold pulled up along body skinfold lines
Suprailiac	1 cm above and 2 cm medial to anterior superior iliac spine, child standing†

* Conventionally left side of body used.
† Cameron, 1984. Durnin and Rahaman (1967) use mid-axillary vertical fold just above iliac crest. Whichever used, consistency is important.

Skinfold calipers are designed to exert constant pressure on tissue however wide their gape. Nevertheless, there are problems measuring very fat skinfolds. The fold may be too wide for the gape of the calipers. It may be difficult to pull a fat fold away from the underlying tissue in the severely obese and to apply calipers to the full thickness of skin and subcutaneous tissue. Often calipers slip off the fold gradually and no constant reading is obtained. Fat folds in the obese who have lost a little fat are easier to measure and provide more repeatable readings than those of the unaffected obese.

Nomograms (Ney, 1984) and regression formulae can be used to relate the percentage of body weight that is fat (%BF) derived from experimental density or inert gas with skinfold thickness measurements (Durnin and Rahaman, 1967; Brook, 1971). Other methods use calculations of the relative size of different parts of the body and the contribution of skinfold thickness in these areas to total body fat (Dauncey, Gandy and Gairdner, 1977). The various methods are outlined in *Table 19.3*. The value of these methods is questionable since the inaccuracies and inter-method variation in results are so large that the results probably have little real meaning (Hager, 1981).

Percentage body weight that is fat (%BF) in childhood

Table 19.4 outlines the varying proportions of fat in the body according to age as determined by a variety of observers and methods. Values vary widely with sex and age and, as discussed above, the method used. Values may not be precise, but trends are discernible. After birth, infants gain fat very rapidly so that at the age of 4–5 months they are probably fatter than they will be at any other stage in their lives.

Table 19.3 Indirect methods of measuring body fat

Age group	Reference	Method
Infancy	1	Measures weight of fat in body (g) from combination of estimates of volume and fat thickness of body
Childhood	2	Uses regression lines derived from comparison of body density by distribution of deuterium oxide with sum of triceps, biceps, subscapular and suprailiac skinfoolds (TSFT) to measure body density. Density: 1.1690 − 0.0788.log TSFT, boys 1.2063 − 0.0999.log TSFT, girls $\%BF = \left(\dfrac{4.95}{density} - 4.5\right) 100$
	3	Nomograms relating triceps, subscapular skinfolds to density and %BF (9–12 yr)
Adolescence	4	As with (2) except: Density: 1.1533 − 0.0643.log TSFT, boys 1.1369 − 0.0598.log TSFT, girls
	3	As with (3) above except different nomograms (ages 13–16 yr)

1. Dauncey, Gandy and Gairdner, 1977.
2. Brook, 1971.
3. Ney, 1984.
4. Durnin and Rahaman, 1967.

Table 19.4 %BF with age

Age	%BF M	%BF F	Reference
28 weeks gestation	1	1	Widdowson
Term infant	11	13	Dauncey, Gandy and Gairdner, 1977
Years:			
0.25	24	24	Dauncey *et al.* 1977
0.38	22	22	Dauncey *et al.* 1977
0.77	21	23	Dauncey *et al.* 1977
5.0	17	15	Poskitt and Cole, 1977
10.0	18	16	Rauh and Schumsky, 1968
15.0	11	23	Rauh and Schumsky, 1968

Many mammals have similar but more dramatic deposition of body fat ('puppy fat') after birth (infant seals of different species double their birth weight in times ranging from 4 days to 2 weeks and tissue deposition is largely fat). In late infancy, %BF in humans falls, and by the age of 5 most children are relatively thin. There is then a prepubertal build-up of fat prior to the growth spurt in boys and a continuing deposition of fat in girls around, and after, puberty. There seems a natural tendency of the body to deposit fat prior to periods likely to demand energy: infancy; puberty in boys; the post-puberty possibilities of pregnancy and lactation in girls.

It is not without interest that the prevalence pattern of obesity follows the pattern of fat deposition. Thus when children are depositing fat rapidly, some appear to escape the normal controls on fat deposition and become very obese. When children are slimming naturally much of this excess fat is lost. Most fat infants slim to normal weight children (Poskitt and Cole, 1977). The age at which children begin the gradual increase in %BF prior to puberty (the adiposity rebound) may indicate the likelihood of obesity developing and persisting to adult life. Early adiposity rebound, for example, leads to more persistent obesity (Rolland-Cachera et al., 1984).

Types of obesity

There have been many attempts to classify obesity and to relate epidemiology to different characteristics. None of these methods seems particularly useful or meaningful in childhood and probably the only important differentiation to be made in childhood obesity is to distinguish those children who have a recognizable 'pathological' and sometimes treatable cause for their obesity from those where the cause is so far unrecognized and not requiring specific management other than fat loss therapy ('simple' obesity) (Taitz, 1983).

Table 19.5 lists conditions where obesity is associated with other pathology. Most of these conditions are obvious on clinical examination or readily diagnosed by relatively simple investigations. Cushing's syndrome and growth hormone

Table 19.5 Some recognizable clinical conditions commonly presenting with obesity (pathological obesity)

Congenital:	
Chromosomal	Down's syndrome
	Klinefelter's syndrome
	?Prader-Willi syndrome*
Genetic	Laurence-Moon-Biedl syndrome
	Pseudohypoparathyroidism
	Carpenter's syndrome
	Alstrom's syndrome
Acquired:	
Hypothalamic	Hydrocephalus
	Cerebral trauma: injury, asphyxia, meningitis, neoplasm
	Craniopharyngioma†
Endocrine	Growth hormone deficiency
	Hypothyroidism
	Cushing's disease
	Insulinoma
Drug induced	Steroids
	Valproate
	Excessive insulin in diabetics
Immobility	Spina bifida
	Duchenne muscular dystrophy
Slow growth	Skeletal causes for short stature

* Perhaps 50% of those with Prader-Willi syndrome have abnormalities of chromosome 15; could be classified as hypothalamic obesity.
† These children usually have growth hormone and thyroid deficiency as well as hypothalamic problems.

deficiency may require more complicated investigation, but usually physical signs and – in growth hormone deficiency – marked short stature separate these children out from cases of 'simple' obesity. The features of these syndromes usually cause the children to present to general paediatricians, endocrinologists or mental handicap specialists before there is real concern for obesity. With the exception of Prader-Willi and Laurence-Moon-Biedl syndromes, obesity is rarely gross in these children. The fattest children – with the possible exception of children with these two named syndromes – are those for whom no cause for obesity is recognized. The lack of a recognized cause represents our ignorance of obesity rather than that obesity has no explanation.

Causes of simple obesity

To the layman, obesity is caused by over-eating. Thus must be true for individual needs, yet the evidence that 'simple' obesity is solely a reflection of dietary intake and that obese children eat more than their peers is not impressive (Rolland-Cachera and Bellisle, 1986). Certainly some obese children do eat enormous quantities of food, but many do not. Widdowson (1947) showed that the range of energy intakes for children of the same age was such that at any age some children would be consuming, on average, twice as much energy as other children and yet were not necessarily taller or fatter. Several studies suggest that children today eat less in terms of energy (although admittedly rather different diets) than 20 years ago, and yet are fatter. Many are less active, generally healthier and living in warmer houses.

Children with 'simple' obesity have not only increased fat but also increased lean body mass. Their obesity must arise from an excess of energy intake over energy output at some stage in life. Early deposition of fat secondary to high energy intakes may be followed by a balancing of intake and output yet with maintenance of the excess fat. The obese child or adult would then remain fat but eat normally, thus further confusing the relation of energy intake to obesity. However, growth and changing total fat in childhood suggest that if such a balance developed, the excessive weight of fat in young children would cease to be excessive in older children. Thus it is likely that there are explanations other than the persistence of the effects of earlier excessive intake for obesity in childhood. If the obese do not invariably eat more than the non-obese, it must be assumed that there are differences in energy utilization in obese and non-obese. This may be so, although appropriate explanations have not yet been provided. Familial differences in resting metabolic rate do not correlate well with familial differences in fatness (Bogardus et al., 1986). Various theories of obesity have been developed (adipose cell theory; brown fat theory, etc.) but none is wholly satisfactory. Thus the investigation, management and treatment of obesity remain clinical and empirical.

Environmental risk factors for obesity

Table 19.6 lists recognized risk factors for childhood obesity. Obesity in parents is extremely common. In infancy, correlations between infantile obesity and parental obesity are relatively weak, but the chances of an obese infant becoming an obese child are increased about six times if one or both parents are obese when compared

Table 19.6 Recognized risk factors for childhood obesity

Hereditary factors:
  Certain racial groups: West Indians, Indians, Amerindians, Aboriginals, etc.
  Parental obesity: highly significant after infancy

Socio-economic:
  Low social class
  (upper social class in Third World)

Family dynamics:
  Single child
  Single parent
  Large family

with the risks for obese infants without obese parents (Poskitt and Cole, 1978). Amongst children attending obesity clinics, about 80% have one parent obese and about 30% have both parents obese (Poskitt, 1986).

Parental obesity can be explained on environmental factors assuming that the family all share the same abnormal eating or activity patterns. However, twin and adoption studies (Borjeson, 1976; Stunkard et al., 1986) suggest that there are genetic factors contributing to familial obesity. The lifestyles of young children are very different from those of adults, so genetic predisposing factors seem likely since correlations with parental obesity are strong from early childhood. Some studies even suggest that the children of obese parents who are themselves not yet obese eat less than the children of normal-weight parents, but at the same time have lower energy expenditure (Griffith and Payne, 1976; Poskitt and Cole, 1978; Roberts et al., 1988).

The explanation for the association of obesity with single-child families is not clear unless obesity is regarded as optimal growth occurring undeterred by other factors such as sibling rivalry. Single parenthood is often associated with poverty and thus the explanation for this association may be the same as that for low social class. Little is known about the relation of the quality of food to the development of obesity, but studies suggest that, despite expectations to the opposite, lower social classes in Britain have, on average, higher energy intakes than the upper social classes; but the food eaten is different in quality with possibly higher fat and carbohydrate content. It is our impression that many obese children in Britain have very faddy appetites and eat diets high in carbohydrate and fat, but low in fibre, meat, fruit and vegetables. In developing countries, where standards of living are lower than in Britain, it is the children of upper social class families who develop obesity.

Clinical features of obesity

Children with simple obesity are characteristically well and without pathological disease. Some have mild psychological disturbance with difficulty making friends, reluctance to go out and reluctance to participate in sports. It is difficult to know whether these psychological changes predate the obesity or are consequent upon the obesity. In most cases it seems that the children who suffer significant psychological disturbance are those whose obesity may well have arisen because they are relatively inactive and are reluctant to take part in activities that require mental or physical effort. These children are usually poor dieters despite the fact that they and their families use obesity as an excuse for their lack of involvement in peer group activities.

The majority of children with obesity are remarkably normal in general affect and general healthy. Above-average stature is characteristic of obesity in childhood prior to puberty. The great majority of obese children are above the 50th centile height for age and many are above the 90th centile. Some of these children have advanced linear growth, advanced bone age and early maturity with early pubertal growth spurt and epiphyseal fusion. Thus they tend to achieve only average or relatively short stature in adult life (Lloyd, Wolff and Whelan, 1961). This pattern of growth is not always seen. Some girls who have an early pubertal growth spurt only become obese after their early growth spurt. These girls stop growing at an age when their peers are eating to accommodate rapid growth and maturation and they may follow their peer group's eating habits rather than their own diminishing needs. Early maturation may predispose to – or be associated with – obesity as an adult (Garn *et al.*, 1986).

Estimates of lean body mass in the obese suggest that these children have increased lean body mass compared with normal-weight children of the same height and age. The increase in lean body mass may be secondary to the increased weight and the need to support this weight, but these obese children may be those with a genetic pattern of exuberant growth both in lean and fat tissue. The importance of the raised lean body mass is that even when they have lost their excess fat, these children may have relatively high weight for height.

Complications of obesity

Obese children show few physical problems as a result of their great weight. The commonest problem is genu valgum secondary to fat thighs and weight of the body on the knees. Slipped femoral epiphysis is a more important complication and is particularly likely if the obesity is associated with hormonal abnormality such as hypothyroidism or growth hormone deficiency and delayed maturation of the femoral epiphyses. Intertrigo and skin conditions resulting from fat folds rubbing together are fairly common, although less common than in obese adults. Striae – pinkish or white compared with the thin purple striae of Cushing's syndrome – are also common around buttocks, thighs, lower abdomen and upper arms.

Pickwickian syndrome

The most worrying condition associated with obesity in childhood is the occasional presentation of children with Pickwickian syndrome (named after the fat boy in Charles Dickens' *'The Pickwick Papers'* who was forever falling asleep). In this condition, hypoventilation in association with obesity gives rise to hypercapnia (raised carbon dioxide in the blood) with drowsiness secondary to the hypercapnia. Oxygen deficiency provides the respiratory drive. Ultimately the hypercapnia leads to pulmonary hypertension and cor pulmonale. Pickwickian syndrome is difficult to manage since giving oxygen leads to respiratory depression and further dangerous hypercapnia or exacerbated right-sided heart failure.

Pickwickian syndrome is the only significant emergency in obesity. Diagnosis is made on suggestive history of obesity and excessive somnolence and by finding polycythaemia, hypercapnia, hypoxia and pulmonary hypertension. Children should be admitted to hospital for vigorous weight reduction. Although the condition usually occurs in the severely obese, it is nevertheless very uncommon in childhood (Ward and Kelsey, 1962) and its occurrence is not entirely related to the degree of obesity. It seems that the weight of fat in the chest wall or abdomen inhibits the depth of respiration so hypoventilation results with rapid shallow respiration and consequent poor ventilation and hypoperfusion of the lungs.

Other complications

Children show few of the complications of obesity but, since many obese children become obese adults, obesity in childhood probably predisposes to hypertensive cardiovascular disease, maturity onset diabetes and cerebrovascular accidents in later life. Hypertension in obese children is a relatively unusual finding if efforts are made to measure blood pressure appropriately. Most paediatric sphygmomanometer cuffs are inappropriately small for the obese child's arm. Ideally the width of the cuff should be two-thirds the length of the child's upper arm and the inflatable balloon in the cuff should wrap completely around the arm. In older children this means that the use of an adult leg cuff folded so as not to exceed two-thirds upper arm length is necessary in order to fulfil these requirements. Blood pressure in childhood varies with age and may be more labile than in adult life. A diastolic measurement above 80 mm Hg in any child demands repeating and levels in small children should be less than this.

Hyperlipaemia is rarely a problem in childhood obesity. Relative weight and fatness seem to account for only a small part of the variation in plasma lipid level (Berenson, 1980). Hyperglycaemia and insulin-resistant diabetes are not common in obese children in Britain, although stated to be fairly common amongst the obese children of the United States (Drash, 1973). Many obese children do, however, show hyperinsulinaemia and abnormalities of glucose tolerance even if they have no overt glycosuria (Brook and Lloyd, 1973). *Table 19.7* outlines the investigation of children with suspected complications to their obesity.

Table 19.7 Investigation of simple obesity for possible complications

Bony problems secondary to excessive weight?
    X-ray hips: slipped femoral epiphysis
    Knees: genu valgum

Insulin-resistant diabetes mellitus?
   Urine for glycosuria
   Blood glucose; haemoglobin A1c
   Glucose tolerance test
   Plasma insulin levels

Pickwick syndrome?
    Blood gases: hypercapnia
    Chest X-ray   enlarged heart
    Electrocardiograph: right ventricular hypertrophy

Hypertension
   Chest X-ray for cardiac size
   Blood urea and creatinine
   Urine for proteinuria

In adult women the complications of obesity are particularly associated with those in whom fat is deposited predominantly periabdominally ('apple' or android obesity) rather than those where fat is distributed more generally and particularly deposited in the upper thighs ('pear' or gynaecoid obesity). So far there is no evidence that these differences apply to childhood obesity.

Management of obesity

The treatment of obesity has such a reputation for failure that it has been suggested that there is no point in trying to treat obesity. In childhood, growth is so demanding of nutrition that there are fears that the treatment of obesity will result in slowed growth and loss of lean tissue mass and should therefore be avoided. These arguments are valid, but the misery caused by obesity is such that there should be some attempt to help those who ask for help. Although very rapid weight loss may be associated with slowed growth rates (Brook, Lloyd and Wolff, 1974) this is not true of slower weight loss where the main tissue lost is fat. There are advantages to obese children if some of their overweight is lost, even if restoration to normal weight is not possible. If the obese can move more comfortably, buy fashionable clothes more readily and excite less teasing, weight reduction – even if incomplete – is worthwhile. Reduction in the degree of obesity may be beneficial to later health, but this has not been proven. There is, however, little sense struggling to treat those obese where neither child nor family have any particular interest in slimming. Helping the well-motivated obese is sufficiently difficult to make it undesirable expending effort on those who are not motivated.

The treatment of obesity depends on motivating children (and their families), reducing their energy intake and increasing their energy output. The only practical way of increasing energy output is to increase activity. This alone may be effective in reducing mild degrees of overweight, but it is ineffective by itself in reducing significant obesity. Obese children are often reluctant to make efforts over activity until they have lost some fat and are generally more mobile, at which time they may take a renewed interest in sport and activity. Thus the mainstay of treatment of significant degrees of obesity remains dietary management.

Motivation

Methods of achieving motivation to slim vary widely and always depend strongly on the interest, attitudes and experience of those running the slimming programmes.

Motivation may be achieved through:

1. Clinical history and physical examination to provide reassurance that there is no underlying cause for obesity.
2. Detailed dietary history including likes and dislikes so any dietary discussion can be individually tailored.
3. Explanation of benefits that may accrue from some weight loss.
4. Explanation that 'normal' weight for height may never be established because of either high lean body mass or gross obesity, but that some weight loss would improve comfort, appearance and mobility.
5. Explanation that 'fat loss' does not necessarily involve weight loss if children are growing rapidly and that weight gain will ultimately occur for all growing children even those who are slimming satisfactorily.

6. Provision of strict but realistic diet so that if it is followed fat loss will occur – thus increasing motivation.
7. Frequent follow-up to reiterate dietary advice and reinforce motivation.

Children with obesity deserve initial examination by a doctor with wide clinical experience of paediatrics to exclude pathological causes for the obesity. It is otherwise not necessary for medical involvement in slimming programmes. Those who are involved must understand growth and nutrition of children since there are considerable risks that restrictive diets will limit nutrients to a dangerous level unless careful dietary assessment is made and results are related to the children's needs and unless growth is monitored closely. Fat loss in childhood is not necessarily equivalent to weight loss because of the effect of weight increments associated with growth, so the emphasis of adult slimming clinics on weight loss must be tempered with understanding of body composition changes in childhood.

Diet

Children and their parents should be asked to itemize the children's diets by 24-hour recall and by asking how the previous 24 hours differed from other days. Specific questions concerning the frequency of intake for sweets, crisps, chips, nuts, biscuits, ice cream, 'pop' and sweetened drinks and added sugar, as well as the amount of bread and milk consumed each day, must be asked so that a picture of the children's eating habits can be obtained. Particular 'likes' and 'dislikes' should be recorded. It is then possible to advise on diets where the intake is reduced but, hopefully, the pattern of eating and the family's social life are not disturbed unnecessarily. Since children's energy intakes are so variable, this approach is probably more appropriate than the prescription of specific 'calorie' diets.

Most children eat three substantial meals interspersed with further snacks. Some seem to exist off almost continuous snacking and few cooked meals. Stopping snacks alone may be effective in slimming some obese children, and control of snacking is important since the obese need to learn to have their mouths empty for most of the day. Chewing gum should be avoided. Even in its sugar-free form, it encourages constant chewing and searching for food when there is no more gum available. Snacks usually consist of the so-called 'junk foods' such as sweets, crisps, biscuits, 'pop' – foods with little nutrient quality apart from their relatively high energy content. Removal of these foods reduces energy intakes without affecting intakes of other nutrients significantly. Thus the first dietary recommendation is to avoid all sweets, crisps, chips, sweetened drinks, cakes, biscuits and ice cream. It seems more likely that children who try to diet will keep the intake of these foods low if the instructions are to avoid them altogether. If these foods are excluded from the diet there is no need for these foods to be available. Often the rest of the family are obese, and the excuse that other members of the family must have biscuits to eat should be regarded as evidence of lack of family dedication towards helping the obese child (or themselves). Clearly, if weight reduction is satisfactory when the child returns to the clinic despite an intake of some of these 'forbidden' foods the child should be advised on the importance of keeping intakes of these foods to very low levels, but it is unnecessarily churlish to complain that the diet has not been strictly kept. Alternatively, if the child is not losing weight and still eating these foods this is an obvious area for further advice.

Similarly, all fried foods and added fats (except for very thin scrapings of butter or margarines – preferably low-energy versions – on bread) and all added sugar in drinks and on cereals should be avoided. It is particularly important to stress the need to reduce fat intake since the high energy density of fats and oils is not always recognized.

Bread and potatoes, rice and pasta are other foods which should be regulated in quantity. Children need considerable amounts of energy for growth and these are fairly filling as well as fattening forms of energy. Eaten in excess they will prevent slimming. One helping of boiled, mashed or baked (mashed and baked without added butter) potatoes or one helping of rice or pasta per day is sufficient. Three rounds of bread are sufficient for most children trying to slim although teenage boys who are dieting and also going through their growth spurt may be able to slim very effectively with considerably higher intakes than this. Children who ate fewer than three rounds of bread before dieting may require less bread when dieting although, if their diet is rationalized so they are eating meals rather than snacks, they may require bread where previously they had eaten crisps or cakes or biscuits.

Milk intakes should be no more than 1 pint daily and three-quarters of a pint in post-menarche girls who have little, or no, growth left. Some young obese drink large quantities of milk a day, and this should be controlled. Skimmed milk is lower in energy but lacks vitamins, especially A and D. The use of skimmed milk should only occur with medical supervision in children aged under 5. Vitamins should be provided if there is doubt about the adequacy of vitamin intake.

Table 19.8 outlines the sort of diet that result from the policies outlined. Whilst it is impossible to give particular energy intake recommendations to be followed in all cases of childhood obesity, most children of school age require diets in the region of 4.2–5.0 MJ (1000–1200 kcal) to slim effectively. Younger children may have normal intakes around this level and thus require less, although their increased requirements for growth mean that proportionately smaller reductions in energy intake may be effective in producing fat loss. Adolescent boys undergoing their growth spurt may slim effectively on much higher energy intakes and it is difficult to prescribe specific energy intakes which would be adequate, but slimming, for these boys since their needs for growth are so high for short periods of peak height

Table 19.8 Outline slimming diet

Breakfast:	Glass natural unsweetened orange juice Cereal, milk, no sugar, or toast from ration* Tea or coffee, no sugar
Break:	Apple, milk from ration*
†Dinner:	Meat, vegetables, no potatoes or Salad – no bread, no potatoes Fresh fruit or slimmers' yoghurt
Home:	Cup of tea
Teatime:	Meat and vegetable and boiled potato. 1 piece bread Fresh fruit or (low energy) yoghurt
Bedtime:	Toast/fruit or small helping cereal and milk from ration

* Bread ration : 3 rounds per day.
   Milk   : 1 pint per day.

† *See* text for advice on school dinners.

velocity. If their bread intake seems excessive it should be reduced and similarly excessive milk intakes should be controlled. They should avoid fried foods, added sugar, and 'junk' foods and concentrate their eating to meal times and recognized snack periods with foods of varied nutrient quality.

Many people trying to slim concentrate on reducing their carbohydrate intake. Fats are, however – per unit weight – more fattening and, as butter, lard, oil or margarine, come in concentrated form. Thus guidance on reducing fat intake is probably more important, particularly since children do need carbohydrate energy to support growth and many carbohydrate foods (such as cereals, bread and potatoes) do contribute to the satiety of a diet. Fat-reduced foods and changing cooking methods to reduce fat intake may affect satiety little but greatly reduce energy intake.

School dinners

One of the problems with obese children is that school dinners rarely provide opportunities for the child to choose slimming foods. Liaison with school authorities is important when trying to slim children since a school in which teachers and catering staff are interested in helping obese children can be extremely helpful. Sadly, the practical difficulties of supervising individual children in large schools and the difficulties of adapting school meals to be more appropriate to children's needs mean that children who continue to eat full school dinners rarely succeed in losing noticeable amounts of weight for any length of time. Therefore, if the children stay at school for dinner provision must be made for dieting. There are three main possibilities for school dinner:

1. Salad with cold meat, chicken, hard-boiled egg or cheese (preferably cottage cheese), no salad dressing, no potatoes, no bread. Either no pudding or fresh fruit or low-energy yoghurt.
2. School cooked meal without potatoes or pastry and without pudding. Either fresh fruit or low-energy yoghurt.
3. Packed lunch of 'salad in a box': plastic box with cold meat, hard-boiled egg or lump of cheese. Fresh salad vegetables: lettuce, tomato, celery, raw carrot, cucumber. Low-energy yoghurt or fresh fruit. Low-calorie soup in a flask if desired in cold weather.

Unfortunately, obese children often do not like vegetables and salads. Thus even when suitable foods are available, modification of school dinners may be difficult. 'Packed' lunches of sandwiches, crisps, etc. are frequently as energy rich as full school dinner.

Increasing activity

An activity history should be obtained in much the same detail as dietary history. Usually there are simple measures that can be taken to increase children's activity. Walking to or from school is possible for some, provided they get out of bed sufficiently early to allow time to walk to school. Insecurity on the streets does not always make walking to and from school possible or acceptable to parents, particularly during the winter. Car and bus journeys should be avoided whenever possible and walking encouraged. Children should be encouraged to take part in school sports and to play outside and go for walks in the evenings and at weekends. Interest in hobbies is useful since even if they are not particularly energetic hobbies, they may prevent boredom. Boredom is a common cause of children feeling hungry and taking unnecessary food. Evenings spent watching television should be avoided since this is the sort of circumstance when children may eat almost continuous snacks.

Most children assume a more positive attitude to their own appearance and health and spontaneously become more outgoing and active when they have lost some weight. These are rarely the children who present because obesity is affecting their behaviour, probably because most of these latter children have problems in relating to other children despite, rather than because of, their obesity. If disturbed obese children are prepared to accept psychiatric help this may provide support for dietary therapy, but behavioural and psychiatric management without dietary advice rarely produces significant weight reduction.

Behavioural methods have been used in combination with dietary methods for the management of obesity in children without obvious psychiatric disturbance. Eating can be made a formal procedure so that no eating occurs except in the dining room with the table fully set for a meal. The irony of eating a boiled sweet or a 'Mars' bar with a knife and fork may prevent the more sophisticated obese partaking of these foods at all. Less co-operative children simply break the rules. Behavioural practices are most likely to be followed by those children who have good motivation and are likely to succeed without such behavioural intervention.

Group therapy has also been used in the management of obesity. Again, without an effective dietary regimen, group therapy does not seem to be particularly effective. It is only an adjunct to the management of obesity and to dieting, but does not provide a cure of itself (Court, Johns and Wilson, 1977).

Follow-up

Children are much more likely to stick to diets if they are reviewed soon after the onset of a slimming regimen. Delay in initiating the diet and reluctance to persist with dieting are likely unless children are reviewed within 2 or 3 weeks. Management at follow-up clinic is probably important for further motivation:

1. Frequent regular attendance.
2. At each attendance:
   (a) Dietary recall – for previous 24 hours and more general enquiries.
   (b) Specific questions about non-meal food items, also bread; milk; potato intakes.
   (c) Weight.
   (d) Height.
   (e) Skinfolds.
   (f) Plot weight and height against centiles and explain significance to child and family.
   (g) Reiterate dietary advice. Arrange to review soon.

It is wise to take a dietary history to find out what the child is eating in as much detail as possible before the child knows whether or not he or she has lost weight. Otherwise those children who have not lost weight may be tempted to pretend that they are dieting more strictly than is the case. Feedback is important in that children should be able to see that they are slimming (if this is the case) by showing them their position on the weight and height charts, or by telling them how much weight they have lost or by plotting their percentage expected weight each time they come. It is particularly important to stress that slimming in childhood may occur even if there is no weight loss. This should, however, not be used for false congratulations of those who clearly have not been dieting and consequently have been losing neither weight nor fat. Following the first re-attendance, further follow-up should be arranged according to clinic size, the distance the family have to travel to get to the clinic, how effective the child is at dieting, how much school they are missing in coming to the clinic and other similar factors. On the whole, the more frequently children are seen, the better they stick to the diet.

Most children will lose some weight, but few children stick to a strict enough diet for a long enough period to get their weight down to normal. Many attend irregularly or for short periods only, and it is these children particularly who make management of the obese seem so unsuccessful.

Long-term assessments of treatment for obesity are difficult to achieve and consequently a few studies influence knowledge. It has to be remembered that the children who attend for treatment of obesity are those who are likely, either by disposition or by constitution, to be fairly resistant to slimming since many children probably slip in and out of obesity during childhood without medical interference (Poskitt, 1986). For the same reasons, children most resistant to slimming and staying slim are likely to be those who have been obese longest. Nevertheless, there is no definite evidence that age of onset of obesity is influential in response to dieting although age at adiposity rebound in early childhood may provide some indication (Rolland-Cachera *et al.*, 1984). If obese children can change not only dietary habits but activity levels and also develop interests in sport or other hobbies, the younger, still-growing children may remain slim. To this author, it is always worth trying to slim willing and significantly obese children.

Pathological obesity

In many of the conditions listed in *Table 19.5* obesity is only part of a syndrome of which the other features are more obvious and which present long before obesity is a problem. Distinction of most of these fat children from those with simple obesity is usually not difficult. Many of the obesity-provoking conditions are associated with short stature, mental retardation, or both. Thus it is appropriate that obese children showing these features should be studied carefully for possible underlying recognizable cause for their obesity.

The great majority of simple obese children under 10 years old are above the fiftieth centile height for age. Those with height below the twenty fifth, and particularly below the tenth centiles for age should probably be investigated for hormonal or other pathological cause for their obesity. In our experience, unless there are other suggestive features on clinical examination or clinical history, further investigation is most unlikely to reveal any underlying condition. In other words, it is very rare indeed for a child with pathological obesity to be diagnosed by investigation when the diagnosis has not been obvious from clinical examination.

Table 19.9 outlines possible investigations in the child with suspected underlying condition causing obesity. It is not necessary to do all investigations on every child, and for the reasons outlined above it is appropriate to be very selective with investigations. Most children, if it is suggested that their obesity might be due to a cause other than simple overeating, diet only very reluctantly. Investigations should be carried out as quickly as possible after first attendance and reassurance

Table 19.9 Investigation of children suspected of pathological or complicated cause for obesity

Biochemical:
  Thyroid function tests and thyroid stimulating hormone
  Blood glucose – random and fasting or glucose tolerance test
  Morning and evening cortisol: check normal diurnal rhythm
  Free urinary cortisol
  Post-exercise growth hormone levels: if low proceed to growth hormone release studies

Chromosomes

Radiological:
  Bone age: retarded bone age suggests endocrine abnormality
  Skull X-ray: craniopharyngioma; hydrocephalus?
  Skeletal survey if suspected cause of poor linear growth
  CAT scan if evidence suggests intracranial problem

Urine:
  Glucose
  Protein
  Water deprivation test: urine and plasma osmolality

Other:
  Visual perimetry studies: hypothalamic lesion?
  Retinitis pigmentosa?

and dietary advice provided as soon as results show no other course of action necessary.

Management of obesity in the child with predisposing condition varies with the condition. Where the problem is a treatable endocrine condition, obesity may resolve on modified food intake and hormonal therapy. A typical example is the obesity of hypothyroidism which is usually eminently responsive to thyroxine. Where the basic condition is untreatable and involves either handicap and reduced activity or mental retardation the outlook for successful treatment is not good.

Guy (1978) studied children in a physically handicapped school and found that 30% of those with Duchenne muscular dystrophy and 60% of those with spina bifida were obese. Encouraging activity in these children was almost impossible owing to their physical disabilities. Thus slimming depended on successful dieting. In our experience many of these children have very faddy appetites making it almost impossible to devise diets that are slimming and yet balanced. The physical and (often) mental handicap and the dismal long-term outlook make families and friends reluctant to restrict intakes of sweets, crisps, etc. Dietary compliance by the children is usually poor for the same reasons. Intake has to be restricted quite severely because of the low output in activity. Thus handicapped children are a very difficult group of obese children to treat.

The problems of slimming handicapped children makes it vitally important to prevent obesity in these children. Certain handicapping conditions (e.g. spina bifida, Duchenne muscular dystrophy and Down's syndrome) are very likely to be associated with obesity. Other handicapping conditions such as spastic and choreoathetoid cerebral palsies where the children have to exert great physical effort to move limbs effectively are more likely to be associated with failure to thrive. Parents of children with obesity-prone handicapping conditions should be advised about controlling the children's food intake and watching weight progress closely at the time of diagnosis, so that obesity can be prevented or at worst treated before it is so severe that it is exacerbating the physical handicap. The same applies for children with skeletal causes for short stature although the requirements for growth are a sufficiently small proportion of intake after infancy to make this group less at risk of obesity than those who have severe motor handicap.

Prader-Willi syndrome

Prader-Willi syndrome (PWS) is a condition of unknown aetiology associated with the development of severe intractable obesity after infancy. Clinical diagnosis is not easy in the early years since diagnosis is dependent on clinical features. Micropenis and cryptorchidism may draw attention to the diagnosis in boys. Features in girls are even less specific. Early infancy is often characterized by failure to thrive and feeding difficulty but after infancy weight gain is excessive and appetite may be pathologically large. Some children have partial deletions of chromosome 15 but this is not a consistent finding (Leadbetter et al., 1981). Diagnosis is from the combination of signs which include early hypotonia, mental retardation and obesity, although probably not all children are significantly mentally retarded (Holm, 1981).

Table 19.10 Clinical features of Prader-Willi syndrome

Facies:
  Almond shaped eyes, anti-mongoloid slant
  Narrow forehead
  Triangular upper lip, micrognathia, carp-like mouth
  Squint

Growth and nutrition:
  Failure to thrive in infancy
  Gross obesity developing after 1 year
  Short stature
  Micropenis, cryptorchidism
  Poor pubertal development

Central nervous system:
  Mental retardation (IQ 40–70)
  Hypotonia
  Stubborn affect

Skeletal:
  Scoliosis
  Small hands and feet, tapering fingers, clinodactyly fifth finger
  Genu valgum
  Congenital dislocation of the hips
  Dental decay and enamel defects

Table 19.10 outlines the clinical features of PWS. No distinct anatomical, biochemical or histological abnormality has been demonstrated in this condition although the combination of intellectual deficit, abnormal appetite and weight control and gonadal developmental problems suggests the condition is a disorder of hypothalamic function. These children do appear to have very low energy requirements for their age and length; and unless energy intakes are severely restricted, weight control will fail. Holm and Pipes (1976) estimate that children with PWS require only 7–8 kcal (28–33 kJ) per cm height for weight control and continued linear growth. Unfortunately it is usually difficult to maintain such an intake throughout childhood and into the years of adolescence when a poor pubertal growth spurt exacerbates the short stature and low food requirements for age. Stubborn personalities, deceit over food intake and stealing food, hamper successful weight control and precipitate disturbing family battles.

The outcome for PWS is dismal (Laurence, Brito and Wilkinson, 1981). Many of these children become grossly obese and very inactive. Few are employable and most live at home or require sheltered accommodation. Death from cor pulmonale secondary to Pickwickian syndrome is common. Insulin-resistant diabetes mellitus is also fairly common and adds to the difficulties these children face.

The classical cases of PWS have distinctive features including mental retardation. Some grossly obese children show the hypotonia, tapering fingers and carp-like facies of PWS without low intelligence or sometimes without short stature. As with so many conditions where diagnosis is purely clinical, it is difficult to know whether these are 'formes frustes' of PWS or totally different conditions.

Laurence-Moon-Biedl syndrome (LMB)

This condition has many similarities with PWS (*Table 19.11*) but usually follows an autosomal recessive inheritance and includes the specific features of diabetes insipidus and retinitis pigmentosa. The easily recognizable feature of polydactyly is

Table 19.11 Clinical features of Laurence-Moon-Biedl syndrome

The classical pentad:
  Obesity – from first year onwards
  Mental retardation
  Polydactyly or syndactyly
  Retinitis pigmentosa
  Gonadal hypoplasia

Associated features:
  Short stature
  Diabetes insipidus
  Renal abnormalities
  Congenital heart disease
  Bony abnormalities

only present in about two-thirds of those with this condition. Incomplete forms of LMB are quite common. Early diagnosis may therefore be difficult even in the presence of a known family history. There have been attempts to subdivide the condition into separate entities according to the systems involved. Subdivision of LMB contributes neither to understanding of the condition nor to management. As with PWS the condition is very difficult to treat. The development of visual handicap in these children only increases the sadness with which the condition is regarded and tends to make it even more difficult to get co-operation from family and friends with dieting. Diabetes insipidus usually develops in adolescence and presents a further complication for children who are already severely handicapped.

Anorexia nervosa

Anorexia is often considered along with obesity as a disorder of appetite regulation. This superficial resemblance and the fact that both conditions tend to be most problematic in adolescent girls are virtually the only similarities or even connections between the two conditions. Nutrition is important in the management of anorexia but attempts to provide appropriate nutrition are liable to be thwarted by the psychological and behavioural problems inherent in the disease process.

Classically, anorexia nervosa is a disease of adolescent girls manifest by pernicious failure to eat, sometimes heavily disguised under a superficial pleasure in food, cooking and apparently eating; severe wasting; amenorrhoea; hirsutes; and restlessness out of proportion to the degree of wasting. Thyrotoxicosis must be excluded since that may also present with weight loss, restlessness and sometimes anorexia and vomiting. In anorexia nervosa pulse rates tend to be slow and the periphery is cool in comparison with the hyperdynamic circulation and warm vasodilated periphery of thyrotoxicosis.

It is sometimes difficult distinguishing early cases of anorexia nervosa from girls with dieting fads which are not pathological. How much the former arises from obsession with the latter is difficult to know but the modern prevalence of anorexia has been blamed on cultural views that slim is beautiful and on widespread interest in dieting and slimming. The American Psychiatric Association criteria for diagnosis of anorexia are:

1. Refusal to maintain minimal normal body weight.
2. Over 25% loss of pre-illness body weight.
3. Disturbance of body image (describing previous state as fat when normal, and current wasted state as average or normal).
4. Intense fear of obesity.
5. No other condition to account for these features.

To these could be added disordered eating patterns since anorexics are either wilful, successful dieters and exercise enthusiasts or they indulge in bulimia which is gorging followed by vomiting and purging to overcome the effect of gorging. Bulimics are liable to fluid and electrolyte inbalance consequent upon these habits. They may also suffer specific nutritional deficiencies as a result of bizarre gorging habits. Anorexics tend to have a generally balanced diet which is deficient in total energy particularly from fat.

Some bulimics are normal weight and, although psychologically disturbed, have less severe personality disorder than bulimic anorexics. Nevertheless, chronic vomiting leads to nutritional disturbances, water and electrolyte loss. There is also the risk of choking over vomit, particularly if gorging has resulted in food being swallowed improperly chewed. Dental erosions may occur due to frequent vomiting.

Management of anorexia nervosa is important since perhaps 10% of these individuals die of malnutrition or overwhelming infection whilst severely malnourished. Others commit suicide. Management consists of admission to hospital with behavioural and psychological management to persuade affected individuals to eat, together with the provision of a nutrient-dense diet so that, although the quantity consumed may be low, the quality of the diet is optimal.

Effective treatment of anorexics is urgent. These individuals are often on the verge of death before they can be persuaded to enter hospital. If the patient is unwilling to eat under supervision there are two alternatives: nasogastric feeding or parenteral nutrition. Some co-operation is required for both these forms of management since self-manipulation of the intravenous line may result in serious complications. Tube feeding uncooperative but weak and wasted individuals runs major risks of aspiration of food and death. Individuals with more than 40% bodyweight loss will probably require nasogastric or intravenous alimentation.

Initially, the aim of dietary management should be to provide energy and nutrients to meet basal requirements for actual weight and then increase energy intake gradually as diet is accepted. The energy density of foods rather than their protein content is important. Vitamin and mineral supplements must be provided (Ketovite liquid and tablets, Paines & Byrne; Metabolic Mineral Mixture, Scientific Hospital Supplies).

Water and electrolyte imbalances must be corrected urgently in the severely wasted anorexic. For the nasogastrically or intravenously fed patients the aim should be to provide energy and protein for height and age rather than weight so as to encourage weight gain since their clinical state is perilous. A number of 'complete' fluid diets are available commercially (*Table 19.12*) and liquidized meals can be enhanced by the use of fat or glucose polymer preparations (*see* Chapter 15). Most commercial preparations are made up to solutions of approximately 4.2 kJ/ml (1 kcal/ml) although some (*Table 19.12*) have higher carbohydrate and fat and consequently higher total energy.

Table 19.12 Some liquid feeds suitable for older children*

Approximately 420 kJ (100 kcal)/100 ml feed:
  Clinifeed range (Roussel)
  Ensure (Abbott)
  Fortisip Standard (Cow & Gate)
  Fortison Standard (Cow & Gate)
  Isocal (Mead Johnson)
  Nutrauxil (KabiVitrum)

Approximately 630 kJ (150 kcal)/100 ml feed:
  Ensure Plus (Abbott)
  Fortisip Energy Plus (Cow & Gate)
  Fortison Energy Plus (Cow & Gate)

*These preparations should not be treated as complete feeds. Extra vitamins and minerals may be necessary. Best used as nutritional supplements to ordinary diet.

Sadly, perhaps, in view of their distorted body image, anorexics tend to deposit fat more readily during recovery than other previously starved individuals. Yet it is difficult to believe that these adolescents are basically obesity-prone individuals who have slimmed successfully. Indeed they seem the very opposite. Obese adolescent girls who restrict their diets conscientiously frequently lose weight despairingly slowly. Their metabolism seems totally different from that of their excessively successful (at slimming) anorexic peers.

References

BERENSON, G. S. (1980) *Cardiovascular Risk Factors in Children.* New York: Oxford University Press
BOGARDUS, C., LILLIOJA, S., RAVUSSEN, E., et al. (1986) Familial dependence of the resting metabolic rate. *New England Journal of Medicine,* **315,** 96–100

BORJESON, M. (1976) The aetiology of obesity in children. A study of 101 twin pairs. *Acta Paediatrica Scandinavica*, **65**, 279–287

BROOK, C. G. D. (1971) Determination of body composition of children from skinfold measurements. *Archives of Disease in Childhood*, **46**, 182–184

BROOK, C. G. D. and LLOYD, J. K. (1973) Adipose cell size and glucose tolerance in obese children. *Archives of Disease in Childhood*, **48**, 301–304

BROOK, C. G. D., LLOYD, J. K. and WOLFF, O. H. (1974) Rapid weight loss in children. *British Medical Journal*, **ii**, 44–45

CAMERON, M. (1984) *The Measurement of Human Growth*. Bristol: Croom Helm

COLE, T. J. (1979) A method for assessing age-standardised weight for height in children seen cross sectionally. *Annals of Human Biology*, **6**, 249–268

COURT, J. M., JOHNS, M. and WILSON, M. (1977) Obese children and their families: a study of a discussion group. *Australian Paediatric Journal*, **13**, 170–175

DAUNCEY, M. J., GANDY, G. and GAIRDNER, D. (1977) Assessment of total body fat in infancy from skinfold thickness measurements. *Archives of Disease in Childhood*, **52**, 223–227

DRASH, A. (1973) Relationship between diabetes mellitus and obesity in the child. *Metabolism*, **22**, 337–344

DURNIN, J. G. V. A. and RAHAMAN, M. M. (1967) The assessment of the amount of fat in the human body from measurements of skinfold thickness. *British Journal of Nutrition*, **21**, 681–689

GARN, S. M., LAVELLE, M., ROSENBERG, K. R. and HAWTHORNE, V. M. (1986) Maturational timing as a factor in female fatness and obesity. *American Journal of Clinical Nutrition*, **43**, 879–883

GARROW, J. S. (1971) *Energy Balance and Obesity in Man*. Amsterdam: North-Holland

GRIFFITH, M. and PAYNE, P. R. (1976) Energy expenditure of small children of obese and non-obese parents. *Nature*, **260**, 698–700

GUY, R. (1978) The growth of physically handicapped children with emphasis on appetite and activity. *Public Health (London)*, **92**, 145–154

HAGER, A. (1981) Estimation of body fat in infants, children and adolescents. In *Adipose Tissue in Childhood*, edited by F. P. Bonnet, pp. 49–56. Boca Raton, Florida: CRC Press

HOLM, V. A. (1981) The diagnosis of Prader-Willi syndrome. In *The Prader-Willi Syndrome*, edited by V. A. Holm, S. Sulzbacher and P. L. Pipes, pp. 27–36. Baltimore: University Park Press

HOLM, V. A. and PIPES, P. L. (1976) Food and children with Prader-Willi syndrome. *American Journal of Diseases of Children*, **130**, 1063–1067

LAURENCE, B. M., BRITO, A. and WILKINSON, J. (1981) Prader-Willi syndrome after 15 years. *Archives of Disease in Childhood*, **56**, 181–186

LEADBETTER, D. H., RICCARDI, V. M., AIRHART, S. D., STROBEL, R. J., KEENAN, B. S. and CRAWFORD, J. D. (1981) Detection of chromosome 15 as a cause of Prader-Willi syndrome. *New England Journal of Medicine*, **304**, 325–329

LLOYD, J. K., WOLFF, O. H. and WHELAN, W. S. (1961) Childhood obesity – a long term study of height and weight. *British Medical Journal*, **ii**, 145–148

NEY, D. (1984) Nutritional assessment. In *Manual of Pediatric Nutrition*, edited by D. G. Kelts and E. G. Jones, pp. 99–124. Boston: Little Brown

POSKITT, E. M. E. (1975) Defining malnutrition in the young child. *Lancet*, **ii**, 343

POSKITT, E. M. E. (1986) Obesity in the young child: whither and whence? *Acta Paediatrica Scandinavica*, **Suppl. 323**, 24–32

POSKITT, E. M. E. and COLE, T. J. (1977) Do fat babies stay fat? *British Medical Journal*, **i**, 7–9

POSKITT, E. M. E. and COLE, T. J. (1978) Nature, nurture and childhood overweight. *British Medical Journal*, **i**, 603–605

RAUH, J. L. and SCHUMSKY, D. A. (1968) Lean and non-lean body mass estimates in urban schoolchildren. In *Human Growth*, edited by D. B. Cheek, pp. 242–252. Philadelphia: Lea and Febiger

ROBERTS, S. B., SAWAGE, J., COWARD, W. A. et al. (1988) Energy expenditure and intake in infants born to lean and overweight mothers. *New England Journal of Medicine*, **318**, 461–466

ROLLAND-CACHERA, M-F., DEHEEGER, M., BELLISLE, F., SEMPE, M., GOUILLARD-BATAILLE, M. and PATOIS, E. (1984) Adiposity rebound in children: a simple indicator for predicting obesity. *American Journal of Clinical Nutrition*, **39**, 129–135

ROLLAND-CACHERA, M-F. and BELLISLE, F. (1986) No correlation between adiposity and food intake: why are working class children fatter? *American Journal of Clinical Nutrition,* **44,** 779–787

STUNKARD, A., SORENSEN, T. I. A., HANIS, C. *et al.* (1986) An adoption study of human obesity. *New England Journal of Medicine,* **314,** 193–198

TAITZ, L. S. (1983) *The Obese Child.* Oxford: Blackwell Scientific

WARD, W. A. and KELSEY, W. M. (1962) The Pickwickian syndrome. *Journal of Pediatrics,* **61,** 745–750

WIDDOWSON, E. M. (1947) A study of individual children's diets. *Medical Research Council Special Reports Series,* No. 257. London: Her Majesty's Stationery Office

WIDDOWSON, E. M. (1971) Changes in body composition with growth. In *Scientific Foundations of Paediatrics,* edited by J. A. Davis and J. Dobbing, pp. 153–164. London: William Heinemann

WORLD HEALTH ORGANISATION (1983) *Measuring Change in Nutritional Status.* Geneva: World Health Organisation

Chapter 20
Adolescence

It may seem unnecessary to treat adolescence separately from the rest of childhood. Several of the conditions discussed in earlier chapters (diabetes, obesity, anorexia, Crohn's disease) are problems more typical of adolescents than of infants or young children. But apart from being a period of transition from the pattern of disease typical of childhood to the pattern of disease of adult life, adolescence presents nutritional problems related to the rapid growth rates and turbulent emotions and lifestyle of this age group. Nutrition is liable to be strained not by disease but, as in infancy, by the high nutrient requirements of growth and physical development.

Nutrient requirements in adolescence are uncertain. As with the adolescent growth spurt, mean values for age can be assessed and 'smoothed' values presented. For individual adolescents, however, growth and nutrient requirements change much more rapidly and more sharply than suggested by these average curves. Requirements are strongly related to growth rates, and the age at which peak height velocity occurs varies from about 12½ to 16 years in boys and 10½ to 14½ years in girls (Marshall and Tanner, 1974).

In girls the most rapid period of adolescent growth is early in pubertal development. Peak height velocity has passed when menarche occurs. In boys the growth spurt is more prolonged, takes place later in puberty and is nutritionally more demanding. In girls early growth is lean tissue and there may be slight slimming but the main body compositional changes at puberty are deposition of fat. In boys there is a tremendous increase in lean tissue with not only lowering in the percentage of body weight as fat, but often actual reduction in total fat to meet the demands of growth.

Table 20.1 outlines recommended daily intakes of energy for adolescents derived from several national and international recommendations. There is a wide range of uncertainty in recommendations particularly at the ages of expected peak height velocity. As at other ages there is also wide inter-individual variation.

In her study of children's diets in the 1930s, Widdowson (1947) found that the peak average daily calorie intake for boys occurred at the age of 15 and was 3440 kcal (14.4 mJ)/day but the range of daily intakes at that age was from 2457 kcal (10.3 mJ) to 5395 kcal (22.7 mJ). In girls peak average daily calorie intake was a year earlier at 14 and daily intakes at that age ranged from 1901 kcal (8.0 mJ) to 3617 kcal (15 mJ), although the wider range (1706–3736 kcal/day; 7.2–15.7 mJ/day) actually occurred at 13 years. These figures serve to illustrate how varied the adolescent diet may be in a single quantitative aspect of nutrition. It is easy to see how varied it may be in quality as well. Unfortunately, Widdowson (1947) could

Table 20.1 Range of recommended mean energy intakes in adolescence*

Age years	Boys MJ	Boys kcal	Girls MJ	Girls kcal
10–12	9.6–11.3	2280–2700	8.6–9.9	2050–2350
13–15	11.1–12.1	2640–2900	8.8–10.5	2100–2490
16–19	12.1–12.9	2880–3070	8.8–9.7	2100–2300

Ranges developed from FAO/WHO; Food and Nutrition Board, USA; and Department of Health and Social Security, UK (Lentner, 1981).

not relate her peak energy intake values to the timing of peak height velocity in these children since the study was cross-sectional.

Appetite in adolescence is usually capable of meeting the nutrient needs for growth when food is available, but taste and selection do not always encourage needs to be met. Peer group activities, publicity on the importance of being slim and determination to show independence by avoiding eating with the family, all contribute to poor quality diets and low intakes of some nutrients in adolescence. Truswell and Darnton-Hill (1981) have listed the specific dietary habits of adolescence outlined below.

Missing meals
Breakfast and lunch are the meals most likely to be missed. Children eating breakfast consume, on average, 20% total energy at this meal and are more likely to meet recommended dietary requirements than those not eating breakfast. The numbers of children skipping meals varies widely in different societies but meal-skipping seems less common in the higher socio-economic groups (Cresswell et al., 1983).

Snacking
Snacking is common at all ages in childhood but the relative financial and social independence of adolescents compared with younger children enables them to snack more liberally. Although snacks have a reputation for being 'junk' foods of no nutritional value other than as a source of energy, this reputation is not wholly justified (Thomas and Cull, 1973). Packed school lunches may even have higher nutrient content than the school dinners (Nelson and Paul, 1983). Adolescent snacks vary widely and may include substantial meals of pies, cereal and milk, milk, chips, nuts, toast, as well as the more familiar sweets, crisps and 'pop'. Many have a very high sugar content. Sixty three per cent (74.8 g/day) of all the sugar intake in one study of English adolescents was taken in snacks (Rugg-Guna et al., 1986). Snack foods will probably be low in vitamin A, iron and calcium except that some adolescents consume large volumes of milk and thus maintain high calcium intakes. Many schools in Britain provide school meals that are quite expensive yet unattractive. It is common for children to snack from food available in local shops or the school snack-bar at lunchtime.

High consumption of 'fast foods'
Many of the criticisms of these foods may be more aesthetic than nutritional. Foods available at 'fast food' stores are very variable. If a beefburger, chips and milk are

consumed, for example, the nutrient density of the meal may be adequate for nutrients other than vitamin A. Chips and a soft drink would be much less satisfactory. Concern over the food available in these shops relates more to the excesses in the foods on offer than their deficiencies. If (*see* Chapter 21) high consumptions of saturated fats, salt, refined sugars and little fibre are undesirable, 'fast foods' fail badly in quality. The energy density of these foods and their lack of satiety are also likely to encourage over-eating and obesity.

Unconventional meals
Conforming with family habits and traditional practices is not the adolescent style. Meals may be huge, eccentric in timing, eccentric in composition – often as adolescents experiment with their own culinary abilities – and new foods may be tried simply because they have been advertised on the television and 'everyone' is eating them. As with toddlers, favourite foods may not be favourite for long and something exciting one week is 'boring' the next.

Alcohol and cigarette use
Most children begin to try alcohol in their teens. This in itself is not necessarily undesirable since those who later have difficulty controlling their intakes are significantly more likely to be either those who have been prevented from drinking because of strong parental pressure and therefore drink in parental defiance, or those who have drunk from early childhood and may even have alcoholic parents. The association of beginning to drink and taking up driving and motor cycling is a matter of great concern. Accident statistics show that death and injury due to road accidents is high in young drivers and motor cyclists and has a very strong association with previous indulgence in alcohol. Whilst cigarettes hardly count as food, the introduction of smoking at this, or even pre-adolescent, age is another health problem which in the long term has even less to recommend it than alcohol consumption. Advice on the risks of smoking must be incorporated with general preventive health education (*see* Chapter 21). Smoking affects nutrition and encourages low weight for height both by reducing appetite and increasing metabolic rate (Hofstetter *et al.*, 1986).

High consumption of soft drinks
In her study of children's diets in the 1930s, Widdowson (1947) commented that the greatest change in the diets of children over the previous 200 years had been in the beverages they drank. In the eighteenth century the staple drink of children was 'small beer' whereas in the 1930s it was tea. In her survey, Widdowson found that 10% of children drank some lemonade and 2% drank other soft drinks. In a study of 5-year-old children in Dudley in the mid-1970s we found that, on any one day, approximately 65% of the children had drunk some fruit squash and about 25% had drunk some aerated drinks (unpublished observations).

In adolescence, canned drinks are consumed – almost certainly – much more frequently. Canned drinks deserve the term 'empty' calories more than other foods since they contain sugar, saccharine, rarely vitamin C, but no other nutrients of significance. Cola drinks contain caffeine. Truswell and Darnton-Hill (1981) suggest canned drinks should be regarded as 'fun' foods. There are, however, some concerning aspects to high soft-drink consumption:

1. Many are cariogenic.
2. They may satisfy appetite without providing nutrients other than energy and thus may discourage an adequate diet.

3. Children may spend their 'dinner money' on these, rather than on foods.
4. Some canned drinks contain food colourants which have been associated with IgE-mediated-like reactions.

Other unusual adolescent dietary patterns revolve around the erratic nature of the adolescent diet. Intakes may be very high one day and very low the next. Preferred foods are often eaten in very large quantities, especially if they are sweets, biscuits, bread or milk. In Britain, intakes of iron followed by intakes of thiamine and riboflavin are the most likely to be less than recommended (Bull, 1985). In the United States, vitamin A, riboflavin, thiamine, calcium and iron intakes are likely to be inadequate. Vitamin D intake may be low but can be replaced by adequate sunlight.

The tendency for some teenagers to diet unnecessarily is also a problem (*see* Chapter 19) and can lead to significantly inadequate energy intakes. Most diets are concerned with 'improving the figure' either because the individual is, or because the individual imagines herself, fat. Occasionally the diets are followed to reduce acne or to improve athletic performance. Teenage is also a time of strong beliefs and emotions. A number of adolescents adopt vegetarian diets from concern about animal welfare or environmental issues. Without dieting advice, they may adopt very incomplete diets which avoid animal products but do not substitute good quality vegetable protein mixes instead. These children need dietary guidance rather than being forced to eat meat.

Despite all the adverse dietary habits described, it is unusual for adolescents in Britain to show evidence of dietary deficiency other than obesity and, in post-menarcheal girls, iron deficiency. In the United States, deficiencies of riboflavin, iron, calcium, thiamine and vitamin A have been demonstrated (Thomas and Cull, 1973). And it is of course impossible to determine whether adolescents have suffered diminution in their growth spurt and thus limited their adult height because of nutrient inadequacy during their growth spurt. The taller stature and earlier age at menarche of girls in the Western world have been attributed to improved nutrition, although many other public health aspects may have been equally important – for example, reduction in atmospheric pollution due to the Clean Air Act, so that vitamin D nutrition is less impaired. Trends to greater height and earlier menarche with succeeding generations seem to have slowed (Dann and Roberts, 1973) although they are probably still demonstrable amongst the less advantaged sections of society in Britain. If the nutrition of children was as 'bad' as media coverage sometimes appears to suggest, we might expect to see a reduction in adult stature and delay of age at menarche again.

In Britain the adolescent groups most at risk of nutritional deficiency are the children of immigrant families, particularly those from the Indian subcontinent who are liable to vitamin D deficiency, rickets and iron deficiency; vegetarian groups, particularly those of Caribbean extraction who adopt the strict vegetarianism of Rastafarian followers; and those pregnant.

Adolescent pregnancy

Whilst it could be argued that the adolescent who becomes pregnant at a young age is still growing and thus the process of pubertal growth is disturbed by having pregnancy thrust upon it, girls have to reach a certain stage of pubertal development and physical maturity before they can become pregnant. It is not the chronological but their 'gynaecological' age that determines whether they can become pregnant. Although the onset of menarche may seem to indicate gynaecological maturity, most girls have anovular cycles for months or years postmenarche and will not become pregnant until some time later. Peak height velocity has occurred by the time menarche is reached and thus linear growth is unlikely to be noticeably curtailed. Pregnant teenagers do not increase in height whilst pregnant. Whether the less mature ones begin to grow again after delivery is not known, but this seems unlikely. The high oestrogen levels of pregnancy will cause epiphyseal fusion and inhibit further growth.

Weight increments are still high in the first years postmenarche and the effect of pregnancy and lactation on the acquisition of pubertal fat in girls who become pregnant in early postmenarche years is unknown. Studies from Peru, where nutritional problems are common and girls' nutrition is likely to be suboptimal, suggest that for the same intrapregnancy weight gain, young teenage mothers have lower birthweight infants than older teenage mothers (Frisancho et al., 1985). In the immature mothers weight gain during pregnancy may be a combination of gain due to the pregnancy and the fetus and gain occurring as part of normal adolescent fat deposition. If this is so, the fetus is likely to receive a lower proportion of available nutrition than the fetus in a woman who has stabilized weight and height post adolescence.

The young pregnant teenager is also more likely to be deficient in iron and folate owing to recent demands of pubertal growth. Whilst these girls do not require special diets or therapy, they should be given extra encouragement to eat a varied and adequate diet. Weight gain and nutritional status during pregnancy deserve special attention (Rees and Worthington-Roberts, 1984).

Sporting activity in adolescence

Some adolescents are notorious for their inactivity and idleness. Others are remarkable for their physical fitness and high levels of activity. Even inactive teenagers may have periods of lazing interspersed by periods of tremendous activity in disco dancing or formal sports.

Sport is often taken seriously for the first time in the teenage years. Training becomes a formal process. Significant increases in activity brought about by training programmes and vigorous sporting programmes demand increased nutrient intakes. Some training programmes put great emphasis on special diets. However, the important demands of activity are for greater amounts of *all* nutrients (McArdle, Katch and Katch, 1981). Energy is of great importance. Protein in excess of normal needs does not build up body protein. Body protein is built up by activity and muscle use. It is wasteful to take protein in excess of the general increase in dietary intake with vigorous activity, since the protein will be converted to energy and the waste nitrogen products demand increased fluid intakes for excretion, not necessarily desirable in prolonged activity where sweat fluid loss is high. Diets should therefore follow intakes at other ages or in less active teenagers with 50–55% total energy as carbohydrate, 30–35% as fat and 10–15% as protein. Vitamin supplements are unnecessary but iron nutrition is important. Deficiency of iron leads to low haemoglobin and impaired performance. But, particularly in long-distance running and jogging, low-grade anaemia due to iron deficiency may develop possibly secondary to low-grade haematuria associated with these sports.

Fluid intakes prior to sport are important. Fluid losses due to sweating in vigorous activity are high. Salt intake – contrary perhaps to traditional practices of feeding salt prior to activity – is relatively less important since sweat is always slightly hypotonic and sodium loss proportionally less than water loss. During sustained activity fluid loss should be replaced with dextrose–saline solution since this is well absorbed and provides salt and an energy source as well as fluid.

In brief activity, such as sprinting, muscle glycogen stores are the main source of energy. In more sustained activity, carbohydrate stores – muscle glycogen – are important initially but as activity is sustained fatty acid metabolism provides a higher proportion of the energy and may be providing 80% of the energy towards the end of sustained activity. Various programmes of diet and exercise have been devised to try to build up muscle glycogen stores and thus increase the amount of glycogen readily available for prolonged activity. These programmes are not advisable in childhood. They are associated with fluid retention and may cause muscles to seem stiff and rigid initially. Chest pain, ECG abnormalities and myoglobinuria have all been reported in relation to their use. These seem undesirable. In adolescent athletes, carbohydrate-loading programmes must be used only on advice from a doctor experienced in managing athletes.

Nutrition education

The most important aspect of nutrition in adolescence may be that at this time children are breaking away from parental habits and experimenting with eating. Habits that continue into adult life may be acquired. It is important, therefore, that adolescents are provided with information on looking after themselves in adult life and on nutrition for healthy living. Nowadays, through publicity and the media, there is plenty of opportunity for adolescents to derive nutritional advice from unqualified or unscrupulous people. The onus is therefore on those who can assess and present nutritional knowledge backed by scientific evidence, to point out what is known, what is uncertain but advisable, and what is without substance in nutrition, so that adolescents have a chance of developing good eating practices in adult life (Moody, 1982; Wheeler, 1982). Hopefully, they will then pass good dietary practices on to their own children.

References

BULL, M. L. (1985) Dietary habits of 15 to 25 year olds. *Human Nutrition: Applied Nutrition*, **39A**, Suppl. 1, 1–68

CRESSWELL, J., BUSHBY, A., YOUNG, H. and INGLIS, V. (1983) Dietary patterns of third year secondary schoolgirls in Glasgow. *Human Nutrition: Applied Nutrition*, **37A**, 301–306

DANN, T. C. and ROBERTS, D. F. (1973) End of the trend? A 12-year study of age at menarche. *British Medical Journal*, **ii**, 265–267

FRISANCHO, A. R., MATOS, J., LEONARD, W. R. and YAROCH, L. A. (1985) Developmental and nutritional determinants of pregnancy outcome among teenagers. *American Journal of Physical Anthropology*, **66**, 247–261

HOFSTETTER, A., SCHUTZ, Y., JEQUIER, E. and WAHREN, J. (1986) Increased 24 hour energy expenditure in cigarette smokers. *New England Journal of Medicine*, **314**, 79–82

LENTNER, C. (1981) Geigy Scientific Tables, Volume I. *Units of Measurement, Body Fluids, Composition of the Body, Nutrition*, pp. 232, 234. Basle: Ciba-Geigy

McARDLE, W. D., KATCH, F. I. and KATCH, V. L. (1981) *Exercise Physiology: Energy, Nutrition and Human Performance*. Philadelphia: Lea & Febiger

MARSHALL, W. A. and TANNER, J. M. (1974) Puberty. In *Scientific Foundations of Pediatrics*, edited by J. A. Davis and J. Dobbing, pp. 124–151. London: William Heinemann Medical Books

MOODY, R. (1982) Priorities for nutrition education in the secondary school. *Human Nutrition: Applied Nutrition*, **36A**, 18–21

NELSON, M. and PAUL, A. A. (1983) The nutritive contribution of school dinners and other midday meals to the diets of schoolchildren. *Human Nutrition: Applied Nutrition*, **37A**, 128–135

REES, J. M. and WORTHINGTON-ROBERTS, B. (1984) Adolescence, Nutrition and Pregnancy: Interrelationships. In *Nutrition in Adolescence*, edited by L. K. Mahan and J. M. Rees, pp. 221–256. St Louis: Times Mirror: Mosby

RUGG-GUNA, A. J., HACKETT, A. F., APPLETON, D. R. and MOYNIHAN, P. J. (1986) The dietary intake of added and natural sugars in 405 English adolescents. *Human Nutrition: Applied Nutrition*, **40A**, 115–124

THOMAS, J. A. and CULL, D. I. (1973) Eating between meals – a nutrition problem among teenagers? *Nutrition Reviews*, **31**, 137–139

TRUSWELL, A. S. and DARNTON-HILL, I. (1981) Food habits of adolescents. *Nutrition Reviews*, **39**, 73–88

WHEELER, E. F. (1982) Teaching nutrition in schools: Can real data be used? *Human Nutrition: Applied Nutrition*, **36A**, 11–17

WIDDOWSON, E. M. (1947) *A Study of Individual Children's Diets*. Medical Research Council Special Report Series No. 257. London: HMSO

Chapter 21
Children's nutrition and later health

The importance of nutrition in childhood for health in later life is a topic that has aroused considerable interest and argument over the past 15–20 years. The depth of interest and the data that arouse the interest are new, but the concept that the way a child is fed has long-term consequences is not new. In Europe and North America in the past (and in many traditional societies today) early feeding has been considered a determinant of later character as much as of later growth and health. Such considerations were not always well substantiated although widely accepted. Thus, feeding eggs made children thieves and wet nurses transmitted their personalities to the children they suckled through their milk (Fildes, 1986). Current beliefs on the relation of childhood diet to later health and development may seem more scientific but are – at present – equally unsubstantiated by hard clinical evidence.

Some long-term complications of childhood nutrition that can be substantiated are well understood. Rickets may be responsible for long-term bony, particularly pelvic, deformity. Energy deficiency may lead to small size and poor physical ability in adult life. But can diets of nutritional *adequacy* contain long-term risks? This is one of the dietary questions that most concern epidemiologists, nutritionists and primary health care specialists today.

Virtually all that we know about dietary excess in childhood leading to health problems in adult life is circumstantial evidence derived from population studies and unsubstantiated by individual correlations. Parameters of nutrition in adult life can be correlated with risks for morbidity and mortality. Childhood is implicated by association. Thus, populations adopting Western high-fat, refined carbohydrate, low-fibre diets show increased prevalence of obesity, hypertension, coronary heart disease, diabetes mellitus, large bowel cancer and several other problems. Is the seed for these problems planted in childhood? We do not know.

Controversy continues to rage over the risks a particular dietary habit may present, even in adult life. Correlations between certain intakes and particular diseases are possible when comparing populations, but calculation of the risks for individuals will probably never be possible. Genetic and non-nutritional environmental factors affecting individuals are risk factors as well.

Obesity

This is perhaps the most obvious situation which provides a health risk and which may be present, and preventable, in childhood. 'Sudden death is more common in those who are naturally fat than in the lean' (Hippocrates: Lloyd, 1978). There has been debate over whether mortality rates are lower in individuals at ideal body weight or slightly above ideal body weight (van Itallie and Abraham, 1985) but the grossly obese are unnaturally liable to sudden and early death. How much obesity *per se* contributes to early death and how much is contributed by frequently associated conditions such as hypertension and diabetes is not clear. However, since obesity exacerbates these conditions this is a rather spurious argument (Taitz, 1983).

The relationship between nutritional state in childhood and adult life is definite in obesity. One-third of obese adults were obese in childhood (Mullins, 1958). Although this study is quite old and the actual proportions may have changed, the basic conclusion is not questioned. Studies showing that obesity, even in childhood, is rarely cured are also old (Lloyd, Wolff and Whelan, 1961; Abrahams, Collins and Nordsieck, 1971).

Those of us treating childhood obesity readily admit that the children who *present* for advice and help for their obesity tend to stay fat. This may not mean that those slipping into obesity at some point in childhood are inevitably going to stay fat. Less intractable obesity may resolve spontaneously or with little effort and never be referred for medical advice (Poskitt, 1986).

Obesity should be preventable in childhood. There is, however, no convincing evidence that childhood obesity has been prevented successfully by controlled, long-term projects. Prevention could be effected by advising all the population to eat less and to worry about their weight. Alternatively, the population could be screened and only 'at risk' children advised on weight reduction. The rise in incidence of anorexia nervosa in teenage girls has been attributed to excessive exposure to slimming advice. Thus, intervention policies directed at the overweight may be safer than those directed at the whole population. Obesity is nevertheless so prevalent that all children (and adults) should practise lifestyles that encourage maintenance of normal weight.

Children should be screened for overweight and obesity when seen by doctors or community health workers at home, the surgery or in school clinics. Unless overweight is gross, when therapeutic rather than preventive advice is indicated, we would suggest the following general advice as a weight control programme.

1. Encourage activity through:
   (a) Walking rather than taking cars, buses, elevators.
   (b) Participating in field sports, swimming, jogging, especially in 'out of school' hours.
   (c) Developing outdoor hobbies.
2. Modify intake by:
   (a) Avoiding fried foods and sugar and fats added to foods (except for modest amounts of margarine on bread).
   (b) Confining eating to recognized meals and snack periods.
   (c) Increasing 'whole food' content of diet to improve satiety.

Whether such policies will be effective in preventing obesity is not known. They have the potential for inducing anxiety and even anorexia in many who are not obese; but they reflect an organized, disciplined lifestyle which may actually induce a healthier mental outlook as well through positive self-help. That is speculation!

In adults, weight reduction of the overweight has been associated with reduced incidence of coronary thrombosis. Hopefully, weight control in childhood will have a similar effect in later life.

Hypertension

Blood pressure rises with age through childhood and adult life. It also increases with increasing weight for height. In adult life, obesity and hypertension commonly occur together. We find hypertension rarely in the adolescent obese we see.

The combination of obesity with hypertension greatly contributes to morbidity and mortality. The increased cardiovascular stress caused by left ventricular wall thickening and concentric decrease in left ventricular diameter in adults with obesity highlights this (Messerli, Sundgaard-Riise and Reisin, 1983). Weight reduction in adults is helpful in lowering blood pressure and in improving the cardiovascular changes described in adults (MacMahon, Wilcken and MacDonald, 1986). Whilst weight reduction may be helpful in controlling hypertension in obese adolescents, Abraham, Collins and Nordsieck (1971) found that the normal and underweight children who later became obese were the adults with most severe hypertension.

Other aspects of Western diets besides obesity correlate with hypertension. Studies of different populations show correlations between levels of sodium intake and prevalence of hypertension (Dahl and Love, 1954). These conditions are not upheld by relating individual sodium intake to blood pressure (Laver et al., 1976). Nevertheless, lowering the sodium intakes of many hypertensive individuals produces falls in mean blood pressure. It is argued that some people are genetically susceptible to sodium and respond to moderately high sodium intakes with hypertension. Thus it has been recommended that where national diets are moderately high in sodium the intake of sodium should be reduced and potassium and calcium intakes increased. (Potassium and calcium intakes seem to relate inversely to the prevalence of sodium-influenced hypertension.)

The high-sodium diet of unmodified cows' milk formula and salt-rich weaning foods in the early 1970s was a disaster to many infants because of the hypernatraemia it caused. No epidemic of hypertension as a result of feeding high-salt weaning diets has been recognized, and it seems unlikely to develop. Nevertheless, there is no indication to add sodium to weaning foods or to children's diets. Avoiding added sodium may encourage reduction of hypertension in the genetically (?) susceptible population. The relevance of this policy is debatable but it would seem to us that, even if the case is not proven, in normal climates healthy children are unlikely to suffer from restriction of added salt on their foods.

Atherosclerosis and coronary heart disease

This is a controversial area for dietary intervention particularly in relation to any action which should be taken in childhood (Ahrens, 1985; Glueck, 1986; Committee on Nutrition, 1986). The adoption of Western diets is associated with a rise in the mean serum cholesterol of a population. Individuals with familial hypercholesterolaemia have greatly increased risk of morbidity and mortality from coronary thrombosis and atherosclerosis related problems. Fatty streaks can be demonstrated in the great vessels of normal children and young adults brought up on Western type high animal fat diets but the actual relationship of these fatty streaks to thrombotic complications later is questioned (Holme, Enger and Helgeland, 1981). Postmortem studies on young people in the United States (a large population study looking for hypertension and atherosclerotic-related disease epidemiological factors) found the extent of aortic and coronary artery fatty streaks related to antemortem levels of total cholesterol and low density lipoprotein (LDL) cholesterol (Newman et al., 1986). These findings fit in with current views that it is the levels of LDL cholesterol in the blood that present a risk for atherosclerosis and that levels of high density lipoprotein (HDL) cholesterol have relative protective effects (Miller et al., 1977).

What part does diet play in determining cholesterol levels and fractionation of cholesterol? In population studies LDL cholesterol levels in the blood are related to intake of saturated fats and inversely to the ratio of polyunsaturated to saturated fatty acids (James, 1982). The body produces cholesterol endogenously, and lowering dietary cholesterol in these and in other individuals with hypercholesterolaemia has only a modest effect on circulating cholesterol levels. By contrast, the Expert Committee of the World Health Organisation recommend that dietary energy derived from saturated fatty acids should be less than 10% of total energy and energy from all fat should be no more than 30% total energy (Health Education Council, 1984). To accommodate these changes, increased carbohydrate intakes will be necessary but these should be of fibre-rich complex carbohydrates since simple sugars contribute energy with little satiety and thus encourage obesity.

These are recommendations for adults. What should be recommended for children? If there is a strong family history of coronary heart disease and atherosclerosis the child's – and the rest of the family's – lipids should be measured. Those with LDL cholesterol on or above the 90th centile for age and with a bad family history should be given every encouragement to follow the dietary recommendations above. Cholesterol-lowering resins should be considered as well (see Chapter 13). There is no indication in the COMA Report (Committee on Medical Aspects of Food Policy, 1984) of when dietary modification should begin. However, if parents are following these dietary recommendations, this is likely to influence the way the children are fed. Thus, perhaps, recommendations should be that the children participate in the adult diet to the extent of consuming less saturated fat and eating more unrefined carbohydrates. The consumption of lowish fat and high unrefined carbohydrate diets may present problems to weanlings by making it difficult for the child to obtain adequate energy. Strict adherence to the regimen above is not indicated for young children without cardiovascular risk factors. Any restrictive dietary policy needs to be pursued with care in the very young.

United States recommendations have suggested that coronary prevention measures should begin at 2 years of age. The recommendations have been questioned by the American Academy of Pediatrics (AAP) Committee on Nutrition (1986). They suggest that restricted diets in the first two decades of life should be avoided. Children should receive good quality mixed diets with 30–40% total energy per day from fat to provide sufficient energy for growth and development. It is pointed out by the AAP that all the reports on coronary prevention discuss recommended measures that are theoretical, and there is no convincing evidence that they protect against coronary artery disease, particularly when they are begun in childhood.

In Britain, recommendations for young children are fewer. Breast feeding is advised. The addition of salt and sugar to weaning foods is not recommended. But skimmed milk – an easy way of lowering fat intake by food substitution – is NOT recommended for children aged under 5 without medical supervision. It may encourage deficiency of fat-soluble vitamins and inadequate energy intakes. Where families are using *semi*-skimmed milk, this may be introduced into the diets of children over 2 years provided the diet as a whole is inadequate (DHSS, 1988).

The trials of diet in coronary prevention continue. We all await further evidence.

Gastroenterological problems

The adoption of a Western diet and lifestyle appears to be associated with increased problems from constipation, appendicitis, diverticulitis, haemorrhoids and, more catastrophically, large-bowel cancers. Burkitt and Trowell (1975) demonstrated differences in transit time and faecal weight between African and British schoolchildren with, on average, much greater stool weights and shorter transit time in African children. This correlated with differences in fibre intake of the diets. There was enormous individual variation in stool output in both groups of children. The differences in faecal weight between different populations is now recognized as related to differences in intake of cereal fibre.

Fibre covers a wide range of poorly digested complex plant carbohydrates–polysaccharides and lignins. Digestion of fibre by bacteria in the large intestine promotes growth of bacteria there. Short-chain fatty acids are produced but rapidly absorbed. Thus the effects of fibre seem to be a combination of increased bacterial bulk and of water retention in the gut lumen by trapping within the cellular structure of undigested fibre (Stephen and Cummings, 1979). This latter effect is prominent with bran which is a relatively poorly digested fibre (James, 1982).

Plant foods vary in their fibre content and in the laxative effect of the fibre they contain. Bowel function is affected more by bran and other cereal fibres and less by vegetable and fruit fibres. This makes the consumption of breakfast cereals and wholemeal bread relevant to bowel function in children.

Constipation may be relieved by high-density fibre intake and this may indirectly reduce diverticulitis and haemorrhoids in adult life. The connections between diet and appendicitis and diet and colonic cancer prevalence are more difficult to explain. The former provided the point of interest which stimulated some of Burkitt's studies (Burkitt and Trowell, 1975) but remains unexplained (Royal College of Physicians, 1980). The latter may be related to bile acid and protein metabolism in the large bowel. Reduction of the time contents stay in the large bowel may reduce the opportunity for production of potential carcinogens (James, 1982).

Are there any other advantages in high fibre intakes? The relation of the fibre content of the diet to blood sugar control in diabetes has been discussed in Chapter 18. Whether lowered fibre intake makes diabetes more likely to develop in those genetically at risk is only speculation. We do not know why diabetes has increased prevalence with Westernization although the high intakes of refined sugars and starches are often blamed.

Fibre, in some cases, reduces bile acid reabsorption and may lower serum cholesterol concentration and influence atherosclerosis. But fibre also has disadvantages. It may affect absorption of nutrients in the small intestine. Increased extraction of the flour in Ireland during World War Two appeared responsible for increased prevalence of rickets in young weaned children (Robertson et al., 1981). Poor absorption of vitamin D or of calcium or phosphate may have resulted from increased binding of these nutrients in the gut. High fibre intake from traditional flour may contribute to the prevalence of rickets amongst Asians in this country. Trace nutrient absorption may also be affected by binding to cereal fibre.

What dietary recommendations can be made for children to encourage later health?

The recommendations that can be made with some certainty of influencing health are those that are not specifically nutritional. All health education programmes should include education on avoiding or stopping smoking. Heavy alcohol intake should be discouraged, not only because of its long-term direct effects of health (which are significant) but because of its relation to accidents and social and domestic stability. Other general advice should encourage weight control and fitness by activity continuing at moderate levels throughout life.

Beyond these general statements it is difficult to itemize recommendations for the normal healthy child population. It seems reasonable to encourage diets that are varied in taste, texture and nutrient content since acceptance of varied foods is more likely to meet adequacy for all nutrients and less likely to include excessive intakes of any food. A child who is not fussy about diet is much easier to feed – a point of importance in family life.

We cannot demonstrate that the following will actually improve adult health and longevity but they would seem safe and reasonable dietary practices which take into account current anxiety about our Western diet:

1. Avoid adding salt to foods at table. If salt is used in cooking use it sparingly.
2. Avoid adding sugar to drinks and to other foods where this is not essential to the recipe.
3. Aim to eat whole foods wherever possible: fresh fruit, fresh vegetables, wholemeal breads.
4. Avoid unnecessary addition of fat in cooking. Grill rather than fry. Use predominantly polyunsaturated margarines and oils for cooking and on bread.
5. Eat breakfast of cereal with milk but no added sugar, or of wholemeal bread (toast).
6. Organize meals so that children eat at meal times and recognized snack periods. Avoid constant chewing and eating.
7. Provide snacks of wholefoods – fresh fruit, wholemeal bread sandwiches – rather than low satiety 'junk' foods.
8. Include fish and poultry amongst meats to reduce saturated fat and cholesterol intake.

To many, these measures will be little different from the policies of healthy eating they have always pursued. On a nation-wide scale, sudden adoption of even the modest recommendations outlined above could have dramatic effects on food manufacturing firms, farmers and retailers (James, 1980). It is easy to conceive the effects of a massive drop in butter sales, for example. Any nutritional advice felt to be wise for the nation to follow must be backed up by availability of suitable foods at acceptable prices; by provision of these foods at school meals; and by school and public health education programmes that promote the same policies. Otherwise the policies will fail. Educational guidance and financial support to initiate the changes may be necessary for farmers, manufacturers, schools, retailers and health workers as well as for the general public. Such changes will take time and money. Hence perhaps the hesitation of governmental bodies to adopt and support nutritional programmes which have no guarantee of success?

References

ABRAHAM, S., COLLINS, G. and NORDSIECK, M. (1971) Relationship of childhood weight status to morbidity in adults. *Public Health Reports*, **86**, 273-284

AHRENS, E. H. (1985) The diet-heart question in 1985. Has it really been settled? *Lancet*, **i**, 1085-1087

BURKITT, D. P. and TROWELL, H. C. (1975) *Refined Carbohydrates, Food and Disease*. London: Academic Press

COMMITTEE ON MEDICAL ASPECTS OF FOOD POLICY (1984) *Diet and Cardiovascular Disease*. Department of Health and Social Security. Report on Health and Social Subjects No. 28. London: HMSO

COMMITTEE ON NUTRITION (1986) Prudent life style for children: dietary fat and cholesterol. *Pediatrics*, **78**, 521-525

DAHL, L. K. and LOVE, R. A. (1954) Evidence for a relationship between sodium (chloride) intake and human essential hypertension. *Archives of Internal Medicine*, **94**, 525-531

DEPARTMENT OF HEALTH AND SOCIAL SECURITY (1988) *Present Day Practice in Infant Feeding: Third Report*. Report on Health and Social Subjects, No. 32. London: Her Majesty's Stationery Office

FILDES, V. A. (1986) *Breasts, Bottles and Babies*, p. 30. Edinburgh: Edinburgh University Press

GLUECK, C. J. (1986) Pediatric primary prevention of atherosclerosis. *New England Journal of Medicine*, **314**, 175-177

HEALTH EDUCATION COUNCIL (1984) *Coronary Heart Disease Prevention. Plans for Action*, p. 59. London: Pitman Publishing

HOLME, I., ENGER, S. C. and HELGELAND, A. (1981) Risk factors and raised atherosclerotic lesions in coronary and cerebral arteries: statistical analysis from the Oslo Study. *Arteriosclerosis*, **1**, 250-256

JAMES, W. P. T. (1980) Towards implementing a good food and nutrition policy in Britain. *Postgraduate Medical Journal*, **56**, 597-603

JAMES, W. P. T. (1982) Diseases of Western civilisation. *Textbook of Paediatric Nutrition*, 2nd edn., edited by D. S. McLaren and D. Burman, pp. 413-435

LAVER, R. M., FILER, L. J., REITER, M. A. and CLARKE, W. R. (1976) Blood pressure, salt preference, salt threshold and relative weight. *American Journal of Diseases in Childhood*, **130**, 493-497

LLOYD, G. E. R. (1978) *Hippocratic Writings*, p. 212. Harmondsworth: Penguin Books

LLOYD, J. K., WOLFF, O. H. and WHELAN, W. S. (1961) Childhood obesity: A long term study of height and weight. *British Medical Journal*, **ii**, 145-148

MacMAHON, S. W., WILCKEN, D. E. L. and MacDONALD, G. J. (1986) The effect of weight reduction on left ventricular mass. *New England Journal of Medicine*, **314**, 334-338

MESSERLI, F. H., SUNDGAARD-RIISE, K. and REISIN, E. D. (1983) Dimorphic cardiac adaptation to obesity and arterial hypertension. *Annals of Internal Medicine*, **99**, 757-761

MILLER, M. E., TAELLE, D. S., FORDE, O. H. and MJOS, O. D. (1977) The Tromso heart study. *Lancet*, **i**, 965-970

MULLINS, A. G. (1958) The prognosis in juvenile obesity. *Archives of Disease in Childhood*, **33**, 307-314

NEWMAN, W. P., FREEDMAN, D. S., VOORS, A. W. et al. (1986) Relation of serum lipoprotein levels and systolic blood pressure to early atherosclerosis. *New England Journal of Medicine*, **314**, 138-144

POSKITT, E. M. E. (1986) Obesity in the young child: Whither and whence? *Acta Paediatrica Scandinavica*, **Suppl. 323**, 24-32

ROBERTSON, I., FORD, J. A., McINTOSH, W. B. and DUNNIGAN, M. G. (1981) The role of cereals in the aetiology of nutritional rickets: lesson of the Irish National Nutritional Survey 1943-8. *British Journal of Nutrition*, **45**, 17-22

ROYAL COLLEGE OF PHYSICIANS (1980) *Medical Aspects of Dietary Fibre*. Tunbridge Wells: Pitman Medical

STEPHEN, A. M. and CUMMINGS, J. H. (1979) Water holding by dietary fibre in vitro and its relationship to faecal output in man. *Gut*, **20**, 722-729

TAITZ, L. S. (1983) *The Obese Child*, p. 182. Oxford: Blackwell Scientific

VAN ITALLIE, T. B. and ABRAHAM, S. (1985) Some hazards of obesity and its treatment. *Recent Advances in Obesity Research, IV*, edited by J. Hirsch and T. B. Van Itallie, pp. 1-19. London: John Libbey

Appendix

Addresses of British organizations that act as sources of information, research and support for professionals and/or families, with some of the conditions described. Addresses are listed according to the alphabetical order of the relevant conditions.

National Childbirth Trust,
9 Queensborough Terrace,
London W23 3TB
(Interested in breast feeding promotion amongst other activities.)

Coeliac Society,
PO Box 220,
High Wycombe,
Bucks HP11 2HY

National Association for Colitis and Crohn's Disease,
3 Thorpefield Close,
Marshalswick,
St Albans, Herts

Cystic Fibrosis Research Trust,
Alexandra House,
5 Blyth Road,
Bromley,
Kent BR1 3RS

British Diabetic Association,
10 Queen Anne Street,
London W1M OBD

Child Growth Foundation,
2 Mayfield Avenue,
London W4 1PW

Association for Children with Heart Disorders,
20 Chadwell Springs,
Cottingley,
Bingley,
Yorkshire BD16 1QE

Infantile Hypercalcaemia Foundation,
37 Mulberry Green,
Old Harlow,
Essex CM17 0EY

Research Trust for Metabolic Disease in Children,
9 Arnold Street,
Nantwich,
Cheshire CW5 5QB
(A useful group for information on many inborn errors of metabolism.)

Association for the Study of Obesity,
50 Ruby Road,
Walthamstow,
London E17 4RF
(For professionals working with obesity.)

National Society for Phenylketonuria and Allied Disorders,
26 Towngate Grove,
Mirfield,
Yorkshire

British Nutrition Foundation,
15 Belgrave Square,
London SW1X 8PS

The Nutrition Society,
Grosvenor Gardens House,
35–37 Grosvenor Gardens,
London SW1W 0BS
(For professionals working in the nutrition field.)

Prader-Willi Association,
30 Folletts Drive,
Abbots Langley,
Herts WDF 0LD

Xerophthalmia Club,
c/o Dr D. S. McLaren,
Department of Medicine,
The Royal Infirmary,
Edinburgh EH3 9YW

Index

Abetalipoproteinaemia, 208
   see also Hyperlipidaemia
Acrodermatitis enteropathica, 120, 207–208
Additives, intolerance to, 188–190
   and hyperactivity, 189–190
Adolescence, 275–281
   activity, sporting, 279–280
   diabetes in, problems of, 246
   dietary habits, 275–278
      and alcohol/cigarettes, 277
   education, nutritional, 280
   growth demands, 275
   pregnancy in, 278–279
Adult health and early nutrition, 282–288
   atherosclerosis/coronary heart disease, 284–285
   dietary recommendations, 287
   gastroenterological problems, 286
   hypertension, 284
   obesity, 282–283
Alactasia, 194
Albumin, *see* Hypoalbuminaemia in intravenous feeding
Alcohol and adolescents, 277
Alcoholism and maternal folate deficiency, 17
Allergy, 186–187
   to foreign proteins in weaning, 75
   cow milk protein, 195–197
   see also Intolerance, food
Allopurinol for hyperuricaemia, 180
Alphacalcidol for rickets, 149–150
   and immobilization, 150–151
Ameloblastic activity
   intrauterine, 161
   post-natal, 162
Amino-acids
   in formula feeds, 43
   in milk, human, 30
   in parenteral nutrition, 222
Anaemia
   cows' milk feeding, 48
   and folic acid deficiency, 138
   in infants, low birth-weight, 67–68
   and intravenous feeding, 227–228

Anaemia (*cont.*)
   iron deficiency
      clinical, 117–120
      and coeliac disease, 199
      and cows' milk feeding, 48
   in malnutrition, 107–108
   pyridoxine-dependent, 137
   and renal failure, 237
Anorexia
   and failure to thrive, 84
   and infection, 87
   nervosa, 271–272
   in renal failure, chronic, 233
Anthropometry, 6–9
   interpretation, 8–9
   in malnutrition classification, 96–97
   obesity measurement, 254–255
      skinfold thickness, 255
   techniques, 7
Antibiotics, after gastrointestinal resection, 213
Apnoea, infant, and enteral feeding, 56
Arginase deficiency, 179
Asthma, and food intolerance, 187
Atherosclerosis, 182
   and diet, 284–285

Beri-beri, 133–134
   congenital, 15
Bile, *see* Cirrhosis, biliary, in cystic fibrosis
   see under Cholestyramine
Bilirubin, *see* Hyperbilirubinaemia and breast milk jaundice
Biopsy, jejunal, for coeliac disease, 199
Blood
   testing in diabetes, 249–250
   transfusion, and iron overload, 119–120
Bonding and breast feeding, 31
Bone disease
   and copper deficiency, 123
   in infants, low birth-weight, 64–65
   in jaundice, cholestatic, 207
   osteomalacia, maternal, and fetal development, 16
   see also Rickets; Rickets, nutritional

Index

Bottle feeding, 41–50
  and infection risk, 158
  'nursing bottle' syndrome and caries, 164
  and weaning, late, 158
Bowel disease, chronic inflammatory, 209–212
  colitis, ulcerative, 211–212
  Crohn's disease, 209–211
    elemental diets, 210–211
    elimination diets, 211
    high-energy diets, 210
    nutritional problems, 210
Brain
  growth/development
    and iodine, 17
    and malnutrition, 12–13
  function, and deprivation, 13
  see also Mental development
Breast feeding, 24–40
  advantages, 26–31
    bonding, 31
    composition, vs cows' milk, 28–31
    infection protection, 27–28
  and atopic history, 187
  disadvantages, 31–36
    drug transmission, 34–35
    failure to thrive, 32–33
    infection transmission, 35–36
    intake measurement, 31–32
    jaundice, 34
    vitamin K deficiency, 34
  encouragement of, 38–39
  establishing, 26
  history, 24
  infant growth, 37
  and milk banking, 36–37
  with oral rehydration therapy, 192–193
  physiology, 24–25
    oxytocin, 25
    prolactin and milk output, 24–25
  practical problems and advice, 25–26
  prolonged, 37–38
  socio-economic factors in, 24
  water supplementation, 33
  see also Bottle feeding; Formula feeding; Infants, low-birthweight

Cadmium, 128
Calcium in intravenous feeding, 223–224
  see also Hypercalcaemia and vitamin D; Hypocalcaemia
Carbohydrates
  in diabetic diet, 241–243
  in formula feeds, 43
  in intravenous feeding, 221
Cardiac problems, see Heart
Caries, dental, 162–163
  and fluorine, 127–128, 164–165
  and heart disease, congenital and neurological handicap, 91
  and 'nursing bottle' syndrome, 164
  Carnitine deficiency

Caries, dental (cont.)
  in infants, low birth-weight, 65
  and intravenous feeding, 227
Casein and cows' milk feeding, 46
Catecholamines, and failure to thrive, 93
Cerebral palsy, spastic, and failure to thrive, 90–91
  see also Brain
Cholecalciferol, 142–143, 148–149
Cholestatic jaundice, chronic, 206–207
Cholesterol, and atherosclerosis/coronary thrombosis, 284–285
  see also Hypercholesterolaemia, familial
Cholestyramine, 182–183
  for bile acid binding, 213
Chromium deficiency, 125–126
Cirrhosis, biliary, in cystic fibrosis, 205
Coeliac disease, 198–200
  diagnosis, 199
  and failure to thrive, 84–85
  management, 200
  presentation, 198–199
Colitis, ulcerative, 211–212
Collagen, and vitamin C deficiency, 140–141
Colostrum
  composition, 28–29
  immunoglobulin in, 28
Constipation, 215–216, 286
Convulsions and pyridoxine deficiency, 136
Copper
  accumulation, fetal, 121
  deficiency, 121–124
    in infants, low birth-weight, 66
    and iron metabolism, 122
    stores, 121
    symptoms/signs, 122–123
    treatment, 124
  formula feed supplementation, 122
  intake/absorption, 122
Coronary heart disease
  diet recommendations, 284–285
  and hyperlipidaemia, 182
Cows' milk
  for infants, 45–48
  in emergency, 45
  protein intolerance, 195–197
    allergy, 187
    presentation, 196
    recovery, 197
Cretinism and thyroid deficiency, 17, 127
Crohn's disease, 209–211
  elemental diets, 210–211
  elimination diets, 211
  high-energy diets, 210
  nutritional problems, 210
  parenteral nutrition, total, 211
  and vitamin B_{12} deficiency, 139
Cyclosporin A, and transplant catch-up growth, 238
Cystic fibrosis, 200–205
  diabetes in, 205

Cystic fibrosis (*cont.*)
  diagnosis, 201
  and failure to thrive, 84
  management, 201–202
  nutritional problems, 203–205
    elemental diets, 205
    hyponatraemia, 204
    meconium ileus, 204
  prognosis, 202, 205
Cytomegalovirus, and breast milk, 35

Dehydration
  hypertonic, and cows' milk feeding, 47
  and phototherapy, neonatal, 33
Deprivation, psychosocial
  and development, 13
  and failure to thrive, 91–95
    clinical features, 92
    and environment, 94
    hormones in, 93
    management, 93
  see also Socio-economic factors
Development
  body composition, 4–5
  and diet, 4
  ear, inner, and iodine, 17
  and iron deficiency, 118–119
  and thiamine deficiency, 15
  see also Mental development
Diabetes, 239–253
  adolescence, problems in, 246
  brittle diabetes, 247
  complications, long-term, 251–252
  in cystic fibrosis, 205
  diet
    carbohydrate, 241–243
    fat, 244
    protein, 244
  and failure to thrive, 85
  hypoglycaemia management, 247–248
  infancy, problems in, 245–246
  ketoacidosis management, 248–249
  management
    advice, 244
    complications, 239
    dietary restraint, 240
    insulin maintenance, 240, 244–245
  Mauriac syndrome, 251
  monitoring, 249–250
  and obesity management, 250–251
  Somogyi effect, 251
Dialysis
  protein loss in, 236
  for renal failure, acute, 231
  for urea-cycle defects, 178–179
Diarrhoea
  acute, 191–193
  and failure to thrive, 88–89
  and nutrient absorption, 89
  toddler, 215

Diets
  adequacy, 11
  of adolescents, 275–278
  and coronary heart disease, 284–285
  and development changes, 4
  diabetic, 241–244
  eccentric, excessive vitamins, 158–159
  elemental
    for Crohn's disease, 210–211
    for cystic fibrosis, 205
  elimination, 187–188
    for Crohn's disease, 211
  Feingold, 189
  and gut resection malabsorption, 213–215
  high-energy, 210
  and obesity management, 263–265
  recommendations
    daily amounts, 1–3
    for adult health, 287
  and rickets, racial factors in, 148
  vegetarian, 153–157
    lactovegetarianism, 155–156
    macrobotic, Zen, 156–157
    problems, general, 154–155
    racial minorities in Britain, 157–158
    vegans, 156
  for weaning, from local foods, 110–111
Disaccharide intolerance, 193–195
Double-blind food challenge procedure, 185–186
Down's syndrome, and obesity, 268–269
Drug transmission in breast milk, 34–35
Dwarfism, diabetic, 251

Ear, inner, development, and iodine, 17
Eczema, atopic
  and elimination diets, 188
  and food intolerance, 187
'Elemental diets', in Crohn's disease, 210–211
Elimination diets, 187–188
  in Crohn's disease, 211
  and eczema, 188
Enamel hypoplasia
  intra-uterine, 161
  post-natal, 162
Encephalopathy, Wernicke's, 134
Enteral feeding
  of infants, low-birthweight, 52–59
    complications, 56–57
    mother's milk *vs* formula for, 57–59, 60
    nasogastric, 53–54
    orogastric, 54
    procedure, 55–56
    transpyloric, 54–55
  after parenteral feeding, 228
Enterocolitis, necrotizing, and enteral feeding, 56–57
Ethics in marketing formula feed, 44–45
Eyes and vitamin A deficiency, 132

Failure to thrive, 80–95
  and age, 81
  and breast feeding, 32–33
  and coeliac disease, 84–85
  definition, 80
  and deprivation, psychosocial, 91–95
  and diabetes, 85
  diagnosis, clinical, 80–81, 82
  and diarrhoea, 88–89
  failure to utilize, 85–86
  and heart disease, congenital, 89–90
  increased requirements, 86–87
  in infants, low birth-weight, 69
  and infection, 87–88
  intake inadequacy, 83–84
    parental management, 84
  losses, increased, 85
  malabsorption, 84
  and neurological handicap, 90–91
Famine and fetal development, 18
'Fast foods', 276–277
Fat
  in diabetic diet, 244
  in intravenous feeding, 222
  malabsorption, in jaundice, cholestatic, 206
  in milk, human, 29–30
  see also Hyperlipidaemia; Obesity
Fatty acids
  essential, deficiency
    in infants, low birth-weight, 66
    in intravenous feeding, 226–227
  in formula infant feeds, 43
Feingold diet, 189
Ferritin, 115
Fetus and maternal nutrition, 15–23
  energy intake, 18–19
  growth retardation, 20–22
    placental insufficiency, 21–22
  mineral deficiencies, 17–18
  protein, 19
  vitamins, 19–20
    deficiencies, 15–17
Fibre, 286
Fluorine
  deficiency, 126–127, 127–128
  and dental caries, 164–165
Folate/folic acid deficiency, 137–138
  and fetal development, 16–17
  in infants, low birth-weight, 68
  in malnutrition, 107–108
Formula feeding, 41–50
  'follow-on' formulas, 49
  composition
    modern formulas, 42
    vs human milk, 41
    taurine, 43
    vitamin E, 43
  copper supplementation, 122
  cows' milk formulas, 45–48
    and dehydration, hypertonic, 47
    emergency use, 45

Formula feeding (cont.)
  cows' milk formulas (cont.)
    and hypocalcaemia, 46–47
    and inspissated curd syndrome, 46
    and iron deficiency anaemia, 48
    and vitamin deficiencies, 47–48
  development, recent, 43–44
  goats' milk, 46
  intake requirements, 44
  lactose-free, 194–195
  for low birth-weight, 58–59
  making up, 44
  for malnutrition, 106–107
  marketing, 44–45
  soya based formulas, 48–49
  sucrose/fructose free, 171
  see also Bottle feeding
Fructose intolerance, 171

Galactosaemia, 168–170
  classical, 168–170
  galactokinase deficiency, 170
Gastrointestinal disorders, 191–217
  adult, and early nutrition, 286
  bowel disease, chronic inflammatory, 209–212
    colitis, ulcerative, 211–212
  constipation, 215–216
  cows' milk protein intolerance, 195–197
    allergy, 187
    presentation, 196
    recovery, 197
  diarrhoea
    acute, and oral dehydration, 191–193
    and failure to thrive, 88–89
    and nutrient absorption, 89
    toddler, 215
  disaccharide intolerance, 193–195
    diagnosis, 194
  malabsorption after resection, 212–215
    dietary management, 213–215
  malabsorption syndromes, 197–207
    abetalipoproteinaemia, 208
    acrodermatitis enteropathica, 207–208
    coeliac disease, 84–85, 198–200
    cystic fibrosis, 84, 200–205
    jaundice, chronic cholestatic, 206–207
    lymphangectasia, intestinal, 208–209
  see also Crohn's disease; resection, gastrointestinal, malabsorption after
Genetics, see also Inborn errors of metabolism
Genu vulgum in obesity, 260
Giardia infestation, and failure to thrive, 85
Glucose
  in intravenous feeding, 221
  metabolism, and chromium, 125
  tolerance factor, 125–126
Gluten intolerance and weaning, 75
  see also Coeliac disease
Glycaemia control in infant diabetes, 246
  see also Hyperglycaemia, postprandial, in diabetes; Somogyi effect in diabetes

Glycaemic index, 243
Glycogen storage
　and activity in adolescence, 280
　disorders, 180–181
　　corn starch, uncooked, therapy, 181
　　nocturnal intragastric feeding, 180–181
　in neonates and low birth-weight, 52
Goats' milk for infant feeding, 46
Goitre, 126–127
Growth
　of adolescents, 275
　and age, 4
　brain
　　and iodine, 17
　　and malnutrition, 12–13
　catch-up
　　and low birth-weight, 69–70
　　after transplantation, 238
　cellular, multiplication/growth phases, 12
　of infants
　　and breast feeding, 37
　　and weaning, 73–74
　retardation, and maternal nutrition, 20–22
　and zinc deficiency, 120–121
　see also Development; Failure to thrive

Haematology in nutritional status assessment, 10
Haemoglobin levels in iron deficiency, 117
Handicap, physical, and obesity, 268–269
Heart disease
　coronary
　　diet recommendations, 284–285
　　and hyperlipidaemia, 182
　congenital, and failure to thrive, 89–90
　and dental caries, 91
　failure, and thiamine deficiency, 133–134
　see also Keshan disease
Hepatitis transmission to infants, 35
HIV transmission in breast milk, 35–36
Hormones
　in breast feeding, 24–25
　and failure to thrive, psychosocial effects in, 93
Hyperactivity and additive avoidance, 189–190
Hyperbilirubinaemia and breast milk jaundice, 34
　see also Phototherapy, neonatal, and water loss
Hypercalcaemia and vitamin D, 150
　and immobilization, 150–151
　in Williams' syndrome, 150
Hypercapnia and obesity, 261
Hypercholesterolaemia, familial, 182–183
Hyperglycaemia, postprandial, in diabetes, 243
　see also Somogyi effect in diabetes
Hyperlipidaemia, 181–182
Hypernatraemic dehydration and cows' milk feeding, 47
Hypermethionaemia in tyrosinaemia, 176–177
Hypertension
　and adult health, 284
　and sodium, 76, 284
Hypoalbuminaemia, in intravenous feeding, 227

Hypocalcaemia
　and vitamin D deficiency, 145–146
　in infants, 16
　and cows' milk feeding, 46–47
　low birth-weight, 64
Hypoglycaemia management in diabetes, 247–248
　see also Somogyi effect in diabetes
Hyponatraemia
　in cystic fibrosis, 204
　in infants, low birth-weight infants, 63
Hypophosphataemia in intravenous feeding, 227

Ileal resection, malabsorption after, 213
　see also Meconium ileus in cystic fibrosis
Immunoglobulin in breast milk, 27, 28
　colostrum, 29
Inborn errors of metabolism, 167–184
　fructose intolerance, 171
　galctosaemia, 168–170
　　classical, 168–170
　　galactokinase deficiency, 170
　hypercholesterolaemia, familial, 182–183
　hyperlipidaemia, 181–182
　lacticacidaemias, 180–183
　　glycogen storage disorders, 180–181
　maple syrup urine disease, 177
　and nutritional co-factors, 178
　phenylketonuria, 171–176
　　assessment, 175–176
　　management, 172–175
　　symptoms, 172
　screening, 167–168
　tyrosinaemia, 176–177
　　and vitamin C deficiency, 141
　urea-cycle defects, 178–179
　　arginase deficiency, 179
Indomethacin for patent ductus arteriosus, 57
Infant diabetes, problems of, 245–246
　see also Fetus and maternal nutrition
Infants, low birth-weight, 51–72
　enteral feeding, 52–59
　　complications, 56–57
　　mother's milk *vs* formula for, 57–59, 60
　　nasogastric, 53–54
　　orogastric, 54
　　procedure, 55–56
　　transpyloric, 54–55
　growth, catch-up, 69–70
　nutritional needs, 51–52
　　and glycogen stores, 52
　nutritional problems, 63–69
　　anaemia, 67–68
　　bone disease, 64–65
　　carnitine deficiency, 65
　　copper deficiency, 66
　　fatty acids, essential, deficiency, 66
　　hypocalcaemia, 64
　　hyponatraemia, 63
　　taurine deficiency, 66
　　vitamin deficiencies, 66–67, 68
　　vitamin supplementation programme, 68–69

Infants, low birth-weight (*cont.*)
  parenteral feeding, 59, 61–63
  and osteomalacia, maternal, 16
  sucking/swallowing reflexes, 52
Infections
  and breast feeding, 27–28
    protection, 27–28
    transmission, 35–36
  diarrhoea, 88
  and failure to thrive, 87–88
  from intravenous feeding, 224–226
  in malnutrition
    resistance, 99–100
    treatment, 105–106
  pyrexia, 87
Injury, non-accidental, and copper deficiency, 123
Inspissated curd syndrome and cows' milk feeding, 46
Insulin
  chromium co-factor, 125
  management in diabetes, 240, 244–245
Intellectual development, *see* Mental development
International Code of Marketing Breast Milk Substitutes (WHO 1981), 45
Intertrigo in obesity, 260
Intolerance, food, 185–190
  additives, 188–189
    and hyperactivity, 189–190
  allergic, 186–187
  double-blind procedure, 185–186
  elimination diets, 187–188
    and eczema, 188
  over-diagnosis, 185
  psychogenic, 186
Intravenous feeding, 218–229
  complications, 224–228
    anaemia, 227–228
    infection, 224–226
    jaundice, 222, 226
    nutrient deficiencies, 226–227
  composition of feed, 221–224
    carbohydrate, 221
    fat, 222
    minerals, 223–224
    protein, 222
    vitamins, 222–223
  enteral feeding reintroduction, 228
  at home, 228
  indications for, 219
  of infants, low birth-weight, 59, 61–63
  procedure, 219–220
  team approach, 220
  timing of start, 220
  total, in Crohn's disease, 211
  see also Enteral feeding
Iodine deficiency, 126–127
  and fetal development, 17
Iron
  in human milk, 30
  and lactoferrin in breast milk, 28

Iron (*cont.*)
  overload from transfusion, 119–120
  supplementation for low birth-weight infants, 67
  therapy, in malnutrition, problems of, 108
  see also Iron deficiency
Iron deficiency, 114–120
  in adolescents, 279
  anaemia
    and coeliac disease, 199
    and cows' milk feeding, 48
    and breast feeding, prolonged, 38
  causes, 116
  and copper deficiency, 122
  and development/behaviour, 118–119
  diagnosis, 117
  and iron stores, 117–118
  requirement *vs* intake, 115
  symptoms/signs, 115–116, 118
  transport, 115
  treatment, 119
  and vegetarian diets, 155

Jaundice
  breast milk, 34
  cholestatic
    chronic, 206–207
    with intravenous feeding, 222, 226

Kaschin-Beck disease, 125
Keshan disease, 125
Ketoacidosis, management in diabetes, 248–249
Kidneys, *see* Dialysis; Renal problems
Kwashiorkor, 102–105
  progression to, 104–105
  symptoms/signs, 98
  vs marasmus, 103

Lactalbumin in human milk, 30
Lacticacidaemias, 180–183
  glycogen storage disorders, 180–181
Lactoferrin
  in breast milk, 28
  in colostrum, 29
Lactose
  in human milk, 30
  intolerance, 85, 193–195
Lactovegetarianism, 155–156
Laurence-Moon-Biedl syndrome, 270
Linoleic acid in formula feeds, 43
Lipid, *see* Fat; Hyperlipidaemia
Liver transplant, and jaundice, cholestatic, 206
  see also Cirrhosis, biliary, in cystic fibrosis; Jaundice; Glycogen storage, disorders
Lymphangectasia, intestinal, 208–209

Macrobiotic diets, 156–157
Maize, and niacin deficiency, 135

Malabsorption syndromes, 197–207
  abetalipoproteinaemia, 208
  acrodermatitis enteropathica, 120, 207–208
  coeliac disease, 198–200
    diagnosis, 199
    and failure to thrive, 84–85
    management, 200
    presentation, 198–199
  cystic fibrosis, 200–205
    diagnosis, 201
    and failure to thrive, 84
    management, 201–202
    nutritional problems, 203–205
  jaundice, chronic cholestatic, 206–207
  lymphangectasia, intestinal, 208–209
Malnutrition
  and brain growth, 12–13
  and macrobiotic diets, 156–157
  and weaning, Asian tradition, 158
  see also Protein-energy malnutrition
Manganese, 128
Maple syrup urine disease, 177
Marasmus, 100–102
  vs kwashiorkor, 103
  symptoms/signs, 98, 101–102
Mauriac syndrome, 251
Meadow's syndrome, 186
Meconium ileus in cystic fibrosis, 204
Mental development, 118
  and galactosaemia, 170
  and malnutrition, 111
  and phenylketonuria, 172
  retarded, and failure to thrive, 90–91
Metabolism, see Inborn errors of metabolism
Methionine, see Hypermethionaemia in tyrosinaemia
Milk, human
  banking, 37
  composition, 28–31
    amino acids, 30
    immunoglobulin, 27, 28
  for enteral feeding, 57–58
  production, and prolactin, 24–25
  see also Breast feeding; Colostrum; Cows' milk; Goats' milk for infant feeding; Formula feeding
Mineral deficiencies
  and fetal development, 17–18
  and vegetarian diets, 155
  see also by particular mineral
Molybdenum, 128
Mortality/morbidity, nutrition in, 11
Munchausen's syndrome by proxy, 186
Muscular dystrophy, Duchenne, and obesity, 268–269

Nasogastric feeding of infants, 53–54
Nephrotic syndrome, 232–233
Neural tube defects, fetal, and vitamins, 19

Neurology
  handicap and failure to thrive, 90–91
  signs of vitamin B_{12} deficiency, 140
  see also Mental development
Niacin deficiency, 135–136
'Nursing bottle' syndrome, 164
Nutrition Rehabilitation Units, 109
Nutritional status
  anthropometry, 6–9
    interpretation, 8–9
    in malnutrition classification, 96–97
    techniques, 7
  assessment, clinical, 5–10
  biochemical, 9–10
  physical signs, 6
  see also Adult health and early nutrition

Obesity, 254–270
  and adult health, 282–283
  causes of simple obesity, 258
  clinical features, 259–260
  complications, 260–262
    Pickwickian syndrome, 260–261
  definition, 254
  in diabetes, 250–251
  fat proportion in body, 255–257
  management, 262–267
    activity, 265–266
    behavioural methods, 266
    diet, 263–265
    follow-up, 266–267
    motivation, 262–263
  measurement, 254–255
    skinfold thickness, 255
  pathological, 267–270
    investigations, 267–268
    Laurence-Moon-Biedl syndrome, 270
    management, 268–269
    Prader-Willi syndrome, 269–270
  risk factors, environmental, 258–259
  types of, 257–258
Oral rehydration therapy (ORT), 191–193
Orogastric feeding of infants, 54
Osteomalacia, maternal, infant effects, 16
  rickets, 145
Ovary failure, and galactosaemia, 170
Oxygen consumption, and heart disease, congenital, 90
Oxytocin, 25

Parenteral feeding, see Intravenous feeding
Patent ductus arteriosus, infant, and enteral feeding, 57
Pellagra, 135–136
Phenylketonuria, 171–176
  assessment, 175–176
  management, 172–175
  symptoms, 172
Phosphate
  absorption and neonatal hypocalcaemia, 46–47
  in intravenous feeding, 223–224

Phosphate (cont.)
  supplementation for low birth-weight infants, 65
  see also Hypophosphataemia in intravenous feeding
Phototherapy, neonatal, and water loss, 33
Phytate in flour, and rickets, 148
Pickwickian syndrome, 260–261
Placental insufficiency, 21–22
Prader-Willi syndrome, 269–270
Pregnancy
  in adolescents, 278–279
  copper accumulation, fetal, 121
  see also Fetus and maternal nutrition
Prematurity, see Infants, low birth-weight
Prolactin, 24–25
Protein-energy malnutrition, 96–113
  classification, 96
    QUAC stick, 98
    Shakir tape, 97–98
  and development, intellectual, 111
  infection resistance, 99–100
  kwashiorkor, 102–105
    vs marasmus, 103
    progression to, 104–105
    symptoms/signs, 98
  management, 105–109
    anaemia, 107, 108
    formula feeds, 106–107
    infection treatment, 105–106
    prognosis, 109
    rehydration/electrolyte balance, 106
    response, 108
    vitamins, 107–108
  marasmus, 100–102
    symptoms/signs, 98, 101–102
    vs kwashiorkor, 103
  Nutrition Rehabilitation Units, 109
  prevention, 109–110
    emergency aid, 111
    weaning education, 110–111
Proteins
  for diabetics, 244
  and fetal development, 19
  in formula feeds, 43
  in human milk, 30
  intake in renal failure, chronic, 234, 236
  in intravenous feeding, 222
  losses in nephrotic syndrome, 232
  and vegetarian diets, 154–155
Psychogenic food intolerance, 186
Pyrexia in infection, 87
Pyridoxine deficiency, 136–137

QUAC stick, 98
Quinoline yellow, 189

Radiology for rickets, 147
Rastafarian diet, 156
Reflux, gastro-oesophageal, and enteral feeding, 56

Renal problems, 230–238
  acute failure, 230–232
    diuretic phase, 232
    oliguric phase, 231
  anaemia, 237
  chronic failure, 233–236
    and growth, 233
    management, 234–236
    monitoring, 237
  in infants
    dehydration, 47
    low birth-weight, and hyponatraemia, 63
  nephrotic syndrome, 232–233
  rickets, 236–237
  transplant catch-up growth, 238
  see also Dialysis
Resection, gastrointestinal, malabsorption after, 212–215
Respiratory distress, and enteral feeding, 56
Retinol, 131
Retinol Equivalents, 130–131
Riboflavin deficiency, 134–135
Rickets
  in Asian immigrants, 157–158
  of prematurity, 64–65
  renal, 236–237
  and teeth, 165–166
  see also Rickets, nutritional
Rickets, nutritional
  biochemical findings, 146–147
  clinical features, 145–146
    symptoms, 146
  and immobilization, 150–151
  racial factors, 147–149
    and diet, 148
    environment, 148–149
  radiology, 147
  treatment, 149–150
    non-nutritional, 149–150
    nutritional, 149

Salt
  contraindicated for diabetics, 244
  and hypertension, 76
School dinners and obesity, 265
Scurvy, 140–142
  and teeth, 165
Selenium deficiency, 124–125
  Keshan disease, 125
Shakir tape for upper arm circumference, 97–98
Short gut syndrome, see Resection, Gastrointestinal, malabsorption after
Skin
  losses from and failure to thrive, 85
  pigment and cholecalciferol synthesis, 148
  see also Acrodermatitis enteropathica; Eczema, atopic; Intertrigo in obesity
Skinfold thickness, 255
Smoking by adolescents, 277

Socio-economic factors,
  in breast feeding, 24
  in fetal risk, 15
  and pregnancy energy balance, 18–19
Sodium and hypertension, 76, 284
  see also Hypernatraemic dehydration and cows' milk feeding; Hyponatraemia
Somogyi effect in diabetes, 251
Soya-based infant feed, 48–49
Spina bifida, and obesity, 268–269
Steroids and nephrotic syndrome, 232
Sucrose avoidance and fructose intolerance, 171

Tartrazine, 189
Taurine
  in breast milk, 30
  deficiency in low birth-weight infants, 66
  in formula feeds, 43
Teeth, 161–166
  deciduous, importance of, 161
  and fluoride, 127–128, 164–165
  maternal nutrition and, 161–162
    ameloblastic activity, 161
  post-natal problems, 162–164
    caries, 91, 127–128, 162–163, 164–165
    enamel hypoplasia, 162
    'nursing bottle' syndrome, 164
    recent improvements, 166
  and vitamin deficiencies, 165–166
    rickets, 165–166
    scurvy, 165
Thiamine deficiency, 133–134
  and fetal development, 15
Thrombosis, coronary
  and diet, 284–285
  and hyperlipidaemia, 182
Thyroid and cretinism, 17, 127
Thyrotoxicosis, and failure to thrive, 86–87
Transferrin levels, 115
Tryptophan
  and niacin deficiency, 135
  and pyridoxine phosphate, 137
Tyrosinaemia, 176–177
  and vitamin C deficiency, 141

Ulcerative colitis, 211–212
Urea-cycle defects, 178–179
  arginase deficiency, 179
Urine testing in diabetes, 249

Vegans, 156
Vegetarian diets, 153–157
  eccentric, excessive vitamins, 158–159
  lactovegetarianism, 155–156
  macrobiotic, Zen, 156–157
  problems, general, 154–155
  racial minorities in Britain, 157–158
  vegans, 156
Virus transmission in breast milk, 35

Vitamins
  deficiencies, 130
    and cows' milk infant feeding, 47–48
    and the fetus, 15–17
    and infants, low birth-weight, 66–67, 68
    and teeth, 165–166
  in diets, eccentric, 158–159
  and fetal development, 19–20
  in intravenous feeding, 222–223
  in malnutrition management, 107–108
  in milk, human, 30
  and neural tube defects, infant, 19
  supplementation
    for infants, low birth-weight, 68–69
    in jaundice, cholestatic, 206
  and vegetarian diets, 155
  see also by particular vitamin
Vitamin A deficiency, 130–132
  and eyes, 132
  intakes, 130–131
  management, 132
  and retinol, 131
  sources, 131
  symptoms/signs, 132
Vitamin B deficiencies
  B_{12}, 139–140
    and fetal development, 16
    neurological signs, 140
    and vegetarian diets, 155–156
  folic acid, 137–138
    and fetal development, 16–17
    in infants, low birth-weight, 68
    in malnutrition, 107–108
  niacin, 135–136
  pyridoxine (B_6), 136–137
  riboflavin, 134–135
  thiamine (B_1), 133–134
    and fetal development, 15
Vitamin C
  as additive, 189
  deficiency, 140–142
  and teeth, 165
Vitamin D
  deficiency
    and breast feeding, prolonged, 38
    and fetal development, 16
    and hypocalcaemia, 145–146
    and teeth, 165–166
    and vegetarian diets, 155
  metabolism, 143–145
  nutrition, in jaundice, cholestatic, 206–207
  sources, 142–143
  see also Rickets; Rickets, nutritional
Vitamin E
  deficiency, 151
    anaemia and cows' milk feeding, 48
    in infants, low birth-weight, 66–67
  in formula feeds, 43
Vitamin K deficiency, 151
  and breast feeding, 34
  in infants, low birth-weight, 68
Vomiting and infection, 87

Weaning, 73–79
　allergy and foreign proteins, 75
　　gluten intolerance, 75
　Asian tradition and malnutrition, 158
　from bottle feeding, 158
　in developing countries, 77–79
　　principles, 78–79
　　traditional inadequacy of, 77
　diet for tissue deposition, 74–75
　education and malnutrition prevention, 110–111

Weaning (*cont.*)
　foods for, and acceptance of, 75–76
　　composition, 75–76
　　educative effect, 76
　　lumpiness, 75
　　refusal, 76–77
　　variety, 75
　timing of, 73–74
　　and energy intakes, 74
　　and growth standards, 73–74
Williams' syndrome, 150